NURSING

concepts of practice

NURSING

concepts of practice

Dorothea E. Orem

Savannah, GA

FOURTH EDITION

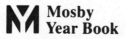 **Mosby**
Year Book

St. Louis   Baltimore   Boston   Chicago   London   Philadelphia   Sydney   Toronto

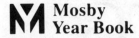
Mosby
Year Book
Dedicated to Publishing Excellence

Editor: N. Darlene Como
Project Supervisor: Barbara Merritt
Designer: Susan E. Lane

FOURTH EDITION

Mosby–Year Book, Inc.
11830 Westline Industrial Drive
St. Louis, Missouri 63146

Library of Congress Cataloging-in-Publication Data

Orem, Dorothea E. (Dorothea Elizabeth)

  Nursing : concepts of practice / Dorothea E. Orem. — 4th ed.

    p. cm.
    Includes bibliographical references.
    Includes index.
    ISBN 0-8016-6064-5
    1. Nursing—Philosophy.   I. Title.
    [DNLM: 1. Nursing. 2. Nursing Process. WY 100 066n]
RT84.5.073 1991
610.73—dc20
DNLM/DLC
for Library of Congress   90-13250
                                                                           CIP

GW/GW/RRD   9   8   7   6   5   4   3   2

PREFACE

The fourth edition of *Nursing: Concepts of Practice* reflects my developing understanding of nursing as a field of knowledge and a field of practice. Areas of nursing knowledge touched on in prior editions are more fully developed. The aim of this edition is to provide nurses and nursing students with a coherent expression of the human and societal foundations for nursing practice.

This edition, like all prior ones, is based on the premise that nursing considered as a field of knowledge and a field of practice has its own domain and boundaries. As in other fields it is the proper object of nursing that defines nursing's domain and boundaries and permits for individuals' growth as they search for understanding of the concrete features of nursing practice.

The contextual and process features of nursing practice are developed in Chapters 1, 2, 5, and 8 through 10. The self-care deficit theory of nursing with its central ideas, presuppositions and propositions, and conceptual structure is expressed in Chapters 3, 6, 7, and 9. The characteristics of nursing as a practical science and a set of applied sciences are represented in Chapter 4. Nursing administration is described in Chapter 11 and its focus is contrasted with that of nursing practice. Chapter 12 represents features of nursing education that have a nursing practice focus. Chapters are so constructed that they can be studied as entities or as units within sequences of chapters formed according to needs and interests at particular times. Exercises which assist in understanding, clarifying, or applying concepts discussed are included in boxes throughout the text.

My search for understanding nursing has been prolonged. My sincere gratitude is extended to all the nurses who have helped me in innumerable ways to be ready to and to engage in the preparation of this fourth edition and to Walene E. Shields for her consistent help in manuscript preparation.

Dorothea E. Orem

CONTENTS

NURSING
concepts of practice

CHAPTER 1

Understanding nursing practice situations

Young children attach meaning to actors and objects introduced into the play situations they create. They set protocols for action and specify relations between and among players and objects, thereby establishing order. Children draw on their own experiences, on stories they have heard or read, and on their imaginations in creating play situations. Children (as well as men and women) when confronted with concrete life situations of types that are disliked or not before encountered may turn away or may elect to enter into them as actors or as participant observers motivated by a desire to know, to experience, or to make events occur.

Concrete situations of human living are complex and are more often lived than understood. There are constituent elements or parts, persons or objects, or environmental conditions. Persons and objects have attributes or properties. Environmental conditions are of various types, physical, social, or biologic; and each type can vary over a range of values. The connections among elements and their properties determine the existent and changing order among situational elements. Since situations of human living are dynamic, changes in elements or relations among them are possible or are predictable. Persons acquire experiential knowledge from concrete life situations and can draw on this knowledge to attach meaning to similar, recurring situations.

Some life situations are outside the usual day-to-day experiences of persons who live together in community. These are situations where specialized knowledge and abilities are required for observing, for attaching meaning and value to judgments about what is, and for developing insights about what can be changed and what should be changed. Nursing situations as described and explained in *Nursing: Concepts of Practice* require specialized knowledge and skills on the part of persons who elect to become able to take action in them, that is, to be nurses with developed capabilities **(nursing agency)** to provide nursing to persons who require it.

NURSES AND NURSING KNOWLEDGE

One essential personal foundation of nurses for the practice of nursing is the specialized knowledge gained through experiences in nursing practice situations (experiential nursing knowledge) and the speculative or theoretical nursing knowledge conceptualized from authoritative sources that is descriptive and explanatory of

1

nursing in a range of types of nursing practice situations. When nurses approach and enter into concrete situations of nursing practice, they are confronted with needs to ask and answer certain questions: What does this situation that involves me with others in this time-place localization mean to me, not just as a person but as a person who is nurse? Why am I here? As nurse what must I know? What do I inquire about? What questions do I need to ask? What meaning do I attach to the information obtained, to the judgments I make? What conclusions are valid? Do I have a language to express what I know so what I know is communicated meaningfully to persons I nurse, to other nurses, and to other health workers? Do I have knowledge of what can be changed through deliberately designed action and what cannot be changed? These questions identify the kinds of specialized, theoretical knowledge that nurses should have as they investigate the nursing-relevant details of concrete nursing practice situations. Without such structured nursing knowledge, nurses rely on their common sense knowledge that is uninformed by nursing science.

Nurses function in community with other nurses, other health workers, and with persons and families who require and can benefit from nursing. The sector of reality that is the world of the nurse must become known to nursing students and nurses if they are to function as effective practitioners of the health service nursing. The world of the nurse includes elements in common with the worlds of other health workers, for example, the persons and families served; but the world of the nurse has a defined domain within boundaries. The domain and boundaries of nursing practice are defined by what nurses are concerned with as nurses within their world and by the way in which they are concerned. Nurses' productive efforts to identify, understand, conceptualize, and express what nurses are concerned with in their world and the ways in which they are concerned lead to the beginning formalization of the content and structure of nursing as systematized and validated knowledge (i.e., as nursing science).

The word nursing

Nursing knowledge is descriptive or explanatory of the situational elements and the relationships among those elements for a range of types of nursing practice situations and to the investigative, decision-making, and production operations of nurses within these types of situations. Nursing knowledge results from inquiry into practice situations and from more formal investigations based on the results of inquiry. Initially, nursing students should inquire about the meaning of the word *nursing* in dictionaries and in writings about nursing.

Nursing is an English language word. It is used as a noun, as an adjective, and as a verbal auxiliary derived from the verb to nurse. Used as a noun and an adjective nursing signifies the kind of care or service that nurses provide. It is the work that persons who are nurses do. The word nursing as used in the statement *I am nursing* is a verbal auxiliary, a participle. To nurse literally means (1) to attend to and serve and (2) to provide close care of a person, an infant or a sick or disabled person, unable to care for self with the goal of helping the person become sound in health and "self-sufficient."* This nominal (lexicographic) definition of nursing identifies that engagement in nursing signifies that persons are:

• Attending to and serving others
• Providing close care of other persons unable to care for themselves
• Helping such persons become sound in health and self-sufficient.

This definition describes nursing in that it signifies the proper use of the word in its broadest sense, but it is not an adequate definition of the *specialized health service nursing*. It does not differentiate persons who require the specialized health service nursing from persons who require nursing in other forms, such as the close care required by and provided for infants. Scholars and theorists in various fields have found that the most productive beginning approach to explain descriptively their specialized fields of knowledge or practice is to identify the **proper object** of the field. **Object** means that toward which or because of which action is taken. **Proper** means that which belongs to the field. Object is used in the philosophic or scientific sense as that which is studied or observed, that to which action is directed to obtain information about it or to bring about some new condition. Object is not used in the sense of something tangible.

The whole reality of human beings — men, women, and children — cared for either singly or as social units, constitute (in the philosophic sense) "the material object" of the activities of nurses, physicians, clinical psychologists, social workers, and others who provide direct care for persons in need. Each of the named human services has its own proper object, which identifies why men, women, or children require each specific service and can be helped through its provision.

A 1958[1] expression of the proper object of nursing answered the following question: What condition exists in a person when judgments are made that a nurse(s) should be brought into the situation (i.e., that persons should be under nursing care)? The answer was expressed in this fashion: The condition is the inability of persons to provide continuously for themselves the amount and quality of required self-care because of situations of personal health. With children it is the inability of parents or guardians to provide the amount and quality of care required by their child because of their child's health situation. **Self-care** is the personal care that individuals require each day to regulate their own functioning and development. Requirements of persons for this day-to-day regulatory care will be affected by, among other factors, age, developmental stage, health state, environmental conditions, and effects of medical care. **Dependent-care** is the continuing health-related personal regulatory and developmental care provided by responsible adults for infants and children or persons with disabling conditions.

---

* From Webster's dictionary of synonyms, ed 1, Springfield, Mass, 1951, G & C Merriam Co, p. 577.

Exercise to assist in the development of a concept of self-care

1. Select an individual (a relative, friend, or associate or an inpatient or outpatient at a hospital) who has a chronic disease, has sustained an injury, has experienced an acute illness, or is pregnant for the first time.
2. In accordance with the individual's ability, interest, and willingness to comply with your request for information, ask the following questions (rephrase if desired) and record the answers.
   a. Since the occurrence of (name the conditioning factor, disease, injury, etc.), do you have to care for yourself differently than you did before its occurrence?
   b. What are some of your new activities or tasks? How did you learn about the need to engage in them?
   c. How do you fit the new tasks into the schedule of your daily activities?
   d. Can you do all of these new tasks by yourself? If not, who helps you?
   e. Did you know how to do these new tasks before the occurrence of (same as in a, above)?
   f. How did you feel about learning to do the new tasks? How do you feel about doing them now?
   g. Of all the things that you know you should do, are there some things that you tend to forget or deliberately decide not to do? If so, why?

This specification of the proper object of nursing makes it possible to conceptualize and express characterizing features of the *specialized health service nursing*. Persons identified in the nominal definition of nursing as "unable to care for self" are now limited to persons who are in this state of inability because of the activity-limiting effects of their states of health or because of the nature and complexity of their day-to-day care requirements that contribute to regulation of their functioning and development. The specialized health service nursing is differentiated not only from other specialized human services, such as medicine, but also from the care of infants and young children and the continuing care of children or adults with illnesses or disabilities by family members. The expressed proper object of the specialized health service nursing is identified as a *subclass* of the *class of persons who are unable to care for themselves*.

Experienced nurses recognize life situations where persons require the specialized health service nursing. Experienced, efficient nurses know when their work of nursing others, caring for others, or helping them care for themselves, produces beneficial results. However, as previously stated, it is essential for nurses to know and be able to express and thereby communicate what they do, why they do it, and the results of what they do. Conceptualizing nursing is a first step.

An expressed conceptualization of nursing

Nursing, a specialized health service, is distinguished from other human services by its focus on persons with inabilities for continuous provision of the amount and quality of time specific care that is regulatory of their own functioning and development whenever inabilities that limit care are associated with their states of health or the complex, specialized nature of required regulatory care measures. Persons who are socially dependent, whether they are children or adults, require the specialized health service nursing when the parents or guardians are unable, because of the health situation of the dependent person, to provide the amount and quality of continuous regulatory care required by the dependent person.

Practitioners of nursing perform estimative, decision-making, and productive operations in order to know what exists in concrete nursing practice situations; to know what can be changed; to make decisions about what can and should be done; and to produce a system(s) of care that will (1) ensure meeting the person's requirements for the regulation of functioning and development now and for some duration, (2) protect developed and developing action capabilities, and (3) regulate the exercise or development of the person's capabilities to care for self or dependents.

The foregoing summary statements about nursing are formally developed in detail in subsequent chapters. The expressed conceptualization of nursing was formulated in a modified form in 1956 (p.85).[2] The expression of the proper object of nursing in 1958 led to further insight about nursing and to the conceptualization of the elements of nursing practice situations and the relations among them and later to the formulation and expression of a general theory of nursing. The subsequent use of the word nursing will refer only to the *specialized health service nursing*.

Nurses knowing nursing

Knowing nursing is a personal achievement of women and men who develop themselves to become and be able to practice nursing. Antecedently (prior to practice) acquired theoretical nursing knowledge enables the search for the answers to previously posed questions that nurses ask when they enter into the life situations of others. Knowledge of the human sciences is essential for nursing practice when properly articulated with nursing facts and points of theory. It is the descriptive and explanatory knowledge of the elements and relationships of nursing practice situations that identify points of articulation with facts and points of theory from the human sciences as well as from the practical science and the applied sciences of medicine.

Theoretical or speculative nursing knowledge from authoritative sources is not to be memorized, but rather understood, conceptualized, and made dynamic in practice situations. Knowledge that gives guidance and direction to action is dynamic in the knower, the nurse. Development of understanding of the features that nursing has in common with other human services, including other health services, is conducive to developing insights about and forming images of the general features of nursing practice situations. Inquiry into nursing as a helping service and inquiry into nursing situations where persons are taken care of should contribute to nursing students' and nurses' understanding of the most general personal and interpersonal features of nursing situations.

UNDERSTANDING NURSING AS A HELPING SERVICE

Considering nursing as a helping service brings to focus the interpersonal features of nursing and some essential differences between and among individuals who need nursing and those who nurse. In helping situations, persons are cast into roles: persons in specific places with needs that must be met at specific times and persons who can help in meeting their needs, helpers. Needs for help arise at specific times under specific circumstances. Television reports of street accidents vividly represent these circumstances as injured persons are helped by trained paramedics who have rushed to the scene.

Helping situations

In daily living, individuals sometimes face situations where they know that existent or emerging needs of others cannot be met without help. Neighbors become ill and are taken to the doctor's office or to the clinic or emergency room. Strangers ask for directions and persons asked try to help them. These types of situations do not require the helping person to have specialized education and training to act in such situations, but they do require knowledge about the other's need, the extent to which they can help, and what is practical and not practical in meeting another's need.

Nurses, physicians, lawyers, and social workers are educated and train themselves to be skilled in specialized types of helping situations. Training in first aid and disaster work represent other types of preparation for helping in specialized situations.

Helping situations are often complex, and taking action is difficult because it demands that one person (the helper) does something to supply what another person with needs should have or do but which the person does not have or cannot do, must not do, prefers not to do, or outright refuses to do. A helping situation is complicated for the helper because the need being met is a requirement of another person. It is complicated for needy persons because they are experiencing an inability to manage and care for themselves and to meet the demands that the situation places on them.

Individuals may be reluctant to accept help from other persons because the positions and the manners and abilities of persons offering help do not fit certain cultural prescriptions or do not inspire the confidence of the person in need. The giving and receiving of help is a process that is affected by the knowledge and skills, personalities, experiences, and life situations of helpers and of persons in need of help. The failure of persons to give help where it is needed may be a function of levels of personal development and maturity. It is more difficult for some persons to engage in processes of helping than it is for others. Helping is basically a practical endeavor demanding insights about what can and should be changed in concrete life situations. Having the desire to help another does not mean that a person has the ability to help.

Persons who need help may be unable to seek it or ask for it. They may lack the necessary information or communication skills. They may be afraid. Sometimes persons believe that they do not have a right to seek and receive help. In such situations, persons need to be "helped to get help" to meet specific existent or emerging needs.

There are similarities and differences in helping situations. The similarities are enabling for understanding some of the basic characteristics of situations where persons are helped through nursing.

Characteristics of helping situations

All helping situations have similar general designs or patterns. The design is engendered by the roles of the persons involved—a person who requires help and a person who is to give help—and by the expected behaviors (roles) of these persons. Ideally, the behavior of the person requiring help is complemented by the behavior of the helper. Consider the following situation:

> Two men have been in an accident. Their car skidded and crashed into a tree. One of the men, the owner and driver of the car, has suffered an injury to his back and hip. He cannot move without severe pain, and he realizes that he can prevent further injury by not moving. His companion, though shaken, is on his feet. He asks about his friend's condition and, recognizing his friend's injured state, extends assurance that help will come. He knows that he should not move his friend, so he stops a passing motorist and asks him to report the accident and request help in the next town. The motorist agrees; soon the police and an ambulance arrive, and the injured man is carefully immobilized, moved onto a stretcher, and taken to the local hospital. The uninjured man, with his friend's approval, arranges through the resident physician for medical care and attends to the details of the admission. He calls the injured man's family, arranges for the removal of the wrecked car, notifies the insurance company, and confers with the police officers.

In this hypothetical situation, the behavior of the uninjured man complemented the role of his injured friend. The man with the helping role communicated with a variety of persons on behalf of his friend. His communications with the passing motorist and with the ambulance attendants, physician, nurses, hospital admitting personnel, garage attendants, insurance agent, and his friend's family contributed to meeting the needs of his friend.

Further examination of the helping activities of the injured man's companion shows that the activities were directed toward achieving four goals: (1) preventing further injury to his friend, (2) securing health services for his friend, (3) taking care of his friend's property—the car—and, (4) attending to his friend's personal affairs—notifying his friend's family and insurance company of the accident. To achieve these goals, the companion had to demonstrate his awareness of his friend's injured state, of the need for immobility and medical attention, and of the legal, financial, and family implications of the accident.

In this example of a helping situation, while a helper actively tried to achieve a goal or goals for another person, he had full knowledge of his actions and his own limitations. In this situation, the helper was aware that he could not give effective

---

Characteristics of helping situations, a summary

There are at least two persons in the situation in different statuses, the status of helper and the status of person in need of help.

The status of the person in need of help is legitimized by meeting two criteria:

There is a need for this person to act to achieve specific purposes immediately or in the future because of prevailing conditions and circumstances.

There are action limitations that make immediate or future action on the part of this person impossible or imprudent or would render action ineffective or incomplete.

The helper's status is legitimized by meeting two criteria:

The helper has identified, has knowledge of, and accepts the demand for the person in need of help to act and the person's action limitations.

The helper knows how to, is willing to, and does act for the welfare of the other in accordance with factors that limit what can and what should be done under prevailing conditions and circumstances.

The actions of the helper:

Complement (or substitute for) the actions of the person needing help in order to accomplish the specific purposes of the person needing help.

Provide and foster conditions to facilitate the development or exercise of this person's capabilities to take necessary actions for achieving specific purposes.

---

health care to his injured friend but could secure such services for him. Thus, the helper first defined and limited what he would do in relation to (1) the condition for which help was required, (2) what he knew how to do and was able to do, and (3) what was considered permissible or advisable under the circumstances.

Helping methods

As men, women, and children live together and help one another, they develop methods for overcoming or compensating for the action limitations that individuals and families have at specific times under specific circumstances to meet existent and emerging needs. Method usually signifies an orderly way of accomplishing something. A helping method from a nursing perspective is a sequential series of actions, which, if performed, will overcome or compensate for the health-associated limitations of persons to engage in actions to regulate their own functioning and development or that of their dependents. There is a limited number of methods that one person can use to help another person perform a task or meet a need. Helping methods are used within the human service occupations and professions and in all situations where bonds of friendship and neighborliness prevail.

There are at least five helping methods through which one person can compensate for or overcome the limitations of others to act for themselves in day-to-day living. In concrete helping situations, the methods are often used in combination. Nurses use all the methods, selecting and combining them in relation to the action demands on persons under nursing care and their health-associated action limitations. These methods are identified as follows:

1. Acting for or doing for another
2. Guiding and directing
3. Providing physical or psychological support
4. Providing and maintaining an environment that supports personal development
5. Teaching

The named helping methods are used in all health services. Selection of helping methods for use singly or in combination rests on the health professionals' insights, judgments, and decisions about what others cannot do, or do effectively, and about what can and should be done in the interests of life, health, and well-being of others. Each helping method has certain characterizing features. For example, the use of some methods under some circumstances demand that helpers be in the physical presence of persons helped, or in physical contact with them, or be continuously available to them in their time-place localizations. The kind and amount of communication varies. Descriptions of helping methods and criteria to validate the selection and use of each method are presented.

Acting for or doing for another

Acting for another is a helping method that requires the helper to use developed abilities toward achieving specific results for persons in need of help. Examples are a nurse positioning a helpless patient or a mother feeding her baby. The person being helped, if conscious, must permit the helper to act for him or her. The method, therefore, cannot be used with a conscious person unless there is a measure of cooperation. Ideally, the helper assists the person in making inquiries, decisions, and plans whenever possible and prudent. The helper should also tell the person being helped what needs to be done, what to expect, and what to report. When the person to be helped is unconscious, incompetent, or unable to participate in making decisions, the helper must act with regard for the rights of the one helped and be clear about the helper's role.

The usefulness and validity of *acting for or doing for another* is determined by the type of result sought. Acting for another is not valid when results depend on internal acts, such as control of one's own behavior. The method is valid, however, in giving care to an acutely ill person or to a physically or mentally incapacitated person according to the nature, degree, and duration of the self-care deficit. In the service professions and occupations, the method of assisting by acting for another is commonly used in situations where scientifically derived knowledge and highly specialized techniques are required for accomplishing a result.

Acting for another is necessary in infant and child care situations, but other methods should be added as soon as the child is ready for them. In the care of the aged or the infirm, acting for another is used in compensating for declining physical and mental abilities. Acting for another often may be gradually replaced by methods of *guiding another, supporting another,* and *teaching.*

Guiding another

Guiding another person considered as a method of assisting is valid in situations in which persons must (1) make choices — for example, choosing one course of action in preference to another — or (2) pursue a course of action, but not without direction or supervision. This method requires that the person extending guidance and the person being guided be in communication with one another. The one being guided must be motivated and able to perform the activities required. In turn, the guidance given must be appropriate, whether in the form of suggestions, instructions, directions, or supervision. For example, a nurse may suggest that an ambulatory patient take a rest from current activity, the nurse may discuss reasons for the limits on the patient's activities, or the nurse may tell the patient how to secure nursing assistance after discharge from a hospital. Guiding another often is used in conjunction with *supporting another.*

Supporting another

To support another person means to "sustain in an effort" and thereby prevent the person from failing or from avoiding an unpleasant situation or decision. It also may enable the person in need of support to do something without undue stress because of the sustaining influence of the helper. Supportive activity is a valid way of assistance when a patient is faced with something unpleasant or painful. The patient must be capable of controlling and directing the action in the situation once psychological or physical support has been received. For example, a nurse may remain with and give support to a seriously ill person who is permitted to be up and to walk for a short period of time. The presence of the nurse and the nurse's words of encouragement and assurance may be needed just as much as physical help when the patient gets out of bed, maintains an erect posture, and walks. The nurse has the responsibility for judging how much the patient being helped can do or endure and when to intervene. Knowing when to step in requires wisdom and understanding. The communication between the helper and the helped (the patient) may not be in words — the helper may convey support by his or her presence, by a look or a touch, or by physical support. In other situations, speech may be necessary. A patient may need both encouragement and physical help. The action to be performed may be practicing a new skill, making a decision, or living through a stressful personal or family situation.

By giving physical and emotional support, the helper is able to encourage another person to initiate or persevere in the performance of a task, to think about a situation, or to make a decision. Support that encourages action is related to both the kind of action the person helped must make and to the stressful effects of the situation.

Parents, teachers, social workers, and nurses frequently use this method. Supporting another is also used extensively in child care and other situations where individuals are in the process of developmental change.

Providing another person with material resources differs from, but is closely related to, the giving of physical and psychological support. This manner of support is used by adults with dependents, by the state with respect to deprived persons, by citizens of one country for citizens of another country in greater need, and by all persons who have concern for their less fortunate neighbors. This type of support is not the specialized work of nurses. Nonetheless, nurses often assist their patients in obtaining resources from institutions or agencies. As a method of assisting, then, supportive activity may include the securing of resources. It is related to and may be a part of providing a developmental environment.

Providing a developmental environment

This method of assistance requires the helper to provide or help to provide environmental conditions that motivate the person being helped to establish appropriate goals and adjust behavior to achieve results specified by the goals. The needed environmental conditions may be psychosocial or physical. It is the total environment, not any single part of it, that makes it developmental. Developmental results include the forming or changing of attitudes and values, the creative use of abilities, and the adjustment of self-concept as well as physical development. Helpers may be required to provide opportunities for interaction and communication with themselves and with other persons, to give both guidance and support, and to use other ways of helping. The essence of this method is the continued and proper relating of selected environmental elements in light of the patient's special needs and the changes being sought in the patient's health state or manner of living.

Environmental conditions conducive to development provide opportunities for persons being helped to be with other persons or to become members of groups where:
1. Care is offered and provided to those with needs.
2. There are opportunities for solitude and companionship.
3. Help is available with respect to personal and group interests and concerns.
4. Individual decisions and pursuits are personal matters; there is no interference except in matters of grave consequence to the individual or others affected by the situation.
5. Respect, belief, and trust are given to others; and developmental potential is both recognized and fostered.
6. Each person expects or strives to earn respect and trust from others.
7. Each person assumes or attempts to assume responsibility for self and personal development.

Physical conditions that contribute to personal growth and development provide the necessities for daily life and for psychosocial and intellectual development. For example, when an individual is tense and frightened because of the demands of daily life, *sufficient resources* — necessities as well as luxuries — *under some circumstances* may enable the person to meet particular life situations and to become better able to accept responsibilities. It must be remembered, however, that elements of the physical environment are closely related to the psychosocial environment and the social positions and roles of individuals. In assisting individuals in their development, it is not enough to supply resources. It may also be necessary to show them how to use these resources and in some instances to share them.

Providing a developmental environment is valid in many areas of living. It should be used in families, in child care institutions, in nursing homes, in schools, in hospitals, and in other organizations where human beings live or work together. The effectiveness of this method of assisting depends in large part on the helper's creativity and his or her appreciation and knowledge of and respect for people. An environment conducive to development is also conducive to learning and participating and is, therefore, of value if used in conjunction with teaching and other helping methods.

Teaching another

Teaching another is a valid method of helping a person who needs instruction to develop knowledge or particular skills. Learning may not take place if the person to be taught is not in a state of readiness to learn, is unaware that he or she does not know, or is not interested in learning.

To use teaching as a method of assisting requires that the helper know thoroughly what the person to be helped needs to know. For example, a nurse cannot help a patient learn how to select foods according to a prescribed diet until the nurse knows whether the patient knows the nutritional components and caloric values of various foods. The ability to make adaptations in light of a patient's food preferences is also required. The nurse must consider the patient's background and experience, lifestyle and habits of daily living, and modes of perceiving and thinking and must have knowledge of self-care requisites in order to be able to impart knowledge to the patient.

In teaching another, appropriate educational experiences must be provided. Teaching is not restricted to classroom activity. A nurse who is near a patient at mealtime is providing the patient with an opportunity to ask questions pertaining to diet. The nurse who explains to a patient how to perform a measure that will eventually be a self-care component (the care of a colostomy, for example) may stimulate the patient's interest in listening, observing, and asking pertinent questions about the activity. Learning to change one's behavior as it relates to self-care may require considerable time and a prolonged relationship with nurses who are able to fill a tutorial role effectively. Under some circumstances, group teaching may be an effective way of helping individual patients become efficient in self-care activities.

The interested patient may learn much from observations of competent nurses who provide care. Learning in such situations almost seems to be a matter of absorption. In other instances, a patient must engage in specific and planned learning experiences, such as reading and discussion. The learning experiences may also be related to solving problems, such as how much bread, potatoes, or rice will supply a specific amount of carbohydrate in a diet. In a self-care situation, a patient may need to recognize certain effects of a prescribed medication, how to adjust the dosage, or when to call the nurse or physician. Frequently, patients in self-care situations must learn to limit their physical activities. Not infrequently, patients must acquire psychomotor skills in applying supportive bandages to an extremity, skill in changing dressings, or skill in measuring and administering medication by injection.

When teaching is the helping method being used, persons being taught ideally see themselves as learners and realize that study, learning exercises, observation of others, and practice are needed. Helpers see themselves as teachers who direct and guide learning activities. Since children and adults approach learning differently, assisting through teaching must be adapted to age as well as to past education and experience.

Methods–individuals and groups

In nursing a single individual in contrast to a group, all the methods of helping may be necessary for effective nursing. What self-care the patient can or cannot manage and the reasons he or she cannot manage it guide the nurse in the selection of appropriate methods of helping. For example, a nurse may decide that the judicious use of *acting for another* and *supporting another* are most appropriate for a patient who is convalescing from a debilitating illness but whose activity must be limited. The nurse would no doubt also use *guidance* and *teaching* and provide appropriate *environmental conditions*. In each specific nursing situation, one or two helping methods will probably be used more frequently than others. A change in what patients can do for themselves would require that the nurse reexamine and adjust the methods.

Specialized adaptations of the helping methods, with the development of appropriate techniques, are essential in multiperson nursing situations. The most commonly used helping methods in these situations are guiding, providing psychological support, providing an environment for personal development, and teaching. In this type of nursing situation, nurses may help family or group members develop proficiency in the use of some or all of the methods of helping. Some adaptations can be identified in the literature on health care for families and groups. Nurses must be aware of the common methods of assisting and select the methods most appropriate under the circumstances.

Summary

Nursing is a specialized helping service. Nurses help others because of action limitations that are within the domain of nursing. Nurses' understanding of nursing's proper object and their dynamic conceptualization of nursing as a health service are basic guides in ensuring fulfillment of their nursing responsibility. In the course of providing nursing, nurses also provide the ordinary kinds of help that members of families and communities give to one another within the context of day-to-day living, for example, securing reading material and sending messages. However, nurses do not cross boundaries of other helping services and attempt to help with matters for which they are not qualified. Nurses enter into personal situations as nurses to provide help in the form of nursing, not to meet all existent and emerging needs of persons under nursing care. Nurses have knowledge of needs that can be met only by other specialized helpers. Nurses help individuals under nursing care to secure needed help from others by referral, by representing needs for a specialized service, or by helping individuals represent their own needs for such services.

INSIGHTS ABOUT NURSING AS CARE

Care signifies different things and situations. The focus here is on care in the sense "to take care of" with some attention to other meanings.

Care as action for others

Take care of means to watch over, to be responsible for, to make provision for, to look after some person or some thing (p. 233).[3] The critical feature is one person's responsibility for something that is discernible with distinguishing characteristics that can be named. Three forms of care are named, described and explained in this text. **Self-care** (continuous looking after and providing for meeting one's own needs for regulation of functioning and development); **dependent-care** (making these same provisions for dependent adults and children for whom an adult is responsible); and **nursing care**. This section treats in a general way interpersonal situations involving at least two persons, one in the role of care agent and the other in the role of one under the care of another.

Care in the sense "take care of" when used with reference to persons or things does not specify why the providing for or looking after is required. Nor does care indicate the kinds of actions or resources required to fulfill the responsibility. It is evident that the *reason for care* and the *characteristics of care* have their origins in whatever is to be looked after or provided for. Fulfillment of responsibilities of persons "to take care of" other persons requires freedom to obtain care-relevant information about others in their time-place localizations and to have access to them as well as knowing how to look after and provide for them. The responsibility can be fulfilled when the care agent — the provider of care — understands what is included under care and can perform actions and use resources to ensure for others a state of being looked after and provided for. A care responsibility for another person includes the provision of "help" throughout the period of care to meet existent and emerging needs of the other, including initiating and performing tasks that emerge at particular times and under particular circumstances.

Various forms of personal care are institutionalized (i.e., established and supported within societies). The human service occupations and professions including health services are formed and maintained to make these forms of care continuously available. Other forms of person-oriented care have their foundations in the general culture of societies or culture groups. Descriptive terms are used to name particular forms of person-oriented care, as in nursing care and medical care; the place of care, as in hospice care and hospital care; or the age of persons cared for, as in infant care and geriatric care.

Situations where pesons take care of others give rise to a number of common questions that require answers because of professional or legal implications for the care agent, as well as for persons needing care. The first question frequently asked is: Can I positively and effectively contribute to providing for or looking after this person(s) under these circumstances? Other questions include: Is it legitimate for me to serve as care agent in this situation? What is the source of my right to be here and to serve? What is the duration of my responsibility if I enter into this situation as care agent? What is the extent of my responsibility? Does my responsibility extend to all aspects of life situations of others or to specific aspects? Nursing students and nurses must be aware of and deal with such questions in each situation of nursing practice. These same questions need to be asked in all helping situations.

Nursing as care

Care is a word in common use by nurses to signify what they do for the benefit of others. It is sometimes used without the descriptive term *nursing*. Some nurses

---

Exercise **to assist in formalization of a concept of being taken care of**

Part A
A Personal Experience. Reflect on experiences when you were taken care of on a particular occasion by a family member or friend or by a health care professional.
1. Select one of these occasions.
2. Identify and describe why you required care or were judged by others to be in need of it.
3. Describe the events that occurred, including:
   a. How contact was effected between you and the care provider
   b. Events following contact
   c. Characteristics of the care provided
   d. The feelings you experienced
   e. Your judgments about the relationship between your perceptions of what you needed and how you were taken care of
4. Describe what you now perceive as short- and long-term results of the experience.
Part B
Experience of Another. Use the instructions in Part A to elicit from a family member or a friend his or her observations and judgments about a care experience.

prefer to refer to what they do as patient care, client care, or health care. Use of these terms in no way identifies what is being done as nursing.

The foregoing discussion of the word *care*, in the sense to take care of another, was presented to aid nursing students and nurses to continue to develop insights about some of the general characteristics that nursing has in common with other forms of health care.

Some of these characteristics are as follows:

1. Care, regardless of type, is for a person(s) in some place(s) and for some amount of time.
2. Care requires a care agent whose responsibility is to watch over, provide for, and look after another person(s).
3. Care of others demands an interpersonal situation(s); care givers must have access to and foster communication with persons whom they take care of and with persons legally responsible for them in the case of dependents.
4. Care includes the care agent's bringing about and maintaining environmental conditions conducive to the personal development of the other for the duration of care.
5. Care demands recognition by the care agent of the essential freedom of the other as a developing person to grasp possible courses of action, to reflect, and to decide, including decisions to function cooperatively with the care agent.
6. Care demands that the care agent view the person being taken care of *objectively* to determine presenting conditions and needs. The objective approach to the other prevails when the focus is on collaboration and understanding with one another with respect to some objectively discernible reality.
7. Care demands that the care agent view the *person being taken care of* as *subject* who lives, experiences, has awareness of self and environment, attaches meaning to what is experienced, and may be accepting or not accepting of the care agent's presence and actions.
8. Care demands that the care agent *respect* and *accept* the person being taken care of as *subject* who has more and more to do with his or her own becoming or developing.
9. Care demands that the care agent view self as subject who lives through the care situation, experiences events and conditions, attaches meaning to them, and is accepting or not accepting of the actions of the other.
10. Care demands that care agents have sufficient theoretical and experiential knowledge to provide care. They must know the persons to be taken care of and why care is instituted, as well as information about events and conditions in the concrete care situation to make judgments and decisions that will be protective of others as persons living and developing with their social group(s).

The foregoing characteristics of taking care of other persons indicate that providing for or looking after another person is a complex and, at times, energy-depleting endeavor for care agents. The extent of the need to be with the other, to provide for the other, to protect the other, to promote the other's personal development, and to meet the other's needs for help, as well as the amount of concern and anxiety generated within the care situation, determine, in part, the demand on the care agent. The availability and adequacy of the resources of daily living also affect what the care agent can do in a situation. Taking care of others during long or short time periods may be exhausting for the care agent and may be a strain and trial as well as exhausting for persons being taken care of. Mutual respect and loving regard of the care agent and the one cared for may ease the burden of the care situation but do not eliminate the need to attend to and provide for the welfare and well-being of the care agent, as well as the person under care.

The person focus is the critical factor in understanding nursing as care. The person focus, when combined with the helping focus, and the nursing focus provide nursing students with one set of foundations for their initial and continued development of understanding of nursing situations (see Fig. 1–1).

Some nurses forget or have never recognized that nursing is provided for persons. These nurses tend to focus on action sequences or tasks that they have learned to perform in nursing situations or on things that persons under care should or should not do. A nurse's task orientation to nursing often disallows a person focus. A person focus will never be explicated if the uniquely human qualities of men, women, and children are ignored.

Other meanings of care

The word care when followed by "for" or "about" in one sense signifies liking, fondness, affection, or having regard for others. In another sense "to care about" has reference to persons' sense of responsibility for the choices and decisions they make and subsequent occurrences as expressed in statements such as "I care about what happens" (p. 223).[3]

Exercise in distinguishing helping features of a child or an adult care situation

Select a situation where adult persons are responsible for a child or a dependent adult.
Secure information about the endeavors of the responsible adults performed for the sake of the child or dependent adult.
Identify endeavors that you judge to be helping endeavors.
What criteria did you use in making the judgments?

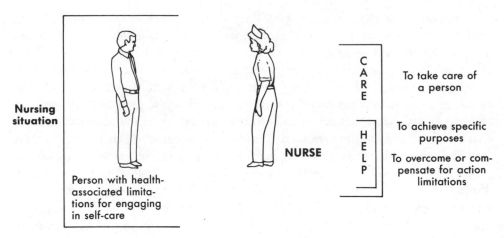

Fig. 1-1 Nursing has taking-care-of and helping features.

Some social philosophers and anthropologists associate caring for or about other persons with men, women, and children living and developing together in their worlds. Their essentially human attributes distinguish them and are enabling for them to develop themselves as *persons in community*. Plattel[4] states that "being-a-person" is revealed to the developing child or adult as "being-together-with-my-fellowmen" (p. 23). The developing child, man, or woman comes to understand his or her relationships to others as conjoined with *person-hood*, leading to a fundamental unity of persons within their world. This according to Plattel is a "personalist conception" of community with a base in "phenomenological anthropology." Its focus is the "entire mystery of the intersubjectivity" of men, women, children and "interhuman communication." This "personalist conception" of community is in accord with the idea that persons who take care of and care for and help others within or outside family units are interested in the welfare of others in their world—that they function to do good for others. Such persons often are viewed as benevolent, as possessing a native kindliness, as persons who act with love and compassion for others.

Care in still another of its lexicographic meanings signifies the "*state of mind* of a person who is wholly occupied and troubled by personal affairs or affairs of others or by conditions within their world" (p. 223).[3] Care signifies a heaviness or oppression associated with burdensome demands. Care in this sense is included in the meaning of the word *concern*, which implies anxious interest in someone or something along with some degree of care.

Nurses use the word care to convey all of the meanings identified in this section. Mastery by nursing students and nurses of the various lexicographic meanings of the word care should aid them in making judgments about the meaning(s) attached to care in the nursing literature and in verbal presentations and discussions. It should aid them in recognizing when to ask speakers or writers: How are you using the word care? What does care signify in this context?

VIEWS OF NURSING

Nursing has been described in prior sections of the chapter as the specialized work of nurses with its own domain and boundaries that distinguish it from other human health services. Nursing has been identified as a form of help or care. A summary of views of nursing are now presented from an historical perspective.

Four views

The word *nursing* in the 1911 historical work *Reminiscences of Linda Richards, America's First Trained Nurse*[5] is used in four different but related ways. In the following three cited quotations from these reminiscences the word *nursing* signifies *care of patients by nurses.*

> Only a small portion of time was given to the care of patients; the household duties were considered of far greater importance than nursing (p. 57).

> Previous to this date, September 1, 1872, nurses had received instructions in the care of obstetrical cases only. Now the work was regularly organized for the definite training of young women in general nursing (pp. 9-10).

> The course was for only one year and embraced training in medical, surgical and obstetrical nursing, but the kind and amount of instruction was very limited (p. 11).

Modifications of the noun *nursing* by the adjectives *obstetrical, medical,* and *surgical* signify specialization of nursing because of the clinical conditions of patients and the kinds of medical care received. In the context of the quotations the term *general nursing* is interpreted as signifying all forms of nursing.

The word *nursing* in Linda Richards' description of her one year of formal preparation for nursing, from 1872 to 1873 at the New England Hospital for Women and Children, signifies a particular kind of knowledge that some persons had, knowledge that could be imparted to others.

> It does not seem quite loyal to my school to tell how little training we received, for everyone in authority gave us of her best nursing knowledge (p. 14).

Linda Richards visited Florence Nightingale at her home in England in 1877. In the reminiscences about the visit the phrase "my nursing years" (p. 38) appears. Implicit in the phrase is the idea of vocation or field of work or occupation or profession.

> The one dream of my nursing years was being fulfilled: I was indeed talking with the one woman whose name and the record of whose good works were known throughout the civilized world (p. 38). (See Stewart and Austin for an account of these "nursing years.")

At the beginning of her reminiscences Linda Richards used *nursing* in a fourth sense. She wrote about her search for a place, a hospital where she could prepare for her "desired vocation," a place where she "could really learn the art of nursing" (pp. 5-6).[5] Since art is a human quality, the reference to nursing as a *particular art* signifies Linda Richards' desire for personal development as a nurse with respect to those qualities of mind required in using practical intelligence in designing and producing nursing for those in need.

Some or all of the senses in which the word *nursing* was used by Linda Richards in reminiscing about her "nursing years" are identified in earlier as well in later works by nurses and others concerned with the condition of or with the advancement of nurses and nursing.

In Florence Nightingale's *Notes on Nursing,* printed in 1859, *nursing* signifies the *care of "sick and well persons"* in their homes or in hospitals by "nurses professional and non-professional."[7] Nursing is "good" or "poor." "Symptoms" and "suffering" result from poor nursing or lack of nursing. Nursing is *knowledge.* There are laws, "canons," or basic rules of nursing. "Laws of health" and "laws of nursing" are said to be the same laws. These laws hold for both the well and the sick. There are "elements" of what constitutes good nursing, and these elements are little understood in relation to nursing the sick or the well. *Notes on Nursing* also specifies nursing as "art" and as a "calling."

The meanings attached to the word *nursing* in the historical material cited are considered to be four different ways of viewing nursing, points of view from which nursing can be examined.

The four expressed points of view are summarized.

1. Nursing is *care provided by nurses* to individuals in their homes or in hospitals, care that varies with the clinical conditions of individuals, care that is good or poor, care that has elements, care designed and produced according to nursing laws.
2. Nursing is a *particular kind of knowledge,* including knowledge of elements of what constitutes good nursing for the well or the sick, and knowledge of the laws or canons of nursing.
3. Nursing is the *particular art,* the *quality of a nurse,* that is enabling for both designing and producing nursing for others.
4. Nursing is a *field of work,* a vocation, occupation, or profession.

The four positions from which nursing can be examined serve the investigations of nurses as well as those of persons from other disciplines.

Examining nursing from a *particular point of view* limits what one must attend to and study and provides organizers for what is said or written. For example, in describing the body of writings about nursing available to nurses in the United States in the early part of the twentieth century, Lavinia Dock's and Isabel Stewart's *A Short History of Nursing* says that "our nursing literature" consists chiefly of manuals on the practice of nursing with "some interesting historical material" (p. 173).[8] The focus here is on the available *body of writings* about nursing with reference to kinds of content.

Practice manuals referred to by Dock and Stewart present accumulated knowledge of what nurses should and should not do in their practice of nursing. This knowledge is properly referred to as *nursing knowledge,* i.e., *knowledge of nursing* essential for use in the practice of nursing. Historical material highlights how nurses and nursing came to be what they are at particular times and over some duration of time. Nursing is attended to in historical material from all four points of view.

Some scholars organize information around one point of view. The social scientist Esther Lucille Brown in the 1930s studied the occupation of nursing with a view toward determining its status as a profession in the United States. Her monograph *Nursing as a Profession* was one of the Russell Sage Foundation's series of monographs on "established" or "emerging" professions.[9]

Nursing as art is a point of view that is recognized in the often-repeated statements "Nursing is an art and a science" and "Nursing is an art but not a science." *Nursing as art* encompasses the point of view of *nursing as care provided by nurses.* Its primary focus, however, is the skilled use by nurses of their practical intelligence in the *creative designing* of care for individuals or groups living under unique and prevailing or changing conditions and circumstances (of which they can have greater or lesser degrees of knowledge) and in the *creative production* of care. The point of view of nursing as art has implicit in it the idea of the nurse as the creator, the maker of nursing under prevailing conditions and circumstances that are or are not subject to regulation or control through nursing.

Nurses as well as others, for example, lawyers in malpractice suits, raise questions at certain times about the *state of the art and the science* of nursing. The reference here is to developing or developed nursing technologies and knowledge for use by nurses in attaining nursing results, the qualifications and capabilities of nurses using the knowledge and the technologies, and to the extent of their use by nurses in geographic areas.

POINTS OF VIEW IN NURSING PRACTICE

The four described points of view are of importance in *nursing practice* where nurses necessarily take and operate from each of them with respect to different matters. The central and enduring point of view in each nursing practice situation, however, is that of *nursing as care provided by nurses.* Nurses take the other three points of view as needed because as nurses they are the essential knowing and skilled human elements of nursing situations with socially designated statuses and roles.

In taking the second point of view, nurses identify in each situation of practice the adequacy of their own nursing *knowledge and skills;* the availability to them of additional knowledge in works of nursing; and the availability to them of nursing consultants, knowledgeable, and skilled nursing experts. Nurses who examine and evaluate not only their own capabilities, including their mastery of nursing science and techniques of practice, but also their own creative approaches to the design and production of nursing under conditions prevailing in specific situations of practice take the third point of view. Finally, nurses who examine their legitimate roles in the *occupation of nursing* as these roles relate to what nurses can legitimately do in particular situations of practice take the fourth point of view.

Nurses who consistently take these points of view in nursing situations meet two basic requirements. First, they accept the *care* point of view as central and enduring in each nursing practice situation. Second, these nurses accept themselves as responsible, knowing, and skilled designers and providers of nursing in specific situations of practice with understanding of their legitimate roles in the occupation and the extent and limits of their nursing capabilities.

Capable and effective nurses understand that their taking the described points of view is a general but necessary way for ensuring their patients' welfare as well as their own. However, the taking by a nurse of any one or all of the points of view, with both discrimination and effectiveness, is not in itself productive of nursing. It is a means used by nurses for *directing and holding their attention* on their patients, on environmental conditions, and on themselves as responsible practitioners of nursing within an occupational field. Appropriate focusing and holding of attention is necessary if nurses are to inquire into the questions associated with each point of view in nursing practice situations. Some questions relevant to each point of view are identified in subsequent paragraphs.

Taking the point of view of *nursing as care provided by nurses* directs nurses' attention to persons under care with concern for questions such as the following:

Is nursing a needed service? If it is, with what human and environmental conditions is the need associated?

What can be and what should be accomplished through nursing?

What kind and amount of nursing will be required and for what time duration?

If this kind and amount of nursing is to be provided, what capabilities must nurses have, and how many nurses will be needed?

Taking the point of view of *nursing as knowledge* directs the nurse's attention to *self,* to *others* who are at more advanced levels of knowing nursing, and to *written works.* The nurse has concern for answering a number of questions, for example:

- Is my nursing knowledge sufficient for the demands for application of particular kinds of knowledge in this situation?
- What are authoritative sources for obtaining knowledge that I lack?
- In what way is my nursing knowledge developing as I work with this person or these persons under nursing care? Have I arrived at new understandings? Should my developing knowledge of elements of nursing and my insights be discussed with nurse colleagues? Should steps be taken toward verification and formalization of this knowledge?

Taking the point of view of *nursing as art* directs a nurse's attention to *self* considered in relationship to the *kind of nursing that should be produced* for each individual under the nurse's care. Inexperienced nurses and nursing students naturally tend to focus on themselves in relationship to isolated tasks that are constituent elements of care. However, experienced nurses can see the dimensions of and a design for the immediate work of nursing this or that individual or group of individuals with understanding of how the work can and should be done creatively and effectively. The question in the art point of view is whether a nurse's mastery of *science* and *technique* is equal to his or her understanding of the work of nursing to be done, for example, can nurses creatively design nursing in light of prevailing conditions and circumstances and produce effective care through which nursing results are obtained? Since the art of nursing subsumes a number of basic arts, nurses must ask questions about their mastery of knowledge and technique with respect to the following basic arts:

The art of talking to reveal what is known by the nurse about the presenting situation and thereby provoke questions about things the nurse has overlooked and to which attention should be given

The art of relating person-to-person to others with recognition of the functions and responsibilities of each in the situation and the kind of experiences each brings to it

The art of coordinating one's actions with those of others whenever the actions of each contribute to or will affect the achievement of some desired result

The art of eliciting cooperation from others in the achievement of a desired outcome

The art of representing facts, positions, needs, desired outcomes, types of action, and results of action to others who are involved in a situation

The arts of discussion and persuasion

These basic arts contribute to the production of nursing because nursing is *care* of some persons by other persons. But the art of nursing is the nurse's quality or habit of reasoning and judging correctly about the design and production of the kind and amount of nursing needed according to the principles or laws of nursing itself. Science and technique are "the first necessary conditions for honest art. (p. 188)"[10] The point of view of nursing as art therefore encompasses the point of view of *nursing as knowledge.*

In taking the point of view of *nursing as a field of work, occupation, or profession,* the nurse's attention is directed to self and to society. The nurse attends to and reflects on self as having a field of work and an occupational status within society and as one among many with the same status or with different but related statuses. The nurse attends to his or her legally and occupationally defined roles and responsibilities and to proscribed types of contractual relationships to persons under nursing care and whenever relevant to an employing institution. Roles and responsibilities may extend to persons nursed, to their next of kin or legal guardian, as well as to an employer or an associate and to persons who serve as helpers to nurses.

From the fourth point of view nurses seek answers to questions such as the following:

- Am I legally and occupationally qualified to take on the roles and responsibilities of nurse in this practice situation?
- Am I personally *capable* and *willing* to be related to this person (or these persons) as nurse and bear and fulfill the nursing responsibility? Now? When predicted changes occur? For what time duration?
- Is this person (or these persons) or the next of kin or legal guardian willing to have me as nurse and enter into a *nurse-patient* or a *nurse-legally responsible person* relationship with me?
- Who are the *nurses* available to me and to persons under my care as *nursing consultants* in the event that nursing matters requiring consultation arise?
- With what other persons participating in the health care or the residential care of this person (or these persons) must I cooperate?
- What is the nature and degree of coordination of nursing with other care providers that is likely to be needed? What are my role responsibilities related to these care providers?

Some nurses from time to time also ask a much broader question that is of deep concern to them. The question is: Can I, on a day-to-day basis, live the occupational aspects of my life with a style that yields good performance, recognition and respect from others, and at times affection (p. 188)[10] and also move within the occupation of nursing in accord with my interests and talents?

Nurses who ask this question more likely than not have a *career orientation to nursing* as their field of work, their profession.

THE NURSE AS AGENT

In the nineteenth century and earlier, the formal education and training of women and in some settings men was recognized by concerned individuals as essential for making nursing available to those who need it. Nursing came to be viewed as an endeavor of women and men who were educated and trained as *nurses*. From an *action* perspective, the educated nurse was recognized as essential for nursing since the *nurse* is the *agent* whose actions are productive of nursing care.

Nineteenth-century advances toward providing nursing were associated with increasing social awareness and concern on the part of individuals and groups for the poor, the homeless, orphans and neglected children, the insane, prisoners, the sick poor, and the hospitalized sick. During this period, the word *nursing* gradually took on the meaning of *care provided by "trained nurses" or by "pupil nurses" in training.*[11]

In the United States in the nineteenth century and into the twentieth century persons with formal preparation for nursing were referred to as "trained nurses." However, training programs varied so in length and in the quality of the experiences provided to "pupil nurses" that Isabel A. Hampton in 1893 speaking to the topic "The standards of education for nurses" remarked that "a trained nurse may mean anything, everything, or next to nothing." (pp. 1-12)[11]

Trained nurses stood in contrast to uneducated and untrained workers assigned or employed to care for the sick in hospitals or in households in a community (pp. 6-7).[5] They also stood in contrast to "born nurses," women described by Linda Richards as having earned the *title nurse* for themselves through "kindness of heart," "cheerful service," "experience," and the "instruction of older women and of the family doctor." These women went outside their homes to provide care to neighbors or others in the community (pp. 3-4).[5]

During the nineteenth century and into the twentieth century nursing was a field to be discovered by those who aspired to its practice. Linda Richards noted that:

> We pioneer nurses entered the school with a strong desire to learn; we were well and strong, we were on the watch for stray bits of knowledge, and were quick to grasp any that came within our reach. What we learned we learned thoroughly, and it has proved a good foundation for the building of subsequent years (p. 14).[5]

The concerned women and men who instituted training schools for nurses and thoughtful graduates of those schools saw nursing as a specific field of practice, however unclear its domain and its boundaries might be. Nursing was being differentiated from the work of untrained and uneducated workers assigned or employed to care for the sick, the suffering, and the helpless. Nursing also was differentiated from housekeeping, welfare services, and medical practice.

Hospital nurses had both housekeeping and nursing responsibilities. These two functions of nurses were distinguished. Housekeeping or household duties were not called nursing (p. 57).[5] District or instructive visiting nurses were not to engage in almsgiving, a welfare service. They were to restrict their work in households to nursing. This included nursing sick members of a household, care of women after childbirth and their infants, and instructing members of households in healthful personal care practices and home nursing and in household sanitation (pp. 127-133).[11]

That nursing was a form of care different from medical care was recognized in the eighteenth and nineteenth centuries by men and women who were concerned about meeting the unmet needs of the sick and injured in hospitals and in their homes. It was known that being under the care of a physician did not meet the continuing care requirements of such persons. Nor did the presence of obstetricians and "sanitary officers" in communities meet the needs of adult household members for instruction about how to care for themselves, their dependents, and their household to prevent death and sickness and maintain the well-being of household members.

In the first quarter of the twentieth century the meaning of the word *nursing* thus became associated with the word *nurse* in the sense of one who *knows nursing* and *can and does produce it*. Additionally, the *action* that is properly named *nursing* was distinguished from action that is not nursing, including actions of untrained persons who attend the sick, housekeeping, welfare service, and medical care.

However, as the twentieth century progressed with an increase in the number of educated nurses and an extension of nursing to more and more people, nurses became burdened not just with housekeeping but with work from other domains. Nursing in its uniqueness as a required human service was overshadowed by the array of duties and tasks from other fields that were showered on nurses. Then nurses began to seek answers to the question: What is nursing? How can one distinguish nursing from other forms of care and service?

REFERENCES

1. Orem DE: Guides for developing curricula for the education of practical nurses, Vocational Division Bulletin N.274, p. 18, Washington, DC, 1959, US Government Printing Office.
2. Orem DE: Hospital nursing service, an analysis, Indianapolis, Indiana, 1956, Division of Hospital and Institutional Services, Indiana State Board of Health, p. 85.
3. The Random House dictionary of the English language, unabridged edition, New York, 1973, Random House, p. 223.
4. Plattel MG: Social philosophy. Pittsburgh, 1965, Duquesne University Press, p. 23.
5. Richards LAJ: Reminiscences of Linda Richards, America's first trained nurse, Boston, 1911, M Barrows and Co, pp. 9-10, 11,14, 38, 57.
6. Stewart IM, and Austin AL: A history of nursing, New York, 1962, GP Putnam's Sons, pp. 142-143.
7. Nightingale F: Notes on nursing: what it is and what it is not, London, 1859, Harrison & Sons.

8. Dock LL, and Stewart IM: A short history of nursing, ed 3, New York, 1931, GP Putnam's Sons, p. 173.
9. Brown EL: Nursing as a profession, ed 2, New York, 1940, Russell Sage.
10. Lonergan BJF: Insight, a study of human understanding, New York, 1958, Philosophical Library, p. 188.
11. Hampton IA, et al: Nursing of the sick 1893, New York, 1949, McGraw-Hill Book Co., p. 1-12, 127-133.

SELECTED READINGS

Backscheider J: The use of self as the essence of clinical supervision in ambulatory patient care, Nurs Clin North Am 1971 6:785-794.
Cousins N: The healing heart: antidotes to panic and helplessness, New York, 1983, Norton.
Entralgo PL: The doctor-patient relationship today. In Doctor and patient, translated from the Spanish by Frances Partridge, New York, 1969, World University Library, McGraw-Hill Book Co.
Nightingale F: Sick nursing and health nursing. In Hampton IA, et al: Nursing of the sick 1893, New York, 1949, McGraw-Hill Book Co.
Plattel MG: Person and community and the mystery of being-together-in-the-world. In Social philosophy, Pittsburgh, 1965, Duquesne University Press.
Roach, Sister MS: Caring: the human mode of being. Implications for nursing, Toronto, 1984, Faculty of Nursing, University of Toronto.
Schmiedling NJ: Orlando's theory. In Winstead-Fry, P: editor: Case studies in nursing theory, New York, 1986, National League for Nursing.
Weiss P: You, I, and the others, Carbondale and Edwardsville, 1980, Southern Illinois University Press.
Wiedenback E: Clinical nursing, a helping art, New York, 1964, Springer Publishing Co., Inc.

CHAPTER 2

Nursing and society

Once a society introduces and establishes nursing as a human health service, persons who seek to provide nursing for others or who seek to prepare themselves to do so must earn and be afforded the status of nurse within the society. The recognition of individual women and men within a social group as nurses affords them the right to represent themselves as able and willing to provide nursing and the obligation to provide nursing in situations which they enter into as nurses. Nursing students and nurses must come to understand, accept, and manage themselves within their public status in social groups. Understanding nursing as an available service in communities and societies emphasizes the societal facets of the relationships of nurses to persons they nurse and to the society that recognizes them as nurses.

The differentiation, development, and maintenance of nursing as a human service in societies and culture groups and the provision of nursing to individuals and groups proceeds within processes of group life and societal relationships. Differentiation and institutionalization of nursing as a health service usually is brought about by concerned persons in locations where people are who need nursing. Movement toward this end occurs at the international and national levels when the need for, the value of, and the means for providing nursing are understood and communicated by innovators and developers.

REFERENCE TERMS

In social groups where nursing is provided, reference terms are used to signify individuals who are accepted as providers of the service nursing, and those who are being provided with the service. In English-speaking countries, the word *nurse* signifies persons qualified through education, training, and experience to provide nursing to persons in need of this special service. Since nursing education in the United States remained outside the national system of education for so many years, the title nurse, as previously stated, signified persons with a wide range of nursing knowledge and capabilities. Reference terms within nursing have changed and will continue to change as nurses continue the development of their science and art.

The term *nursing practitioner* is used in this text to signify persons professionally qualified to practice nursing and who are engaged in its regular provision. At times, the terms *nurse* and *nursing practitioner* are used interchangeably. In the text, the term *nurse* is used to refer to women and men prepared either through high-level technical education or professional level education. However, nursing practitioner is used to refer specifically to professionally educated nurses working at the entry or advanced level of nursing practice. Nurses prepared through high-level technical education work with nursing practitioners or work under established nursing protocols.

The use of the term *nursing practitioner* presumes that within the broad domain of human service and health professions there is a field identified as nursing. The professionally educated nurse knows the field of nursing and may specialize in one or more areas of its practice. Knowing nursing as a field of practice and knowing the relation of areas of specialization to the whole field is one characteristic of persons who function as nursing practitioners.

The term *nursing practitioner* as used in this text is not equated with the term *nurse practitioner*. The latter term came into use to designate nurses with a technical to technological level of preparation for performing selected tasks or managing certain subsystems of operations within the domain of medical practice. Some nurse practitioners function as nursing practitioners who do initial physical examinations and prescribe for common ailments. Other nurse practitioners function within medical protocols with a medical orientation to care sometimes as physician assistants. *Nurse practitioner* is viewed as an *ambiguous term* because it does not indicate what is being practiced by the nurse who carries the title. The settings in which nurse practitioners function may provide clues to what is being practiced.

Persons under the care of nurses, physicians, or other direct health care providers, as well as persons under care in hospitals, have been and are identified by the term *patient*. The same person could be a nurse's patient, a physician's patient, and a hospital patient. The word *patient* means a receiver of care, someone who is under the care of a health care professional at this time, in some place or places.

Some nurses use the term *client* in place of the term *patient*. This effort seems to be directed toward recognition of the contractual nature of the relationships of nurses to persons under their care and to avoidance of the philosophical use of the word *patient* to mean *that which is acted upon*. It is customary to use the term *client* in the practice of law, in business, and trade. In the legal profession, clients are persons who *employ* or *retain* an attorney or counselor for advice and assistance. Clients place their affairs in the hands of an attorney who acts for them in any legal matters. *Client* also means a customer who *regularly* buys from another or receives services from another.

In the health care professions, it would seem that the terms *patient* and *client* are not interchangeable. Persons who are regular seekers of the services of, that is who are clients of, this or that nurse may not be under nursing care at particular times and, therefore, would not have patient status. In child nursing situations or in situations where adults have legally appointed guardians, parents or guardians are the nurse's clients; but it is the child or dependent adult who is the nurse's patient. The terms *patient* or *nurse's patient* will be used to refer to persons under the care of nurses.

Exercise **on nurses' use of reference terms for persons under nursing care**

1. In your contacts with at least five nurses who are engaged in nursing practice determine whether they are willing to respond to a number of questions about their use of general terms in referring to persons under nursing care.
2. If they are willing, ask them already formulated questions to determine:
   a. Whether they use the term *patient* and why.
   b. Whether they use the term *client* and why.
   c. Whether they use other ways of referring to individuals under their care.
3. Express your findings about general terms used by nurses.
4. What conclusion did you reach?

ESTABLISHING AND MAINTAINING NURSING

Nursing as a service is the provision of professional aid that combines features of helping with features of taking care of others when the reasons for the need for help and for being taken care of are within the boundaries of nursing as these boundaries are understood at particular periods in the life of a social group. The initiation and development of a system(s) or method(s) of providing people in communities with nursing include (1) offering education and opportunities for training that are enabling for men and women to prepare themselves to provide nursing and (2) the development of means for persons with nursing requirements to come into relationships with nurses who are able and willing to nurse them. The history of the institution of nursing as a health service in various societies reveals commonalities and differences. Once nursing is instituted, maintaining nursing as an available service within social groups is a continuing problem.

Establishing nursing

The initial establishment of nursing as an organized health service is brought about in societies and social groups because insightful persons recognize the need for it. These enterprising persons provide ways and means to secure and prepare interested women and men to provide nursing. Dock and Stewart (pp. 99-103)[1] note that the foundations for nursing were laid in the seventeenth century by Vincent de Paul and Louise de Marillac and the French women who worked with them to bring nursing first to the people of Paris and later to those in outlying French villages. Men as well as women were active in the initial establishment of nursing in countries throughout the world. In the United States it was recognized that medical care without concomitant nursing care was nonproductive of results sought. The value of nursing was recognized in the Shattock Report of 1850 (pp. 7-17).[2]

The process of distinguishing nursing begins with the recognition that human beings under some range of conditions (1) cannot provide continuing care for themselves or their dependents because of existent situations of personal health and

(2) cannot control internal and environmental factors in such a way as to prevent pathology and maintain, promote, or restore human integrity and well-being. Being physically ill or injured and not having the necessary knowledge and skills were some of the conditions identified by the early developers of nursing. The process of developing nursing continues with the formal preparation of persons to provide a kind of care known as nursing. This is followed, in the sociologic sense, by the institutionalization of forms of nursing education and practice.

The process of distinguishing and establishing nursing begun in several countries at different times during the eighteenth and nineteenth centuries continues. Regardless of the time and place of its initiation, the process is a continuing one and includes at least six sets of actions:

- Recognizing that some persons in their time-place localizations are unable to completely care for themselves or their dependents in whole or in part because of their own or their dependents' states of health and the factors that are conditioning it, or because day-to-day requisites for self-care or dependent-care are novel or complex.
- Naming the help or care that is required nursing.
- Studying conditions under which help or care requirements for nursing arise, including the duration of requirements.
- Identifying and adapting effective and socially acceptable ways for selecting and preparing men and women to provide nursing.
- Identifying and adapting ways to bring about associations between nurses who are prepared, able, and willing to provide nursing, and persons in need of it.
- Extending the work of persons prepared as nurses to more and more individuals who need nursing.

Each of these six sets of actions should be continuously performed because the process of distinguishing and establishing nursing to make it continuously available in a society is never ended. Distinguishing and establishing nursing is a complex process that involves nurses, as well as others who understand the human condition associated with needs of individuals and groups for nursing. Community-based and governmental agencies are also involved.

Maintaining nursing

Initial and continuing efforts to make nursing available depends on societal interest and support and on the willingness of women and men to prepare themselves initially and subsequently through continuing education to function in society as nurses. The strength of nursing in a society does not rest in the number of persons who support nursing, but rather in the ability of practicing nurses to continue to advance their nursing knowledge and capabilities and at the same time to manage and reduce stress associated with day-to-day demands to be with and in communication with others as they provide nursing for an ever changing population of men, women,

Exercise **to compare what a nursing journal publishes by time periods**

1. Select a single issue from a specific year of a national nursing journal for the 10-year periods of the 1940s, 1950s, 1960s, and 1970s.
2. For each issue identify the subject matter, the expressed problem, or the issues that were the focus of editorials.
3. For each issue read the table of contents and the articles as necessary to make a judgment about the subject matter of each article. Make notations about the number of articles by subject matter for each issue selected.
4. Compare and contrast your findings about the subject matter of editorials and articles.
5. Express conclusions about similarities and differences in editorials and articles.

and children in time-place localizations singly or in groups. Nursing's strength also is associated with (1) recognition afforded nurses, (2) satisfaction nurses receive from the effectiveness of their nursing and from their relationships with persons they nurse and with colleagues, and (3) support nurses receive from colleagues and administrators of health care agencies and from their own families. Management of stress involves the development by nurses of realistic expectations of themselves in all aspects of their living including their nursing endeavors.

Maintaining nursing in societies requires deliberate effort by nurses, nursing organizations, community groups, government agencies, educational agencies, and the public. Keeping nursing available and viable is a complex undertaking. The parts or elements of the undertaking must be identified, their meaning and relevance understood, and ways and means instituted to ensure nursing's continued presence and effectiveness. A number of such elements are identified:

- Clear identification of nursing practitioners within social groups along with prerequisites for their practice in types of nursing practice situations
- Clear distinctions between nurses prepared through technical education and persons vocationally trained as aides or attendants
- A public image of nursing practitioners and nurses that is in accord with their contributions to the health and well-being of members of social groups and the responsibilities they bear in a range of health care situations
- Clear distinctions between the contributions of nurses to health care of individuals, families, and communities and the contribution of members of other health professions and occupations with recognition of contributions that are common to all
- Public and private support of university- and college-level educational programs for preparing nursing practitioners and nurses, including requisite access to liberal arts courses directed toward personal development and to science courses that are foundational for understanding nursing

- Assurance that nursing practitioners and nurses are able to effectively represent themselves and their work verbally and in writing to persons they nurse, to other nurses, to other health professionals, to executives of health service agencies, and to the public
- Assurance that nursing practitioners have the freedom to practice nursing for the populations they serve, and that contributions of nursing practitioners and nurses that further the effectiveness of the work of physicians and others be kept within nursing's boundaries
- Maintenance of work environments, conditions of work, and remuneration for nursing practitioners and nurses that is protective of their lives, health, and well-being and conducive to personal and professional development
- Knowledge of existent and emerging or predicted conditions and circumstances of members of communities that are indicators of needed changes in nursing practice and in the number of preparation of nursing practitioners and nurses who work with them
- Development and redevelopment of ways to ensure provision of nursing to men, women, and children that is effective and economical of time, money, and materials, including new ways of offering nursing as in nursing clinics and the development of new nursing positions and titles

Nurses, organizations of nurses, and organizations for the promotion of nursing and nursing education are or should be in the forefront in expenditure of efforts to maintain nursing in social groups. National and state or provincial governments, as well as local governments, community groups, and individual citizens, contribute to ensure nursing's continued availability. Public and private groups under some circumstances and through policy decisions at state and national levels fail to contribute to the maintenance of nursing so that nursing becomes less and less available in communities to persons for whom it is an essential service.

The process of distinguishing nursing from other forms of care and establishing and maintaining its availability in social groups requires both attention and effort. Although this process is distinct from the process of providing nursing to those in need, both are necessary to maintain effective nursing in social groups. Nurses and other concerned persons are involved in ensuring that nursing is available. But it is only the actions of adequately prepared and responsible nurses that result in the kind of care that is named nursing.

THE SERVICE FEATURES OF NURSING

Nursing is a human service in societies in that it meets certain requirements of men, women, and children that arise during day-to-day living. Nursing is but one of an array of human services available to the public in many geographic areas. Like all services, it must be distributed, produced, and financed. The proliferation of services of all types is attested to by the Yellow Pages of urban and rural telephone books.

Nursing meets personal requirements of individual human beings and families andcommunities. It is a direct service for persons singly or in groups.

Nursing's helping and caring features described in the prior chapter express general characteristics of the person-to-person relationships of nurses and nurses' patients. Nursing's service features identify and describe characteristics of nurses, nurses' patients, and nursing that are in the public view. Service features of nursing relate persons who are nurses or aspiring nurses to the larger community and to governmental jurisdictions. These features must be made operative in every situation of nursing practice. Service features of nursing thus provide a societal frame of reference within which nurses function in each situation of nursing practice.

Service connotes action and implies that the results of action or work are beneficial to individuals or groups or whole communities. Services are understood in terms of the functional society where interrelationships come about because of and are dominated by the work performed. One person or group seeks another so that together an objective goal can be attained that could not be attained alone. Plattel (p. 53)[3] states that "in the functional society" relationships between or among persons have "an external character" so that it is possible to talk about "having" or "possessing" a relationship. Individual nurses, their patients, and patients' significant others thus constitute collaborating units within a society.

Service enterprises

The continuous offering of a service (e.g., nursing) to members of a society requires laborious effort, perseverance, persistent exertion, resourcefulness, and the human and material resources necessary to provide the service. Since services offered should be available in accord with the time at which and the ways in which needs for them are revealed, the availability of services must be timed and the nature and quality of services made known to potential users. Specific services may be offered by individuals or collaborating groups as in the private or the group practice of nursing or medicine. Specific and sometimes related services may be made available to the public through controlling bodies, such as hospitals that are incorporated as nonprofit or profit-making entities within a governmental jurisdiction. Also national, state or provincial, or local governments may make specific services available to persons who need and qualify to receive them.

Legally constituted bodies, such as hospitals, sponsor the offering of human services by ensuring, for example, that physicians, nurses, and other essential health professionals are available and ready to practice in situations where their specialized work is required. Such institutions make it possible for health professionals to practice within an enabling environment and for members of the public to seek and receive services within this environment. It is important for nurses and nursing students to understand the functional systems needed for the private or group or the large-scale institutional offering of nursing and other health services.

Functions and functional systems are the same in kind but vary in magnitude of performance for private or group practice or large-scale institutional offering. Before offering service, the legal authority to exist as an enterprise that provides services to the public toward fulfillment of the defined purposes must be obtained. The conditions for receiving this authority must be met initially and conditions for retaining it fulfilled.

In order for human service enterprises to survive and fulfill their reasons for existence in communities, they must have persons engaged in performing three sets of functions: governing functions, executive functions, and essential operational functions. The main subfunctions of each are identified in the following outline.

GOVERNING FUNCTIONS

1. Acting for the enterprise as a whole
2. Leading the enterprise to achieve its end in the society
3. Providing what is needed and correcting what is out of order

EXECUTIVE FUNCTIONS

1. Defining and limiting the purpose of the enterprise in accord with its purpose for existence and the nature of the current and changing requirements of people for services
2. Securing and maintaining essential effort
3. Providing and maintaining a system of communication

ESSENTIAL OPERATIONAL FUNCTIONS

1. Initial and subsequent distribution of opportunities to individuals or multiperson units to partake of available services
2. Production of services in association with continuing acts of distribution over the time period when services are provided to specific individuals or multiperson units
3. Financing of the services distributed to and produced for individuals and multiperson units

These are dimensions of the mainstreams of functioning of human service enterprises.

Fig. 2-1 shows sets of managerial and contributory functions that feed into and out of the three central functional systems. The contributory functions are concerned with the securing, availability, and care of essential resources. The managerial functions are directed to each of the three central functions and focus on the development of designs and plans for execution of each subfunction and on performance evaluation and control.[4] Failure to comprehend the nature of, to provide for performance of, and to perform the identified functions will result in the failure of service enterprises to fulfill their purpose for existence.

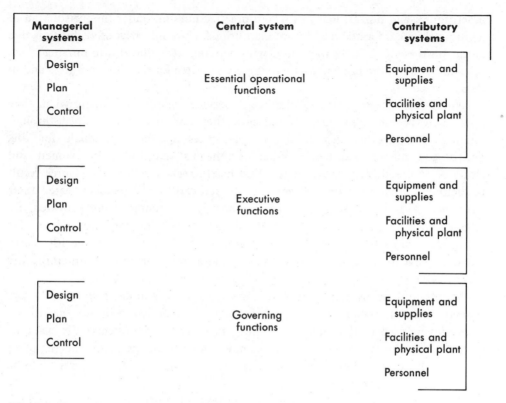

Managerial systems	Central system	Contributory systems
Design Plan Control	Essential operational functions	Equipment and supplies Facilities and physical plant Personnel
Design Plan Control	Executive functions	Equipment and supplies Facilities and physical plant Personnel
Design Plan Control	Governing functions	Equipment and supplies Facilities and physical plant Personnel

Fig. 2-1. Functions of human service enterprises.

Nursing's health service features lend specificity of purpose to the types of enterprises that offer nursing in societies.

HEALTH SERVICE FEATURES

Nurses speak and write about nursing as a health service. Insightful nurses have better understanding of nursing's position in the family of health services than do members of other health professions or the public. From a public perspective, nursing occupies an obscure to invisible position as a specialized health service. The absence of nursing is afforded greater recognition than its presence or its effectiveness as a health service.

Public recognition of health features

Nursing continues to be viewed by health policy makers and others as an adjunct to medical care provided by physicians. Nursing also is viewed by some persons as a hospital or health care agency service and not as specialized work of nursing practitioners and nurses, many of whom practice nursing under the jurisdiction of legitimately incorporated health care institutions. Nursing's lack of visibility is due in part to these traditional ways of viewing nursing. It is due also to nursing's lack of visibility since the provision of nursing is a private affair, visible to nurses and to those nursed.

Nurses are able to articulate the health service features of nursing when they know why people need nursing and how they are or can be helped through nursing. **Self-care** or **dependent care** is necessary for individuals for life, health, and human well-being. When the health states of men, women and children or the characteristics of required health-related self-care measures result in action limitations for engagement in self-care or dependent care, their lives, health, and well-being may be in jeopardy if nursing is not provided. By compensating for or overcoming health-associated human limitations for engagement in self-care or dependent-care, nurses contribute to health maintenance, prevention of disease and disability, and to restoring or maintaining life processes.

Nurses in their practice of nursing know the human and environmental factors that condition (1) persons' self-care requirements and (2) their self-care capabilities. Condition is used in the sense of to affect, to modify, or influence; for example, childrens' developmental states influence how they express their experiencing of an existent self-care requisite, such as the requisite for food intake, or a requisite to be relieved of discomfort or pain.

The term **self-care requisite** is used in this text as required actions through which individuals regulate factors that affect their human functioning and human development. Care requisites may be met through self-care, dependent care, or nursing. Self-care requisites, when formulated, express desired results, the goal of self-care.

Persons in environments

Nurses in concrete nursing practice situations seek nursing-relevant information about both persons who seek or need nursing and their environmental situations. Human beings are never isolated from their environments. They exist in them. For purposes of understanding, environmental features can be isolated, identified, and described; and some environmental features are subject to regulation or control. Human environments are analyzed and understood in terms of physical, chemical, biologic, and social features. These features may be interactive. Certain environmental features are continuously or periodically interactive with men, women, and children in their time-place localizations. As is well known, environmental conditions can positively or negatively affect the lives, health, and well-being of individuals, families, communities; under conditions of war or natural disaster, whole societies are subject to disruption or destruction.

Environmental features

Some environmental features relevant to the values or presence of self-care requisites are listed in three categories:

Physicochemical Features

Atmosphere of the earth
Gaseous-composition of air
Pollutants — solid, gaseous
Smoke
Weather conditions
Geologic stability of earth's crust

Biologic Features

Pets
Animals in the wild
Infectious organisms or agents — virus, rickettsia, bacteria, fungus, protozoa, helminth
Persons or animals, including birds and anthropods, under natural conditions affording subsistence or lodgement to infectious agents
Persons or animals harboring infectious agents with manifest disease or inapparent infection

Socioeconomic-cultural features

Family
Composition by roles and ages of members
Cultural prescriptions of authority, responsibilities and rights for family as a unit, dominant family member, other members
Positions of members within families and culturally prescribed relationships
Time-place localizations of members
Family dynamics
Nature of relationships — familial, contractual, coercive
System of family living
Resources of family as a unit
Resources of individual members
Culture prescriptions for securing, managing, and using resources
Culture elements specifying specific patterns of self-care and dependent care and selection and use of care measures

Community

Population
Composition by family units; by other functional, collaborating social units; and by governmental organs

Availability of resources for daily living of community members and for special
    needs of the community as a whole

Health services

Kind, localization, availability

Openness to individuals, to families

Accessibility

Culture practices and prescriptions about use

Cost costs, methods of financing

Human features

In all situations of human living the health states of involved persons affect what persons do. Health service situations come into being when individuals become concerned about their health states or when they or others perceive changed features or recognize that their health may be in jeopardy. If at the same time they judge that seeking health care and service is a good thing to do and if health services are available, entry to the service is initiated. Existent or projected or potential features of *persons' states of health* are central concerns of health service professionals, including nurses. Nurses view health states of the persons they nurse as a *basic conditioning factor* influencing what persons need to do and what they can do with respect to self-care. Physicians view the health states of persons under their care as a central concern since the focus of medicine is the human potential of persons for health and their subjectivity to ill health, injury, and disability.

Nurses view the health states of individuals in relation to chronologic age and developmental stage. Developmental stages are age related and health states are understood in relation to both development and age of individuals. If health is accepted as a state of being, whole or sound personal health is linked to persons' growth and developmental states which change as individuals age. Clear examples of relatedness is the physiologic difficulties experienced by premature infants and the extraordinary developmental demands on persons of any age who suffer from disabling conditions.

The health states of persons in relation to their ages and their developmental states determine in nursing practice situations (1) the amount and kind of help required, (2) the extent of need to be taken care of as persons, and (3) patient and nurse roles in the process of nursing. Nurses must have accurate and reliable information about the health states of their patients throughout the duration of a nursing situation. Nurses obtain direct information about aspects of patients' health states and use information obtained by physicians and others. Nurses recognize that in concrete situations health states of individuals are at times understood and expressed (1) as all encompassing, well-defined conditions, such as being consciously aware, being rationally conscious, being well, or acutely ill or debilitated; or (2) as specific characterizing features such as recurring events that reveal cardiac or respiratory functioning or the presence of abnormal structures such as tumors.

SOCIETAL ASPECTS OF NURSING PRACTICE

In modern society, adults are expected to be self-reliant and responsible for themselves and for the well-being of their dependents. Most social groups further accept that persons who are helpless, sick, aged, handicapped, or otherwise deprived should be helped in their immediate distress and helped to attain or regain responsibility within their existing capacities. Thus, both self-help and help to others are valued by society as desirable activities. Nursing as a specific type of human service is based on both values. In most communities people see nursing as a desirable and necessary service.

Historical works and the investigations of anthropologists provide evidence that, in the past, societies recognized the social position of nurse and provided ways and means to have nurses. In some situations, persons became nurses because of their position in the family or in the larger society. In other situations, individuals were recruited to become nurses, as is presently done in many countries. Preparation for nursing was both formal, through prescribed systems of training, and informal. Modern society introduced science-based education preparatory to nursing practice. The continued presence of active nurses in a society indicates that nursing is a desired and utilized service.

What is nursing? What are the nurse's contributions to the health and wellbeing of individuals, families, and communities? Is it to give care? Is it to bring about psychological adjustment so that a person will be able to accept and to live with illness or disability and develop personally, using his or her human potential? Is it to implement physicians' prescribed measures of care for the patient? Although the answers to each of these questions is "yes," the answers do not adequately describe how and why nursing is specifically different from other human services.

Requirements for nursing

When do nurses enter into the life situations of individuals or groups? Societies specify the conditions that make it legitimate for its members to seek the various kinds of human services that are provided. These conditions become the criteria that members of the society use in determining whether a particular human service can or should be used. The condition that validates the existence of a requirement for nursing in an adult is *the absence of the ability to maintain continuously that amount and quality of self-care which is therapeutic in sustaining life and health, in recovering from disease or injury, or in coping with their effects.* With children, the condition is the *inability of the parent (or guardian) to maintain continuously for the child the amount and quality of care that is therapeutic.* The word **therapeutic** is used to mean supportive of life processes, remedial or curative when related to malfunction due to disease processes, and contributing to personal development and maturing.

Requirements for nursing cannot be met unless they are recognized. Physicians identify the need for and seek nursing for their patients. Friends and family members also may recognize when a person needs nursing, and adults may recognize their own needs for nursing. The family is often the first line of assistance when its members are in need. When family, friends, or neighbors are unable or unwilling to help, assistance with management or maintenance of self-care may be sought from organized nursing services. Nursing may be provided in the home, or in health care institutions, on an inpatient or outpatient basis. There may or may not be a sufficient number of nurses to provide the needed service. Organization for the delivery of nursing is a need of every community.

Physicians traditionally have had as the focus of their service the health and disease states of individuals. Their concern is with life processes, body structure, and interferences with life and developmental processes. Physicians evaluate health states, determine evidence of the presence or absence of disease, and prescribe and give therapy to maintain health and to cure or control disease or the effects of injury and disease. When able, persons under medical care are expected to manage their own health affairs and maintain the type of self-care they require. When unable, assistance from persons other than the physician is required. Nursing is required whenever the maintenance of continuous self-care requires the use of special techniques and the application of scientific knowledge in providing care or in designing it.

It is an accepted practice for the physician to see patients periodically. The time a physician spends with a patient varies with the patient's health state and the medical care techniques used. Some patients see their physicians once a year, once a month, or more frequently. Physicians do not remain continuously with chronically ill or disabled patients. In the event of serious injury or when life processes or rational processes have been seriously interfered with, the physician may remain with patients for prolonged periods, sometimes working closely with nurses and other health care workers. Patients, nurses, and other specialized workers carry out measures of care prescribed by the physician, and nurses and others assist patients in preparing for measures of care to be performed by physicians. In such instances, a person's self-care becomes linked not only to the medical care given by the physician but also to care or services given by other health personnel, sometimes working as a team. Nurses must often synthesize or unify a variety of care elements into a process of self-care action for the patient.

Nursing as a human service has its foundations, on the one hand, in persons with needs for self-care of a positive, therapeutic quality and limitations for its management or maintenance and, on the other, in the specialized knowledge, skills, and attitudes of persons prepared as nurses. Societies provide ways and means to bring individuals in need of nursing into relationships with qualified nurses. These relationships should be sustained as long as specialized techniques of care are required or until the person or a family member becomes able to manage and maintain the required self-care. Nursing, therefore, has foundations that can be conceptualized as biological, behavioral, and social.

Effecting nursing contacts

Nurses who practice nursing engage themselves in the regular provision of nursing to persons who require it. Nurses function as members of the occupation and profession of nursing in particular geographic areas and governmental jurisdictions. Nurses must be educationally qualified, not exceed their practice capabilities, and be personally willing to provide nursing. Furthermore, nurses must meet standards and conform to regulations that make their practice legitimate in particular jurisdictions.

Although nursing is a valued service in many social groups, it is frequently in short supply for those who need it. A critical factor is the availability ratio: the number of persons in diverse places who require nursing at the same time and the deployment of nurses in relation to those persons. Nurses, as designers and providers of nursing for populations, should be aware of indexes of the objective need for, the demand for, and the supply of nursing.

On a communitywide basis, it is a continual struggle to bring together those who can benefit from short- or long-term nursing and those able and willing to design, put into operation, produce, and manage systems of nursing. This problem should be a concern of social groups that offer nursing as a community service.

A related problem is financing the provision of nursing in social groups. How much does it cost to produce effective nursing for those who need it? How should these costs be distributed within social groups? These questions have not been answered adequately in the United States, where for decades available nursing was produced in large part by nurses-in-training. This practice has changed, but the problem of financing nursing remains partly unaddressed.

Other prerequisites include (1) contact and communication among those who can benefit from nursing and those who are able and willing to produce this service; (2) willingness by those who can benefit from nursing (or others who can legally act for them) and by nurses to enter into and maintain legitimate interpersonal relationships in their respective positions of nurse's patient and nurse; and (3) interpersonal relationships that foster an understanding of how and to what degree nurses' patients can be helped through nursing. These three prerequisites for the production of nursing emphasize a requirement for the social legitimacy of the nurse-patient relationship, a mutual agreement to enter into such a relationship, and the purpose and, therefore, the limits of the relationship.

Contact and communication among persons who can benefit from nursing and persons able and willing to provide it define the first prerequisite for the provision of nursing. Social groups have provided and continue to provide ways and means to effect this contact.

People generally come into contact with nurses in one of two ways: Either they find nurses who publicly represent themselves as being engaged in the private or joint practice of nursing, or they come in contact with nurses through a health care institution that employs nurses. These two methods differ in terms of the way agreements are established and the number and nature of agreements among

Exercise* on use of the words *agreement* and *contract

1. Read about the meanings attached to the words *agreement* and *contract* in:
   a. An unabridged dictionary.
   b. A law dictionary, for example, *Black's Law Dictionary.*
2. Identify and record the meaning expressed for each word.
3. Reflect upon these meanings and think and make judgments about the following:
   a. *Expressions*
      "I contracted with my teacher to do B level work this semester with respect to assignments X, Y, and Z." Express what the verb *contract* means in this context.
      "I contracted with my patient Mr. Jones to reach X goal in two weeks." Express what the verb *contract* means in this context.
   b. *Situation*
      Miss Burns, RN, was designated as nurse for five individuals hospitalized on Unit A. She agreed with the head nurse of Unit A about the designated assignment. Miss Burns, RN, contacted each of the designated individuals, introduced herself as their nurse, and elicited their questions or expressions of their interests or concerns about the relationship. If each of the five patients accepted Miss Burns as his or her nurse, how would you designate the mutual acceptance of the nurse and the five persons on Unit A as a nurse-patient relationship?

individuals and institutions. In the early and middle years of this century, hospitals, state and district nurses' associations, and training schools for nurses maintained registers of nurses in private practice. These registers were the primary means of effecting nurse-patient contacts. Nurses would make their availability known by placing their names on a register; and individuals, families, or physicians whose patients needed nursing would contact nurses directly or through such a register. More recently, nurses have been maintaining their own offices, sometimes in group practice with other nurses or physicians, which has made the office visit another method of effecting nurse-patient contacts.

In the second and more prevalent arrangement, persons who need nursing associate themselves with health care institutions, such as hospitals and visiting nurse associations, where nurses as well as other health workers are available. Under this arrangement, nurses are usually employees of the institution as well as practitioners of nursing. Some of them, however, may be attached to registers.

Where nursing is provided in private or group practice, there is a contract or agreement between the nurse and the patient (or the patient's legitimate representative). Where nursing is effected through a health care institution, there is a contract or agreement between the patient and the institution. In this case, patients have contact with nurses who have been assigned to them by a manager or supervisor, who is usually also a nurse. Individuals who accept care from assigned nurses indicate explicitly or implicitly that they agree to this relationship.

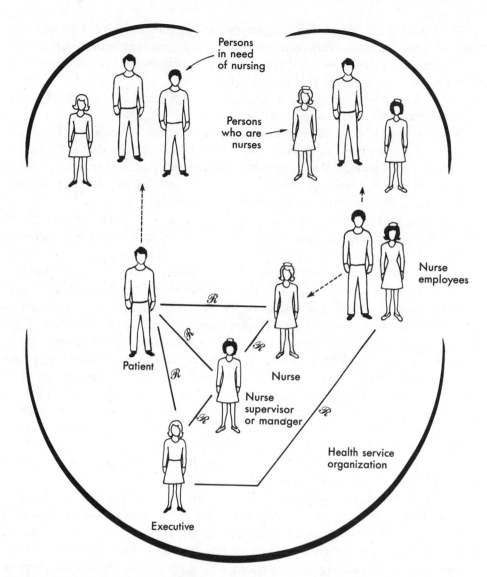

Fig. 2-2 Nurse and patient relationships in health service organizations. R, relationship.

Nurses have not always been aware of the complexity of the relationships in the second arrangement. Nurses who are institutional employees should understand clearly that as members of a social group they occupy two social statuses: that of employee of a health care institution and that of nurse. This situation sometimes creates boundary maintenance problems and role conflict. The legal perspective in such situations is that the person who is the nurse in the status of *employee* is the *agent* (in the legal sense) of the employing institution. Fig. 2-2 illustrates facets of this type of arrangement for nursing.

In both methods of bringing together nurses and persons who can benefit from their care, nurses may go where patients reside or patients may go to the location of the nurse. From this perspective, nursing as a service can be classified into four categories:

- Home nursing—nurse goes to home of patient
- Ambulatory nursing for adults—patient comes to location of the nurse (clinic or office) and returns home after the visit
- Infant and child nursing in clinics or offices—patient is brought by parents or guardians to where the nurse is and returns home after the visit
- Nursing for persons in any age group who are short- or long-term residents of health care institutions, such as hospitals or extended care facilities—nurses come to the institution where patients are in residence

Health care organizations, such as medical centers with hospitals and health maintenance organizations, may offer services in all of these forms and locations.

From an occupational perspective nurses should accept nursing cases in accord with the fit between their individual nursing capabilities and the nursing requirements of those seeking nursing care. Determining whether individuals or groups evidence needs or requirements that nurses can legitimately meet is an essential nursing action. After this determination has been made, nurses should make a more detailed investigation of the nursing requirements of the individual or group. Finally, in light of a precise knowledge of their own nursing capabilities, nurses, as persons responsible for their own nursing acts, must make the judgment that they do or do not have the nursing capabilities required. If the nurse judges that he or she has the requisite capabilities, the nurse can enter into an agreement with the person seeking care (or those acting for the person) about the nature and form of the nursing that will be provided. At this point the nurse in private or group practice or the nurse who is an employee of a health care institution is in a position to negotiate with patients (or those acting for them) about the provision of nursing.

Nurses and persons who are their patients must be aware of the reasons for their relationships. Hospitalized individuals may be unaware that they have agreed to receive nursing when they contract for hospital care. Such individuals are surprised and at times unaccepting when nurses seek information to determine their nursing requirements. On the other hand, persons who expect to receive nursing may be concerned and frightened when they are attended by aides, technicians, or orderlies and have no contacts with nurses. Ideally, nurses foster the development of mutual respect and trust in their relationships with patients. They maintain the frequency of contact and the kind and amount of communication with patients and their families essential in determining and meeting patients' requirements for nursing.

As previously indicated, why individuals require nursing is a critical question to be answered by nursing practitioners. The answer provides nurses with knowledge necessary to identify persons with whom they can have legitimate nursing relationships.

Nurses' previously developed (antecedent) knowledge about the domain of nursing practice, about the elements and relationships of nursing practice situations, and about nursing cases is used in making observations, as well as in judging and making decisions about legitimacy of nurse-patient relationships.

NURSE AND PATIENT ROLES IN SOCIAL GROUPS

Individuals who receive help and care from persons qualified as nurses are referred to as *nurses' patients*. The term symbolizes the social status and roles of persons under the care of nurses. From a sociologic perspective, the terms *nurse* and *nurse's patient* signify related statuses or positions in social groups. Each status carries with it a *role*, that is, a set of prescriptions for organized action through which the status is filled. Nurses must be aware of the professional-occupational prescriptions for their roles as nurses and the role prescriptions for nurses and patients that are part of the general culture of social groups. General cultural prescriptions about nurse and nurse's patient roles may vary from one social group to another. The specific understandings individual nurses and those under their care have about their roles operate as underlying assumptions about the expectations and actions of the nurse and the nurse's patient in each nursing situation.

In nursing situations, nurse's patient roles are specified by the reasons why the nursing is required and by what can and should be done under prevailing conditions. Nurses can help their patients to know and fulfill their roles only when nurses themselves know why and how their patients can be helped through nursing. Nurses' roles become specific in actual nursing situations by their knowledge of why and how an individual, singly or as a member of a family or group, can and should be helped through nursing.

Status and role

The sociological concept of *status-role,* when combined with an understanding of when, why, and how people can be helped through nursing, can aid nurses in their efforts to develop insights about the *fit* or the *relatedness* of their actions to those of patients. A nurse's domain of action within a nursing situation may extend to some or to all or nearly all matters related to the existence and functioning of those under nursing care. How many aspects of the patient's daily life are encompassed in the nurse-patient relationship indicates the *extensity* of the relationship. The extensity of nurse-patient relationships varies with the patient's capabilities for self-care. For example, the extensity of a nurse-patient relationship is great when persons under nursing care have little or no capability for self-care because of their health state and the health-related nature of their continuing self-care requirements. This is so because nurses' roles extend to and encompass matters related to the moment-to-moment existence of such individuals.

The *intensity* of a nurse-patient relationship reflects the meaning that nurse and patient attach to their role relations. A nurse, for example, may know that nursing care can facilitate a patient's movement toward relative self-sufficiency in self-care. The patient, on the other hand, may view some types of help proffered by the nurse as intrusions into his or her life, or a patient may fear to be alone and may desire a nurse's presence continually, or a patient may dread being in the physical presence of a nurse who is rough or verbally abusive. Ideally, in adult nursing situations the extensity as well as the intensity of a nurse-patient relationship has an objective basis in (1) the patient's self-care abilities, limitations, and potential for self-care and self-management and (2) the meaning that nursing care has in relation to the patient's current and future well-being and to the nurse's effectiveness in filling the status of nurse.

Nurses at times have misconceptions about the rights and responsibilities of those who are seeking or who are under nursing care. The nurse-patient relationship is contractual in nature. This means that the functions and responsibilities of nurses are necessarily limited to matters within the domain of nursing, that the help sought is for a limited time, and that nurses are remunerated (directly or indirectly) for the help provided. There should be an initial agreement between the nurse and the nurse's patient or between the nurse and those responsible for the patient's affairs about the general characteristics of the nursing required and the nursing to be provided. The responsible person may be the parents of a child, the legal guardian of an adult, a person with the power to act for an adult, or the next of kin. At times executives of health care institutions employing nurses may need to be informed about these agreements. As previously indicated, each nursing situation requires that nurses must establish that persons or groups who have been represented to them as being in need of nursing are indeed in need of it and that they, as nurses, are able and willing to provide nursing. When nurses are employees of health care institutions, such as public health organizations, hospitals, or nursing homes with which patients have contracts for care, there should be a second, preferably explicit, verbal agreement between the nurse and each patient or individuals acting for the patient about the nurse's willingness to provide nursing and the patient's willingness to receive nursing from assigned nurses. Patients and their families should be informed about the goals to be sought through nursing.

Ideally, in health care institutions, explicit verbal agreements about the nursing to be provided should be made by the nurse who has determined the particular patient's nursing requirements, who has designed a system of nursing assistance, and who bears continuing responsibility for nursing the patient. A number of nurses may contribute to the provision of nursing according to the original or adjusted design; this contributory care includes continuous observation of the patient. These nurses as well as the patient should know their own roles in addition to the role of the nurse who bears nursing responsibility for the patient. Nurses should understand that nursing requirements cannot be met unless they are known. Such knowledge comes only through directed and controlled observation, which necessitates contact and communication with the patient.

Agreements to provide nursing to individuals, families, or groups bind nurses to the provision of nursing in accord with objective nursing requirements. Nurses may be aware that they are not capable of providing the amount and kind of nursing required. At other times they are capable but know that external conditions, including the number of persons requiring nursing, their locations, and the amount and complexity of their care will sometimes preclude the provision of sufficient nursing. When such conditions predominate, nurses, as responsible members of a social group, must be able to represent the existing situation prudently to the patient, to the employing executives, or to their own supervisors by indicating how all involved can best contribute to ensuring the safety and well-being of the patient. Nurses too often remain silent about situations where nursing is inadequate in quality or quantity or where patients have no contacts with nurses but are charged for it. One problem related to nursing charges within health care institutions results from the failure of those institutions to compute the costs of nursing for persons with differing nursing requirements. For example, the cost of nursing in some hospitals has been and continues to be included in a blanket charge for room accommodations. In some instances such charges are made when no nursing has been provided. Health care administrators sometimes seek to keep costs down by employing vocationally trained workers rather than nurses. When it is inadequately designed and planned, nursing can be a very costly service.

The relation of nurse to patient is *complementary*. This means that nurses act to help patients act responsibly for their health-related self-care by (1) making up for existent health-related deficiencies in the patients' capabilities for self-care and (2) supplying the necessary conditions for the patients to withhold, for therapeutic reasons, the exercise of capabilities or to maintain or increase capabilities for self-care in order to maintain, protect, and promote their functioning as human beings.

The complementary nature of nurse-patient relations is a core concept in a nurse's development of insights about nursing and its practice. It is also the reason why nurses and patients or those who act for patients should seek to develop cooperative working relationships. Individuals, families, or groups under nursing care may be receiving other forms of health care, for example, medical care from one or more physicians, sometimes accompanied by a vast array of paramedical services. A nurse's patient, more likely than not, will be in contact and communication with relatives, friends, and work colleagues. The complementary nature of nurse and patient roles is also manifested by nurses' contacts with others who are significant to their patients and who represent a range of statuses.

Nurses require insights about conditions that militate against cooperative working relationships. For example, nurses should seek to understand the cultural elements involved in the prejudicial attitudes or discriminatory practices of social groups. These elements may affect both nurses and patients in their role fulfillment. Such elements include the prevailing attitudes of members of a social group about skin color, national origin, religion, degree of affluence and influence, social status, social deviance, or even being male or female. Such cultural elements can influence how nurses help patients in the development or exercise of self-care abilities.

Patients too are influenced by such factors and may be reluctant or initially refuse nursing care or care from particular nurses. If nurses are to become safe and successful practitioners they must learn to deal with their own prejudices and discriminatory practices. They can learn to recognize such attitudes in their patients, help patients express their difficulties, and at times move to an early resolution of problem situations. Persons as well as societal and interactional features of nursing are summarized in Fig. 2-3.

Role-set

The sociological concept *role-set* can add an essential dimension to nurses' understanding of the complexity of the nurse role in some nursing situations. The term *role-set* stands for the idea that each status, for example, that of nurse or nurse's patient, involves the status-holder not in a single role but in a set of roles that may include contact with persons in other social statuses. The totality of roles is known as the set of roles associated with a specific status.

The concept of role-set, which is associated with a specific status and role, must be distinguished from that of *multiple roles*. For example, a person qualified in a society as a nurse may act to provide nursing care to patients. In addition, this person may also assist physicians in their performance of medical care measures for patients, or may function as a medical care technician, a clerk, or a manager of a total system of health service. That nurses in health care institutions have historically had multiple roles has tended to obscure their central role of providing nursing to those in need of it. The fact that nurses have performed, and in some settings continue to perform, in the roles of physicians' assistants, medical care technicians, clerks, housekeepers, or managers does not make these roles nursing practice roles because they involve activities outside the domain of nursing practice. In organizations, however, combining a number of roles into one organizational position is common.

A related consideration in nursing is that the majority of nurses in health care institutions are employees as well as nurses. The role-set associated with the status of employee differs from the role-set associated with the status of nurse. Nurses' and their employers' failures to recognize the differences in these roles and to effect a legitimate alignment of them have hindered the progress of health care institutions and those nurses who are employed in them.

Nurses' patients as well as nurses may be operating concurrently within a number of other statuses and roles. Nurses and their patients may experience role conflicts in trying to fulfill the responsibilities of two or more roles. For example, a nurse's patient

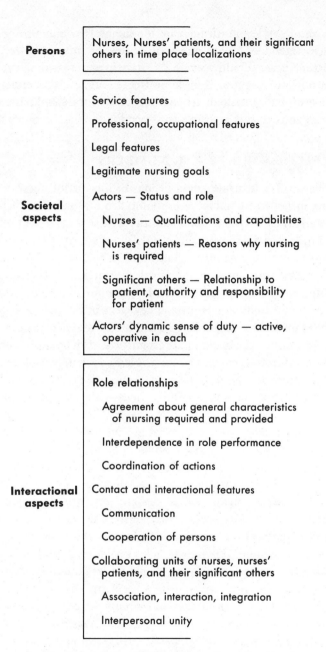

Persons

Nurses, Nurses' patients, and their significant others in time place localizations

Societal aspects

Service features

Professional, occupational features

Legal features

Legitimate nursing goals

Actors — Status and role

　Nurses — Qualifications and capabilities

　Nurses' patients — Reasons why nursing is required

　Significant others — Relationship to patient, authority and responsibility for patient

Actors' dynamic sense of duty — active, operative in each

Interactional aspects

Role relationships

　Agreement about general characteristics of nursing required and provided

　Interdependence in role performance

　Coordination of actions

Contact and interactional features

　Communication

　Cooperation of persons

Collaborating units of nurses, nurses' patients, and their significant others

　Association, interaction, integration

　Interpersonal unity

Fig. 2-3 Persons and societal and interactional aspects of nursing practice.

who is also a mother may find that fulfilling her responsibilities to herself for health-related self-care conflicts with her homemaking role and the role expectations she holds for her husband and children with respect to contributing to the conduct of the household. Persons under nursing and medical care who are confronted with a need to change life-style in order to care for themselves may not be able to do so until they have attended to the pressing duties of another role, for example, occupational role. Nurses should become able to help patients who have the necessary capacities to work out methods to become free enough, and therefore responsible enough, to provide or to manage their own self-care. Nurses and patients must learn to recognize and resolve role conflicts in order for them to achieve nursing goals.

THE PROBLEM OF VARIETY AND NUMBERS

In 1893 Florence Nightingale's descriptions of the "art of nursing the sick" and "health nursing or general nursing" were published and made available to nurses.[5] Nurses historically have served the sick and the well in a variety of settings. Nurses have worked in the homes of persons in need of nursing, in clinics, and in hospitals. They have worked with community groups and in industry in the interests of the prevention of injury and illness and toward the maintenance and promotion of desirable health states for individuals and communities. They have worked to improve sanitary conditions in hospitals. They were in the forefront of recognizing the importance of understanding the social and behavioral dimensions of health care and in caring for individuals based on a recognition of their uniqueness as persons.

It is questionable, however, whether nurses have adequately explored the problems of providing nursing in social groups in terms of (1) the variety of nursing requirements and (2) the numbers of individuals with a range of types of nursing requirements who need nursing at the same time in different locations. The problem of supplying the numbers of people who need or want a service is a perennial problem in all human services. But the combined problem of numbers of people and varieties of requirements is the perennial problem of the health care services.

The ability of nurses to creatively design adequate means for identifying and describing nursing requirements and to design, put into operation, and manage systems of nursing assistance for individuals, families, and groups is one characteristic of the *professional* nurse. Throughout nursing history there has been an inadequate number of nurses who could function to achieve these goals. Traditionally, nurses were trained to relate to individuals or groups under nursing care in order to (1) perform standardized nursing care measures for them and (2) socialize patients to institutional regimens to which nurses and patients were expected to conform. For many years the prevailing forms of education for nursing militated against the availability of nurses who were prepared and willing to accept professional responsibilities. For too long nurses were unable (and some continue to be unable) to make the focus of nursing explicit and to speak knowingly about nursing to patients, co-workers, and health care administrators. How to look at people from a nursing perspective continues to be a problem in nursing circles. This problem will not be solved until nurses are able and willing to ask and answer the question: When and why can people be helped through nursing as distinguished from other forms of health care?

The problem of the variety and numbers of persons requiring nursing in many places at the same time requires the thoughtful and concerted work of both nursing administrators and nursing practitioners. Nursing administrators (for example, nurses who fill positions of supervisor, coordinator, or directors of nursing divisions or units) bear an enabling responsibility which when fulfilled makes it possible for nursing practitioners in particular settings to proceed with nursing persons who have requirements for this service. Persons nursed may be members of relatively stable or rapidly changing nursing populations.

Over the years, organized nursing services, especially in hospitals and other resident care institutions, have tended to emphasize a hierarchy of administrative positions and deemphasize the positions of nursing practitioners. The enabling function of nurses in administrative positions in nursing services centers on the population to be provided with nursing, on the settings in which nursing is to be provided, and on ensuring that nursing practitioners are continuously present, qualified, willing to nurse, and nurse effectively in a manner satisfying to their patients and to themselves.

The enabling function of nursing administrators has been thoughtfully examined and is effectively carried out by some nursing administrators. Some administrators have made and continue to make contributions to developing knowledge about providing nursing for populations.

Particular health care agencies and institutions contract with individuals or groups to supply nursing to them. These same agencies and institutions contract with nurses to provide nursing. If such agencies and institutions contract with aides or technicians to supply *nursing*, steps should be taken to advise institutional administrators that the service provided is an attendant or dependent-care type of service. Nursing practitioners and the profession should protect the name *nursing* as well as the *domain of nursing practice*.

Another dimension of the problem of variety of requirements for nursing and numbers of persons in need of it is the need for continued study of the nursing requirements of populations and their subgroups. On an institution or agency basis this is viewed as a responsibility of nursing administrators. On a local community basis it should be a function of professionally qualified practitioners of community health nursing working in collaboration with nursing administrations. On a state and national basis special projects and programs sponsored by nursing and other health care organizations, including federal agencies, are required. Since the nursing requirements of individual members of populations vary with conditioning effects of factors such as age, developmental state, and health state, studies of nursing requirements of populations must be continuous. Such studies could be articulated with a foundational structure for a developing science of nursing economics.

Role combinations

The primary work of nurses is to provide nursing in accord with the needs people have in assuming responsibility for, in producing, and in managing their health-related self-care. The practitioner of nursing, the nurse, is the designer and provider of nursing in the social group. Nurses cannot become and remain competent practitioners, however, unless they know and are able to apply nursing and nursing-related knowledge in their practice. This knowledge should be continuously formulated and validated through the work of nursing theorists, researchers, and the developers of nursing technologies, techniques, and rules of practice. The status and role of nurse, therefore, should be linked always to that of *student of nursing* and *student of nursing-related disciplines*. Too many nurses remain intellectually impoverished in their chosen field in an age characterized by explosions of knowledge in the health care disciplines and the disciplines related to them. Anyone entering nursing should understand the essentiality of combining the status and role of nursing practitioner with that of nursing student or scholar. The dual role is necessary for the adequate provision of nursing.

Individuals cannot develop themselves as practitioners of nursing and as students of nursing without teachers. Some members of the nursing profession elect to teach nursing students. Ideally, teachers of nursing are prepared and are advancing in proficiency as nursing practitioners while becoming advanced scholars in one or more areas of nursing and in one or more nursing-related disciplines. Some teachers of nursing have not advanced themselves as nursing scholars. It is difficult, if not impossible, for nurses and nursing students to develop as scholars in fields as new as nursing science when they are without adequate guidance from advanced nursing scholars.

Because of the type of education they elect and the roles in which they choose to become proficient, nurses contribute to the maintenance of nursing in social groups in different ways. Nurses who function in the roles of nursing theorists, researchers, developers of nursing technologies, and teachers should be contributing to the advancement and further development of present and future nursing practitioners (see Fig. 4-6). The role of *developer* should be afforded greater recognition in nursing. It is the nurse developer who moves the findings of nursing science researchers into a nursing practice frame of reference by inventing processes, technologies, techniques, artifacts, and rules and by determining their effectiveness and reliability in practice settings. At times, developers invent valid and reliable ways of doing things and only later are the scientific foundations of these new practices identified.

NURSING AS A HUMAN SERVICE

In summary several general statements about nursing practice can be made. The statements may stimulate thought or discussion of nursing as a human service:
1. Nursing relationships in society are based on a state of imbalance between the *abilities of nurses to prescribe, design, manage, and maintain systems* of therapeutic

self-care for individuals and the *abilities of these individuals or their families to do so.* In other words the nurses' abilities exceed those of other individuals. When the imbalance is in the opposite direction or when there is no imbalance, there is no valid basis for a nursing relationship.

- Nursing practice has not only technologic aspects but also moral aspects, since nursing decisions affect the lives, health, and welfare of human beings. Nurses must ask is it right for the patient as well as will it work.
- Solutions proposed to problems of the management and maintenance of therapeutic self-care for patients and families with limited ability to maintain their own care may give rise to other problems, solutions to which may be difficult if not impossible.

REFERENCES

1. Dock LL, and Stewart IM: A short history of nursing, ed 3, New York, 1931, GP Putnam's Sons, pp. 99-103. Also see Stewart IM and Austin AL: A history of nursing, ed 5, New York, 1962, GP Putnam's Sons, pp. 84-87.
2. Roberts MM: American nursing, New York, 1959. The Macmillan Co., pp. 7-17, esp. p. 8.
3. Plattell, MG: Social philosophy, Pittsburgh, 1965, Duquesne University Press, p. 53.
4. Developed in the 1950s, The Division of Hospital and Institutional Services, The Indiana State Board of Health, revised by D. Orem 1975 and 1989.
5. Nightingale, F: Sick nursing and health nursing. In Isabel Hampton A, et al., editors: Nursing of the sick 1893, New York, 1949, McGraw-Hill Book Co., Inc., pp. 24-25.

SELECTED READINGS

Boyer, DC, and Martinson DJ: Intraprenurial group practice, Nurs Health Care 2:29-32, 1990.

Brown EL: Nursing as a profession, ed 2, New York, 1940, Russell Sage Foundation.

Chase RB: Where does the customer fit in a service operation? Harvard Business Review, 56:137-142, 1978.

Lysaugh JP: Action in affirmation: toward an unambiguous profession of nursing, New York, 1981, McGraw-Hill Book Co.

Maglacas AM: Close encounters in international nursing: impact on health policy and research, J Prof Nur 5:304-314, 1989.

Monteiro LA: Florence Nightingale on public health nursing, Am J Public Health 75:181-186, 1985.

Parker AW, Walsh JM, Coon M: A normative approach to the definition of primary health care, Milbank Memorial Fund Quarterly 54:415-438, 1976.

Starr P: Medicine and the waning of professional sovereignty, Daedalus, A New America, 107:175-193, 1978.

Styles MM: Nurse practitioners creating new horizons for the 1990s, Nurse Pract 15:48-57, 1990.

Sutliffe I: History of American training schools. In Hampton IA, et al, editors: Nursing of the sick 1893, New York, 1949, McGraw-Hill Book Co.

The Committee on the Function of Nursing: A program for the nursing profession, New York, 1948, The Macmillan Co.

Walsh M: Accident and emergency nursing, a new approach, London, 1985, William Heinemann Medical Books Ltd, pp. 3-51.

Weston JL: Ambiguities limit the role of nurse practitioners and physician assistants, Am J Public Health 74:6-7, 1984.

Winslow GR: From loyalty to advocacy: a new metaphor for nursing, The Hasting Center Report, June, 1984.

Yarmolinsky A: What future for the professional in American society, Daedalus, A New America, 107:159-174, 1978.

CHAPTER 3

The self-care deficit theory of nursing

A general theory

Valid general descriptive explanations of nursing begin with nurses' conceptualized and expressed insights about dominant features of nursing practice situations known to them through experience and investigation. Insights when formulated as concepts and expressed verbally or in writing constitute static representations of situational features and relationships. Dominant features identified in explored nursing practice situations provide the concrete basis for insights leading to the formulation of theoretical positions about nursing.

Nursing has **form** as well as situational features with which nurses deal as nurses. The form of nursing is expressed in part by its helping and taking care of characteristics, which lay out its interpersonal form. Other aspects of nursing's form arise from the fact that nurses deal with life **situations** where results are sought, that is, where new, not presently existent, conditions are to be brought into existence through the goal-oriented deliberate actions of nurses and their patients. Theoretical positions about nursing include both form and situational features.

DEVELOPMENT OF A GENERAL THEORY IN A PRACTICE FIELD

A general theory in a practice field is descriptively explanatory of the dominant features and relationships that characterize the field's practice situations. General theories structure what is already known and thus provide organized foundations for the continued development, structuring, and validation of knowledge that is of practical value for practitioners in the field. General theories are of particular value in fields such as nursing where nursing knowledge that should be available to nursing students and scholars is relatively unstructured within a nursing frame of reference, as attested by textbooks in various areas of nursing practice. A general theory of nursing is an effective but general answer to the questions: What do nurses attend to and do when they nurse? What do nurses make when they nurse? A general theory of nursing also provides structure for the organization of nursing knowledge.

> **_Exercise_ in examining statements responsive to the question:**
> **What is nursing?**
>
> Select a number of written statements of nurses that are responsive to the question:
> What is nursing?
> Identify why you selected these particular statements.
> 1. Read each statement carefully. Examine it for and identify its structure. Reflect
>   about the meaning of the statement. Reflect about the relationships among the parts
>   of the statement that give it structure.
> 2. Extract the parts of each statement that express elements or features of nursing.
> 3. After working with each one of the statements you selected, compare the statements
>   for similarities and differences as related to expressed elements.
> 4. Discuss the results of your investigation with colleagues in a planned meeting.
> 5. Note and record the questions that arise during the discussion.

The formulation and expression of a general theory of nursing occurs over time. It is based as previously indicated on insights about (1) recurring features of nursing practice situations and (2) relationships between and among features. Analysis of situations of nursing practice and analysis of nursing case material (a nursing case is a particular instance of nursing) yield insights about the recurring features of nursing practice and the relationships between and among them. Identified recurring features, for example, the capability of healthy adults to meet self-care requisites for maintaining adequate intakes of water and food under some conditions but not under others, are investigated. Insights are formulated as concepts and expressed concepts are then validated in concrete practice situations or through analysis of nursing case material. Experiences of members of the Nursing Development Conference Group* in these matters are described in "Dynamics of Concept Development" in the 1973 and 1979 editions of *Concept Formalization in Nursing: Process and Product,* Boston, Little, Brown and Co.

Formulation and expression of a general theory of nursing proceeds as a creative synthesis of the conceptualized recurring dominant features of nursing practice situations and the relationship among them. There is, as indicated, the question of form or structure of the synthesis of nursing features.

Nursing as previously stated has an interpersonal form. But form also is reflective of the practical service nature of nursing, which gives rise to requirements for nurses to perform operations to determine what is and what can and should be and to decide

---

* This voluntary study group had its origins in 1965 as the Committee on the Nursing Model, The School of Nursing, The Catholic University of America, Washington, D.C. The name *Nursing Development Conference Group* will be used regardless of time period.

within the interpersonal frame what will be done and then engage in its production and evaluation. Operations involve the selection and deliberate performance of actions and action sequences by nurses and nurses' patients according to their determined roles. A general theory of nursing is thus a synthesis of postulated entities with an interpersonal form; within the interpersonal structure, there is an operational structure.

Every theory has its beginnings in the concrete world of persons and events, in the world of ideas, and in the world of the theorist. The historical development of the self-care deficit theory of nursing is expressed in terms of its beginnings, the subsequent development of a concept of nursing system and a conceptual framework for nursing, and finally in expression of a general theory of nursing.

Beginning development

American nurses experienced increasing instability in practice situations during the period extending approximately from 1940 to 1960. An outstanding public health physician who worked intensively with nurses, physicians, hospital administrators and governing boards, specialists in public health, and others on state and national levels remarked that "nursing gets much of the blame for poor patient care" in hospitals; and nurses tend to accept the blame for conditions and problems that involve physicians, hospital technical services, and hospital administrators as well as nurses.[1]

This was a period when health care services, especially within hospitals, were affected by conditions that were destabilizing, to say the least. Changes included the following:[2]

* Changes in health care needs of people associated in part with the increasing numbers of individuals with chronic diseases and the decrease in acute communicable disease
* Revolutionary advances in knowledge and technique in medical diagnosis and treatment and in prevention and rehabilitation
* A threefold to fourfold increase in the number of individuals seeking hospital care
* Increase in the number of individuals providing care, an increase in total number and in number from specialized fields
* Changes in public attitudes toward health and increasing awareness of the advantages gained from effective health services for individuals and communities

Nurses became concerned with questions about their proper work, about time available for nursing, and about their relationships to persons seeking and receiving nursing and to members of other health care disciplines. The subtitle to Nightingale's *Notes on Nursing: What It Is and What It Is Not* expressed the concern of many nurses during and beyond this period.

As long as stable conditions prevail in occupations or professions, members usually do not raise questions about their domain of practice. The unstable conditions in nursing practice demanded that nurses begin to deal with domain and boundary problems. However, nurses' endeavors to do so and to advance nursing as a practice field were hindered at times by lack of interest and understanding from persons outside of nursing and at times by direct opposition from within nursing. Some recognized internal barriers to the advancement and development of nursing included the continuing focus of nurses on tasks and procedures, many of which were outmoded; demands of nurses that exceeded their preparation; the unstructured state of nursing knowledge; the inability of many nurses to formulate goals of care specific to nursing; and the inability of many nurses to communicate adequately about nursing with persons under nursing care and their families and with members of other health care disciplines, administrators, and officials of government.

Despite barriers, nurses' achievements during the period contributed to a forward, developmental movement that continued through the 1960s, 1970s, and 1980s. Virginia Henderson's organized, succinct, yet comprehensive statements about nursing's contributions to individuals, sick or well, with an expression of the reason why people need nursing, was published in 1955 (p. 4).[3] Hildegard Peplau expressed her conceptualization of nursing as a "significant, therapeutic interpersonal process" in her 1952 work *Interpersonal Relations in Nursing* (p. 16).[4] During the 1950s my own interest in and insights about the domain and boundaries of nursing began to take on more of a proper nursing focus in distinction to the more global preventive health care focus that previously had characterized them. A beginning formalization of my insights about nursing as a field of practice was expressed in 1956 and followed by a more precise expression in 1959.

From 1949 to 1957 as a nurse consultant with the Division of Hospital and Institutional Services of the Indiana State Board of Health, I had an intensive experience in working with the director and the professional staff of the division, with nurses in Indiana hospitals, and with nurses in the Division of Public Health Nursing. In 1956 I completed a report of study of administrative positions in nursing in one Indiana hospital and appended to the report a chapter entitled "The Art of Nursing." The following quotations are from this chapter (p. 85).[5]

> Nursing is an art through which the nurse, the practitioner of nursing, gives specialized assistance to persons with disabilities of such a character that more than ordinary assistance is necessary to meet daily needs for self-care and to intelligently participate in the medical care they are receiving from the physician. The art of nursing is practiced by "doing for" the person with the disability, by "helping him to do for himself" and/or by "helping him to learn how to do for himself." Nursing is also practiced by helping a capable person from the patient's family or a friend of the patient to learn how "to do for" the patient. Nursing the patient is thus a practical and a didactic art.

In 1958 and 1959, as a consultant in the Office of Education, U.S. Department of Health, Education, and Welfare, I participated in a project to upgrade practical (vocational) nurse training and to identify ways to include in practical nurse curricula an explicit nursing component. Such a component would give nursing meaning to the tasks around which the knowledge and experience components of training programs were organized. All vocational programs extract content from one or more disciplines. Therefore, in curriculum development it is essential that one know how disciplines are structured or organized to extract content of various types without distortion and error. Knowing the relatively unstructured state of available knowledge about nursing practice, I was aware that I must have as a working tool at least a gross conceptualization of elements within the domain of nursing and of the relationships among them. This, I thought, would enable me to make some inferences about the structure of nursing as a field of knowledge necessary for nursing practice.

I proceeded not by reviewing and analyzing components of available statements about nursing, my own and others, but by reflecting on my experiences in nursing. I stated a proposition and asked a question: *Not all people under health care, for example, from physicians, are under nursing care nor does it follow that they should be.* I then asked: *What condition exists in a person when that person or a family member or the attending physician or a nurse makes the judgment that the person should be under nursing care?* The answer to the question came spontaneously with images of situations where such judgments were made and the idea that a nurse is "another self," in a figurative sense, for the person under nursing care.

My insights into the *human condition* associated with *requirements for nursing* were formulated as a concept and expressed as follows: the inability of a person to provide continuously for self the amount and quality of required self-care because of the situation of personal health. Self-care was conceptualized as the personal care that human beings require each day and that may be modified by health state, environmental conditions, the effects of medical care, and other factors. The expressed proper human object of nursing also specified that in child nursing situations, the parent or guardian is no longer able to provide the amount and quality of continuing care required by the child because of the child's health situation. This 1958 expression of nursing's proper object conforms to that expressed in my 1956 statement about nursing and in substance with that in Virginia Henderson's 1955 statement about nursing.

My understanding of the human condition that gives rise to requirements for nursing was both an ending and a beginning. It ended my search for an answer to the question: What is nursing? It brought me to a new developmental stage with respect to knowing and understanding nursing. There was an intellectual readiness to make explicit the elements and relationships that give form and meaning to nursing as a field of practice and a field of knowledge.

A concept and a conceptual framework

My work of theorizing about nursing had its formal beginning in 1958 with my formalization of the proper object of nursing considered as a field of knowledge and a field of practice. My efforts were joined with efforts of members of the Nursing Development Conference Group in 1965.

A concept of nursing system

As a result of combined efforts, a theoretical concept of *nursing system* was formulated, expressed, and revised in 1970. My colleagues and I considered this theoretical position about nursing, as expressed in the box, as a forward step in the development of a model adequate to guide nursing research and further the structuring of nursing as a body of knowledge. Before the expression of the concept of nursing system, its conceptual elements along with the concept self-care had been formalized and then validated in nursing practice situations. The theoretical concept of nursing system expressed group members' insights about the creative end product of the work of nurses and the dynamics of its production.

The term *system* with reference to the 1970 conceptualization of what nurses make is used in its broadest sense. *System* refers to persons or actions or things with relationships between and among them behaving together as a whole with changes in

---

Conceptualization of nursing system

A *nursing system*, like other systems for the provision of personal services, is the product of a series of relations between persons who belong to different sets (classes), the set A and the set B. From a nursing perspective any member of the set A (legitimate patient) presents evidence descriptive of the complex subsets self-care agency and therapeutic self-care demand and the condition that in A demand exceeds agency due to health or health-related causes. Any member of the set B (legitimate nurse) presents evidence descriptive of the complex subset nursing agency which includes valuation of the legitimate relations between self as *nurse* and instances where, in A, certain values of the component phenomena of self-care agency and therapeutic self-care demand prevail.

B's perceptions of the conditionality of A's subset objective therapeutic self-care demand on the subset self-care agency establishes the conditionality of changes in the states of A's two subsets on the state of and changes in the state of B's subset nursing agency. The activation of the components of the subset nursing agency (change in state) by B to deliberately control or alter the state of one or both of A's subsets — therapeutic self-care demand and self-care agency — is nursing. The perceived relations among the parts of the three subsets (actual system) constitute the organization. The "mapping" of the behaviors in "mathematical or behavioral terms" provides a record of the system [4]. (p. 107)

From Nursing Development Conference Group, Orem DE, editor: Concept formalization in nursing: process and product, ed 2, Boston 1979, Little, Brown and Co.

any one of the entities affecting the whole that is the system. A nursing system, however, is viewed as a particular type of system, a self-organizing system. Such systems exist "only when and for the duration that there are self-connecting links between the behavior or state of independent parts or subjects, the connection occurring at some point of conditionality between them (p. 125)."[6]

This view of nursing as a self-organizing system emphasizes that nursing is deliberately produced within time and place frames of reference, that is produced through discrete deliberate actions or sequences of action, and that its existence depends on the bringing about and sustaining of relationships between persons and among actions that they select, decide to execute, and execute. Nursing has no concrete existence except through persons in relationships of nurse and patient and through what they choose and proceed to do or not do within the relationship. A *nursing system* is something constructed through actions of nurses and nurses' patients. It is a product that should be beneficial to persons with patient status in nursing practice situations when the time frame for production fits the time of occurrence of requirements for nursing.

Entities described and synthesized in the theoretical concept nursing system are summarized.

- Persons in the designated statuses of "legitimate patient" and "legitimate nurse"
- Two properties of "legitimate patient," namely, "therapeutic self-care demand" and "self-care agency"
- An inequality of patient properties, therapeutic self-care demand, and self-care agency within an action frame of reference—the demand for self-care (therapeutic self-care demand) exceeds the existent and operational capabilities of a legitimate patient to meet the demand (self-care agency)
- One property of "legitimate nurse," namely, "nursing agency," which includes capabilities to value legitimate relations between self as nurse and the person(s) in patient status under prevailing values of the component phenomena* of self-care agency and therapeutic self-care demand
- Motion or change revealed by events and operations including (1) nurse perceptions of conditionality between patient properties therapeutic self-care demand and self-care agency, (2) nurse insights that change in patient properties, dependent on nurses' creative endeavor, is conditioned on the nurse's own state of development of nursing agency and the nurse's exercise of it, and (3) nurse activation of components of nursing agency to deliberately control or alter the state of one or both patient properties.

---

* The reference here is to the substantive components of these two conceptualized properties that point to concrete features of individuals and their environments.

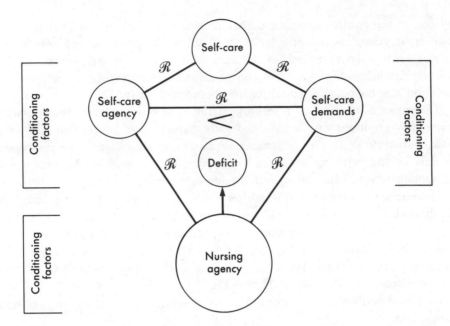

Fig. 3-1 A conceptual framework for nursing. R, relationship; <, deficit relationship, current or projected.

The expressed conceptualization of nursing system can be viewed as an explanatory definition of nursing since it sets forth what nurses do when they nurse others. It can also be viewed as a general model. Meanings of terms used to express conceptual elements within the conceptual model of nursing system are summarized (Fig. 3-1). Four terms are patient oriented; two are nurse oriented.

Legitimate patients of nurses are persons whose self-care agency or dependent-care agency, because of their own or their dependents' health states or health care requirements, is not adequate or will become inadequate for knowing or meeting their own or their dependents' therapeutic self-care demands.

Self-care is learned, goal-oriented activity of individuals. It is behavior that exists in concrete life situations directed by persons to self or to the environment to regulate factors that affect their own development and functioning in the interests of life, health, or well-being. **Dependent care** is activity as described above performed by responsible adults for socially dependent individuals.

Legitimate nurses are persons who have the sets of qualities symbolized by the term nursing agency to the degree that they have the capability and the willingness to exercise it in knowing and meeting the existent and emerging nursing requirements of persons with health-associated, self-care or dependent-care deficits.

Nursing agency is a complex property or attribute of persons educated and trained as nurses that is enabling when exercised for knowing and helping others know their therapeutic self-care demands, for helping others meet or in meeting their therapeutic self-care demands, and in helping others regulate the exercise or development of their self-care agency or their dependent care-agency.

Therapeutic self-care demand signifies a humanly constructed entity. It stands for a summation of measures of self-care required at moments in time and for some time duration by individuals in some location to meet self-care requisites particularized for individuals in relation to their conditions and circumstances. Care measures arise from the selection and application of specific methods or technologies to meet universal, developmental, or health deviation-type, self-care requisites.

Self-care agency is the complex developed capability that enables adults and maturing adolescents to discern factors that must be controlled or managed in order to regulate their own functioning and development, to decide what can and should be done with respect to regulation, to lay out the components of their therapeutic self-care demands (self-care requisites, technologies, care measures), and finally to perform the care measures designed to meet their self-care requisites over time. Dependent-care agency is the complex developed capability of responsible adults to do the foregoing for dependents.

A conceptual framework

Subsequent to expression of the 1970 theoretical concept of nursing systems, its dominant themes or conceptual elements were represented as a conceptual structure, a circle of terms and relationships (Fig. 3-1). This was done to emphasize the relationships of the theoretical concepts among themselves and to the production of self-care. Fig. 3-1 also shows the theoretical conceptualization of nurse and patient properties as being related to factors internal or external to persons who are nurses or nurses' patients that under some circumstances condition the qualitative or quantitative values of patient and nurse properties.

Elements expressed in the concept of nursing system and in the conceptual framework emerged from my own work and that of the Nursing Development Conference Group. All the conceptual elements were formalized and validated as static concepts by 1970. Since then, some refinement of expression and further development of substantive structure and continued validation have occurred, but no substantive change has been made. Each concept continues to undergo development through the identification and organization of secondary concepts that constitute its substantive structure. For example, the conceptualization of three types of self-care requisites — universal, developmental, and health deviation — are secondary concepts within the broad concept therapeutic self-care demand; and each of these secondary concepts has a structure that must be explicated.

The explication of the structure of secondary concepts leads to identification of the component phenomena, the concrete features of conceptualized entities, and combinations of entities.

Secondary concepts establish a framework for integrating facts and segments of theory "from other disciplines and provide some direction to the selection of useful research methodologies (p. 130)"[6] for study of concrete life situations.[6] For example, the secondary concept universal self-care requisites provides for articulation of facts and points of theory from physiology, bioclimatology, psychology, public health sciences, and other disciplines. The substantive (secondary) structure of the concept of self-care agency has been a fruitful base for research oriented to self-care agency in a variety of populations. This also is true for therapeutic self-care demand.

THE SELF-CARE DEFICIT THEORY OF NURSING

The theoretical concept of nursing system is not meaningful in the absence of subsumed concepts of self-care deficit and self-care. These three concepts taken together were understood to be parts of a general concept of nursing. To further formalize the concepts and the relationships between and among them, efforts were expended to express a general theory of nursing constituted from a theory of self-care, a theory of self-care deficit, and a theory of nursing system. Together the three theories constitute a general theory of nursing, named the self-care deficit theory of nursing. Fig. 3-2 identifies that the theory of nursing system subsumes the theory of self-care deficit, which subsumes the theory of self-care. The expression of the theories as they appeared in the third edition of *Nursing: Concepts of Practice* have been refined.

Underlying premises

Five premises about self-evident characteristics of human beings served as guiding principles throughout the process of conceptualizing nursing. They have been

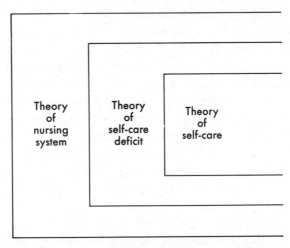

Fig. 3-2 Constituent theories, the self-care deficit theory of nursing.

referred to at times as assumptions. They are more properly referred to as premises since they were and are advanced as true and not merely assumed. The five premises that follow were formalized in 1973 (pp. 3-5).[7]

1. Human beings require continuous deliberate inputs to themselves and their environments in order to remain alive and function in accord with natural human endowments.
2. Human agency, the power to act deliberately, is exercised in the form of care of self and others in identifying needs for and in making needed inputs.
3. Mature human beings experience privations in the form of limitations for action in care of self and others involving the making of life-sustaining and function-regulating inputs.
4. Human agency is exercised in discovering, developing, and transmitting to others ways and means to identify needs for and make inputs to self and others.
5. Groups of human beings with structured relationships cluster tasks and allocate responsibilities for providing care to group members who experience privations for making required deliberate input to self and others.

A general theory of nursing is an account of relationships that serves to organize the outlook of nurses. It also lays a framework that expresses essential variables and relationships and a base for predicting relations. The theory is viewed as descriptively explanatory of the lawlike relationships or universal conditionals implicit in premises 1, 2, 3, and 4, and in premise 5 as this pertains to societies where nursing is established as an available human service.

Overview of the general theory of nursing

The self-care deficit theory of nursing is a synthesis of knowledge about the theoretical entities self-care (and dependent care), self-care agency (and dependent-care agency), therapeutic self-care demand, the relational entity self-care deficit, and nursing agency. This general theory of nursing is expressed in terms of the named theoretical entities and introduces existential statements about them, such as *mature adults engage in self-care.* Indicative and recognitive criteria are required for verification or falsification of such statements within space-time matrices. Indicative criteria would verify that mature adult persons do or do not perform actions to care for themselves in their environmental setting. Recognitive criteria would be developed to establish that the action is self-care and not another form of deliberate action.

In each of the three theories, four categories of postulated entities establish the ontology (pp. 213-227),[8] the realities that are the foci of the theories: (1) persons in space-time localizations, (2) attributes or properties of these persons, (3) motion or change, and (4) products brought into being.

Table 3-1 identifies the reality foci of the theory and names the entities postulated within each of the three theories.

Table 3-1 Postulated entities for the theories of self-care, self-care deficit, and nursing system

Postulated entities	Theory of nursing system	Theory of self-care deficit	Theory of self-care
Persons in space-time matrices	Nurses, patients with S-CD* Clients with D-CD†	Persons not able to know and meet their own or their dependents' health associated TS-CD‡	Persons performing operations to know and meet their own or dependents' TS-CD
Properties of persons	Nursing agency of nurse Nature of patient's self-care deficit	Health-derived or health-related self-care or dependent-care deficit—partial to complete	Self-management capabilities Self-care agency or dependent-care agency Therapeutic self-care demand
Properties of relationships	Legality of relationship Nursing legitimacy Interpersonal unity		
Motion or change	Change in patients' TS-CD or S-CA§ or D-CA‖ Exercise of nursing agency by nurse Role allocation Role acceptance Role fulfillment by nurse, by patient Role change Change of nurses	Self or another—seeking nursing assistance agreeing to receive nursing under specified conditions	No performance to complete performance of self-care or dependent-care operations
Product	Nursing system	Agreement to receive nursing Beginning interpersonal relationship with nurse(s)	No care system or a self-care system or a dependent-care system

* Self-care deficit.
† Dependent-care deficit.
‡ Therapeutic self-care.
§ Self-care agency.
‖ Dependent-care agency.

In subsequent sections, each of the three theories is described by presentation of the central idea of the theory, the presuppositions to the theory that are required preceding conditions, and the propositions that flow from the expressed central idea.

THE THEORY OF SELF-CARE

The theory of **self-care** is presented first because it is basic to understanding the theory of self-care deficit and the theory of nursing system.

Central idea of the theory

Within the context of day-to-day living in social groups and their time-place localizations, mature and maturing persons perform learned actions and sequences of actions directed toward themselves or toward environmental features known or assumed to meet identified requisites for controlling factors that either promote or adversely affect or interfere with ongoing regulation of their own functioning or development in order to contribute to continuance of life, self-maintenance, and personal health and well-being. They also perform such regulatory actions for dependent family members or others. Regulatory requisites are of three types: requisites universally required by all individuals regardless of age, requisites specifically regulatory of human developmental processes, and those that arise from or are associated with persons' health states and associated health care.

Presuppositions

The central idea of the theory of self-care rests on at least four presuppositions.
1. All things being equal, human beings have the potential to develop intellectual and practical skills and maintain the motivation essential for self-care and care of dependent family members.
2. Ways of meeting self-care requisites are culture elements and vary with individuals and larger social groups.
3. Self-care and care of dependent family members are forms of deliberate action, dependent for performance on individuals' action repertoires, and their predilection for taking action under certain circumstances.
4. Identifying and describing recurring requisites for self-care and the care of dependent family members lead to investigating and developing ways to meet known requisites and to form care habits.

Propositions

The following propositions related to the central idea of the theory of self-care serve as principles and as bases for continued investigation.
1. Self-care is intellectualized as a human regulatory function deliberately executed with some degree of completeness and effectiveness.
2. Self-care in its concreteness is directed and deliberate action that is responsive to persons' knowing how human functioning and human development can and should be maintained within a range that is compatible with human life and personal health and well-being under existent conditions and circumstances.
3. Self-care in its concreteness involves the use of material resources and energy expenditures directed to supply materials and conditions needed for internal

functioning and development and to establish and maintain essential and safe relationships with environmental factors and forces.

4. Self-care in its concreteness when externally oriented emerges as observable events resulting from performed sequences of practical actions directed by persons to themselves or their environments. Self-care that has the form of internally oriented self-controlling actions is not observable and can be known by others only by seeking subjective information. Reasons for the actions and the results being sought from them may or may not be known to the subject who performs the actions.

5. Self-care that is performed over time can be understood (intellectualized) as an action system—a self-care system—whenever there is knowledge of the complement of different types of action sequences or care measures performed and the connecting linkages among them.

6. Constituent components of a self-care system are sets of care measures or tasks necessary to use valid and selected means (i.e., technologies to meet existent and changing values of known self-care requisites).

THE THEORY OF SELF-CARE DEFICIT

The theory of self-care deficit is the critical constituent of the self-care deficit theory of nursing. This theory has its origins in the proper object of nursing, namely, human beings as subject to health-derived or health-related limitations for engagement in self-care or dependent care.

Central idea of the theory

All limitations of persons for engagement in practical endeavors within the domain and boundaries of nursing are associated with subjectivity of mature and maturing individuals to health-related or health-derived action limitations that render them completely or partially unable to know existent and emerging requisites for regulatory care for themselves or their dependents and to engage in the continuing performance of care measures to control or in some way manage factors that are regulatory of their own or their dependents' functioning and development.

Presuppositions

Two sets of presuppositions link the central idea of the theory of self-care deficit to the theory of self-care and to the idea of social dependency.

Set one

• Engagement in self-care requires ability to manage self within a stable or changing environment.
• Engagement in self-care or dependent-care is affected by persons' valuation of care measures with respect to life, development, health, and well-being.

- The quality and completeness of self-care and dependent care in families and communities rests on the culture, including scientific attainments of social groups and the educability of group members.
- Engagement in self-care and dependent-care are affected, as is engagement in all forms of practical endeavor, by persons' limitations in knowing what to do under existent conditions and circumstances or how to do it.

Set two

- Societies provide for the human state of social dependency by instituting ways and means to aid persons according to the nature of and the reasons for their dependency.
- When they are institutionalized, direct helping operations of members of social groups become the means for aiding persons in states of social dependency.
- The direct helping operations of members of social groups may be classified into those associated with states of age-related dependency and those not so associated.
- Direct helping services instituted in social groups to provide assistance to persons irrespective of age include the health services.
- Nursing is one of the health services of Western civilization.

Propositions

The following propositions serve as principles and guides for the further development of the theory of self-care deficit.

- Persons who take action to provide their own self-care or care for dependents have specialized capabilities for action.
- Individuals' abilities to engage in self-care or dependent-care are conditioned by age, developmental state, life experience, sociocultural orientation, health, and available resources.
- Relationship of individuals' abilities for self-care or dependent-care to the qualitative and quantitative self-care or dependent-care demand can be determined when the value of each is known.
- The relationship between care abilities and care demand can be defined in terms of *equal to, less than,* and *more than.*
- Nursing is a legitimate service when (1) care abilities are less than those required for meeting a known self-care demand (a deficit relationship); and (2) self-care or dependent-care abilities exceed or are equal to those required for meeting the current self-care demand, but a future deficit relationship can be foreseen because of predictable decreases in care abilities, qualitative or quantitative increases in the care demand, or both.
- Persons with existing or projected care deficits are in, or can expect to be in, states of social dependency that legitimate a nursing relationship.

THE THEORY OF NURSING SYSTEM

The theory of nursing system is the essential organizing component of the self-care deficit theory of nursing because it establishes the form of nursing and the relationship between patient and nurse properties.

Central idea of the theory

All systems of practical action that are nursing systems are formed by nurses through their deliberate exercise of specialized nursing capabilities (nursing agency) within the context of their interpersonal and contractual relationship with persons with health-derived or health-associated deficits for production of continuing, effective, and complete care for themselves or their dependents for purposes of ensuring that therapeutic self-care demands are known and met and self-care agency is protected or its exercise or development regulated. Nursing systems may be formed or produced for individuals, for persons who constitute a dependent-care unit, for groups whose members have therapeutic self-care demands with similar components, or who have similar limitations for engagement in self-care or dependent-care, for families, or for other multiperson units.

Presuppositions

Basic to the theory and providing foundations for it are at least two presuppositions.
- Nursing is the practical endeavors of nurses engaged in for some duration of time for individuals in time-place localizations whenever their action limitations for engagement in self-care or dependent-care are health related or derived.
- Nursing is an institutionalized human health service with a domain and boundaries defined by its proper object or specialized focus in society.

Propositions

Eight propositions are suggested guides for the continued development of the theory of nursing system.
- Nurses relate to and interact with persons who occupy the status of nurse's patient.
- Legitimate patients have existent or projected self-care requisites.
- Legitimate patients have existent or projected deficits for meeting their own self-care requisites.
- Nurses determine the current and changing values of patients' self-care requisites, select valid and reliable processes or technologies for meeting these requisites, and formulate the courses of action necessary for using selected processes or technologies that will meet identified self-care requisites.

- Nurses determine the current and changing values of patients' abilities to meet their self-care requisites using specific processes or technologies.
- Nurses estimate the potential of patients to (1) refrain from engaging in self-care for therapeutic purposes or (2) develop or refine abilities to engage in care now or in the future.
- Nurses and patients act together to allocate the roles of each in the production of patients' self-care and in the regulation of the exercise or development of patients' self-care capabilities.
- The actions of nurses and the actions of patients (or nurses' actions that *compensate for the patients' action limitations*) that regulate patients' self-care capabilities and meet patients' self-care needs constitute nursing systems.

SUMMARY

This general theory of nursing is referred to as the *self-care deficit theory of nursing* because it is descriptively explanatory of the *relationship* between the action capabilities of individuals and their demands for self-care or the care demands of children or adults who are their dependents. *Deficit* thus stands for the relationship between the action that individuals should take (the action demanded) and the action capabilities of individuals for self-care or dependent-care. *Deficit* in this context should be interpreted as a relationship, not as a human disorder. Self-care deficits may be associated, however, with the presence of human functional or structural disorders.

The self-care deficit theory of nursing assumes that nursing is a response of human groups to one recurring type of incapacity for action to which human beings are subject, namely, the incapacity to care for oneself or one's dependents when action is limited because of health state or health care needs of the care recipient. From a nursing point of view, human beings are viewed as needing continuous self-maintenance and self-regulation through a type of action named *self-care*. The term *self-care* means care that is performed by oneself for oneself when one has reached a state of maturity that is enabling for consistent, controlled, effective, and purposeful action. The unborn, the newborn, infants, children, the severely disabled, and the infirm cannot meet any or some of their own requirements for maintenance and for regulation of their functioning.

The theory posits two *patient variables*, namely, self-care agency and therapeutic self-care demand, and one *nurse variable*, nursing agency. In conceptualizations of the theory of self-care deficits, the patient variables are viewed as related, and within the theory of nursing system, nursing agency is viewed as related to both patient variables (Fig. 3-1). Persons with health-related, self-care deficits are designated as legitimate patients. Nurses view their own legitimacy in terms of their capabilities for providing the kind and amount of nursing required by persons under their care.

FUNCTIONS OF A GENERAL THEORY OF NURSING

The self-care deficit theory of nursing is not an explanation of the individuality of a particular concrete nursing practice situation, but rather the expression of a singular combination of conceptualized properties or features common to all instances of nursing. As a general theory, it serves nurses engaged in nursing practice, in development and validation of nursing knowledge, and in teaching and learning nursing.

Eight functions of the self-care deficit theory of nursing are identified:
- To set forth the views of human beings proper to nursing
- To express the specific focus or proper object of nursing in human society
- To set forth the key concepts of nursing considered as a field of knowledge and practice and to establish a system of symbols or language
- To set limits on and orient thinking and practical endeavor in nursing practice, research, development, and education for nursing
- To reduce cognitive load by providing subsumers for incoming information and enable persons who understand the theory to categorize and form concepts from related insights about features of concrete nursing situations
- To allow inferences to be made about the articulations of nursing with other fields of human service and with patterns of daily living of individuals and families in communities
- To generate in nurses and nursing students a style of thinking and communicating nursing
- To bring nurses together as communities of scholars engaged in the continuing development, the structuring, and validation of nursing knowledge

Nurses' mastery of the self-care deficit theory of nursing and the results of their use of its principles to guide their nursing endeavors attests to its usefulness.

Nurses who have mastered and use the self-care deficit theory of nursing and who contribute to its refinement and further development have noted changes in themselves and in other nurses. One experience that nurses express is an increase in their sense of self-value or self-worth as nurses. Other positive changes expressed by nurses over the years since the theory has been in use were compiled in 1987.[9] Changes in the listing have not been subjected to validation procedures. They are offered as an indication of what nurses have expressed in relation to their own or other nurses' use of the self-care deficit theory of nursing.
- Nurses develop their personal styles of practice within the domain and boundaries of nursing set by the theory.
- Nurses focus on providing nursing to persons whose legitimate need for nursing is established through the criterion of the existence of health-derived or health-related self-care deficits. Stereotyping is eventually eliminated.
- Nursing diagnoses become more valid and are expressed within a nursing frame of reference.

- Therapeutic self-care demands and ways to protect and to regulate the exercise or development of self-care agency are determined and prescribed. Nursing care systems are designed.
- Nursing documentation increases and improves.
- There is an increase in and upgrading of the kinds of referrals made by nurses, including referrals to nursing specialists.
- Nurses (and physicians more slowly) recognize the need for nursing discharge of patients separate from medical discharge.
- There is movement toward nurse-managed clinics.
- Nurses recognize that they have a theoretical base that serves them in performing the professional function of design of systems of nursing care. The design function is retained by and specific to the professional person.
- Nurses through their design of systems of nursing bring into focus their own role responsibilities and role functions, as well as those of other nurses, their patients, and members of patients' families who are dependent-care agents.

Such practice changes are most likely to occur in health service enterprises where nursing administration views the self-care deficit theory of nursing theory as one means to aid in efforts to ensure the continuing provision of effective nursing to populations served by the health care enterprise.

REFERENCES

1. O'Malley M: personal communication, 1952.
2. O'Malley M et al: What do we mean, improvement of patient care and how do we implement it. Presented at Tri-State Assembly, Division of Hospital and Institutional Services, Indiana State Board of Health, April 9, 1958.
3. Harmer B: Textbook of the principles and practice of nursing, revised by Virginia Henderson, ed 4, New York, 1955, Macmillan, p. 4.
4. Peplau HE: Interpersonal relations in nursing, New York, 1952, Putnam, p. 16.
5. Orem DE: Hospital nursing service, an analysis, The Division of Hospital and Institutional Services, Indiana State Board of Health, 1956, Indianapolis, p. 85.
6. Nursing Development Conference Group, Orem DE, editor: Concept formalization in nursing: process and product, ed 2, Boston, 1979, Little, Brown Co.
7. Orem DE: A general theory of nursing. Presented at the 5th Annual Post-Master's conference, Marquette University School of Nursing, June 1, 1973.
8. Wallace WA: Essay X: causality analogy, and scientific growth. From a realist point of view. Essays on the Philosophy of Science, ed 2., Lanham, Md, 1983, University Press of America.
9. Orem DE: Changes in professional nursing practice associated with nurses' use of Orem's general theory of nursing. Presented at Le Centre Hospitalier de Gatineau, Gatineau, Quebec, Canada, May, 1987.

SELECTED READINGS

Dickoff J, James P, and Wiedenback E: Theory in practice disciplines, part I, practice oriented theory, Nurs Res 17:415-435, 1968.
Nursing Development Conference Group. In Orem DE, editor: Frames of reference in nursing and nursing: a practice discipline. In Concept formalization in nursing: process and product, ed 2, Boston, 1979, Little, Brown and Co.

Orem DE: Guides for developing curricula for the education of practical nurses, Washington, DC, 1959, US Government Printing Office.

Orem DE: The form of nursing science. Nurs Sci Q 1:75-79, 1988.

Wallace WA: Being scientific in a practice discipline. In From a realist point of view, essays on the philosophy of science, ed 2, Lanham, Md, 1983, University Press of America.

Zderad LT, and Belcher MC: Developing behavioral concepts in nursing, Atlanta, 1968, Southern Regional Education Board.

CHAPTER 4

The practical science of nursing

Nurses in practice situations experience events involving themselves and others. They observe, reflect, reason, and understand as persons who know nursing. Knowing nursing is a cognitional process and not a static condition of a nurse or nursing student. Developing a cognitional orientation to nursing requires both teaching and learning focused on nursing as a field of practice with its developing fields of knowledge. Teaching communicates insights with empirical meaningfulness that are enabling for nurses' understanding of the complexities of nursing situations. Learning results in the accumulation of related insights by nurses and in nurses' movement to spontaneously seek answers to questions that arise when discussions, actions, or thoughts reveal that understanding is incomplete.

Teaching and learning preparatory for nursing practice should have as their organizing center a core of formulated, expressed, and validated concepts that are constituent parts of the *practical science nursing.*

Nurses must be able to think nursing, as well as perform the operations of nursing practice. Nurses who do not develop the ability to think within a nursing frame of reference may tend to be task oriented, viewing persons who require nursing as objects on which work operations are performed. Learning to think as a nurse is facilitated or hindered by the way in which nursing content and experiences are selected and organized in nursing courses in educational programs. The practical science nursing provides the content for courses with a nursing practice focus.

THE FACTUAL AND THE PRACTICAL

Nurses work in life situations with others to bring about conditions that are beneficial to persons nursed. Nursing demands the exercise of both the speculative and practical intelligence of nurses. In nursing practice situations, nurses must have accurate information and be knowing about existent conditions and circumstances of patients and about emerging changes in them. These factual insights provide knowledge of the concrete base for nurses' development of creative practical insights about what can be done to bring about more beneficial relationships or conditions, relationships, and conditions that do not presently exist.

Asking and answering the questions "what is?" and "what can be?" are nurses' points of departure in nursing practice situations. Answers provide foundations for nurses' judgments and decisions about what should and will be done. Speculative or factual refer to knowing the state of things as they are. Practical refers to that which is useful under some set(s) of circumstances in bringing about needed or desired conditions that are not yet present.

Nurses, like persons in other human services or persons engaged in result-seeking endeavors, must be conscious of the consistency between what they know and what they do. To achieve this state, nurses must be cognitively active in each nursing practice situation. Nurses search out characterizing features of situations and the patterns and relationships among identified features, including evidence of what should and can be changed. Observation, including the exercise of highly developed perceptual skills, and reflection and judgment are essential in determining nursing relevant features both factual and practical of situations where persons are under nursing care. Nurses reflect on their practical understanding of what can be done to effect more desirable conditions and make critical judgments about what should be done and what should be avoided. Final decisions about what will be done may or may not be in accord with judgments about what should be done.

Engagement in the foregoing types of intellectual activities demands that nurses and nursing students have prior or antecedently acquired authoritative knowledge from a number of organized fields of knowledge, including nursing science and the sciences foundational to nursing. In the absence of such antecedent knowledge, observations, and judgments made and the courses of action selected will be based wholly on common-sense knowledge of individuals that is uninformed by nursing science and nursing-related science. Nursing is practical endeavor, but it is practical endeavor engaged in by persons who have specialized theoretical nursing knowledge with developed capabilities to put this knowledge to work in concrete situations of nursing practice.

Without knowledge of the practical sciences of nursing, nurses and nursing students are unable to attach *nursing meaning* to what they observe and to the factual information they obtain, to the complex judgments they make about concrete situations, and to the needs for and the possibilities for change that they discern. Situational conditions and relationships among them at times are not known or understood because of nurses' lack of knowledge to guide and attach meaning to observations or because of their inability or failure to observe. At times, persons are moved to and do take action without knowing the appropriateness of what they do and even at times with full knowledge of its inappropriateness.

The complexity of some nursing situations requires that knowing and effective practitioners select courses of action to achieve a sought after result without full knowledge of the situation. At other times, practitioners know conditions and know what situational changes are desirable, but how to effect change is unclear. Measures to effect desired change may be undiscovered, or, if discovered, they are not validated or have limited reliability. In both of the preceding situations, the nurse's rule is to proceed with caution, using controlled trial approaches and acting to prevent harm as action proceeds. Such situations demand the presence of nursing practitioners with sound theoretical and experiential knowledge of nursing.

DELIBERATE ACTION

Deliberate actions of persons are based on their judgments about what is appropriate under existent conditions and circumstances. Arnold states that "psychologically speaking it means that we can do what we judge to be appropriate even though it be neither pleasurable nor appealing" (pp. 169-204).[1]

Nursing as deliberate action

Nursing in every instance of its practice is action deliberately performed by some members of a social group to bring about events and results that benefit others in specified ways. Thinking about and conceptualizing nursing as *deliberate action* is the most general approach that one can take to understanding nursing. It is an exercise in abstraction, the logical process of discovering in the provision of nursing the same elements and properties that will be found together and correlated in some way whenever individuals act to achieve a purpose — to reach a goal.

Deliberate human action includes simple acts like the set of actions performed in turning an electrical appliance, such as a lamp, on or off. It includes complex or compound acts where sets of organized and consecutive actions, individually and together are coordinated to achieve a common end (pp. 47-54).[2] Compound actions can be performed by one individual, as when a person accomplishes the purpose of being in Boston on a particular day by driving there in an automobile, or they can be performed by a number of individuals, as when two individuals coordinate their actions to move a heavy object from one location to another. Nursing is a complex of compound actions.

Nursing is the performance by a nurse or nurses of sets and series of organized, coordinated actions to achieve specified goals. Actions are connected in the sense that this action is made possible or facilitated by another action, or an action may interfere with the performance of a contemplated action.[2] The terms *organized* and *coordinated* thus refer to *relations between and among actions* performed by one or more individuals.

Organized and coordinated actions, for example, of a nurse and the person under the nurse's care, demand that the performer(s) or agent(s) have prior knowledge of the nature, timing, and duration of each action within the coordinated set or series and have the performance skills required.

Knowing what actions to perform and *having the skills to perform the actions* are combined with knowledge of the events and results that should accrue from their performance. For example, in a specific instance the deliberate turning of the ignition key of an automobile to the *on* position brings about a series of events resulting in the

---

***Exercise* to assist in understanding the complexity of practical endeavors**

Select an activity, a course of action, in which you engage to attain or partly attain some desired goal or purpose. It could be a household chore, an aspect of personal care or grooming, or a recreational or craft activity.
1. Identify the concrete circumstances and conditions that exist in yourself or the environment when you decide to engage in the activity.
2. Describe your usual perceptions of what will be changed as you engage in the activity.
3. Describe the actions you perform sequentially. What actions must be deliberately coordinated?
4. How do you know when to stop action?
5. What materials, equipment, and forms of energy do you use?
6. What standards do you use to judge results as action proceeds? When action is terminated?

---

desired and anticipated starting of the motor. This result may be one of a series of results sought, as when the *purpose* of the person who turned the ignition key is to arrive at work by automobile within some time interval. However, if a person's purpose is to determine whether the car battery is dead, then the purpose is achieved when the motor starts or does not start.

In the foregoing examples, the person who turns the ignition key to achieve either purpose would have relevant information about the situation of action. The person knows whether the key is inserted, recognizes when insertion has occurred, and when relevant, considers whether the car is cold, and so on. The agent, the person performing the actions, has incoming *sensory knowledge and awareness* of the reality of the situation of action. The agent *reflects* on the meaning of existent conditions and circumstances for the set or series of actions in process and for attainment of results toward purpose achievement. Reflection terminates in a particular productive situation with the agent's *decision* about the action that will be taken.

Assumptions about human beings

Accepting the generalization that nursing is deliberate human action involving reflection requires the acceptance of human beings as having intrinsic activity rather than passivity or strict reactivity to stimuli. The minimum set of assumptions about human beings would include the following (pp. 193-204).[1]

- Human beings know and appraise objects, conditions, and situations in terms of their effects on ends being sought.
- Human beings know directly by sensing; but they also reflect, reason, and understand.
- Human beings are capable of self-determined actions, even when they feel an emotional pull in the opposite direction.

- Human beings can prolong reflection indefinitely in deliberations about what action to take by raising questions about and directing attention toward different aspects of a situation and different possibilities for action.
- In order to act, human beings must concentrate on a suitable course of action and exclude other courses of action.
- Purposive action requires not only that human beings be aware of objects, conditions, and situations but also that they have the ability to contend with them and treat them in some way.
- Persons, as unitary beings, are the agents who act deliberately to attain ends or goals.

If the foregoing assumptions are accepted, it is possible to identify human and environmental conditions and factors that must be developed and operational if individuals are to appraise, select, and proceed with courses of action. Arnold's position about deliberate action and motivation led in 1987 to the expression of six conditions that may encourage action tendencies for self-care. Since the conditions are general and not specific to self-care they are presented in this section on deliberate action.

- Persons must have available the knowledge necessary to distinguish something as good or desirable from bad and undesirable and to reflect on its desirability or undesirability. The goal and ways to achieve it must be conceptualized or imagined.
- Reasons for selecting certain actions to attain what has been appraised as good or desirable and afforded the tentative status of a goal should be known.
- Time as well as knowledge is required for persons to form ideas about particular actions or to form images of how each action relates to the goal.
- Reflection should be directed to these questions: Is this way of acting good or desirable? Is it more desirable or less desirable than other ways of acting to achieve the goal?
- Reflection about choosing a way of action could go on indefinitely; therefore, reflection should be brought to a close with a decision when the ways of action have been conceived as clear ideas or clear images are formed.
- A person owns his or her appraisal of possible ways of action to attain a goal and his or her decision to act according to one or a combination of these ways, when this way of acting is formalized and incorporated into the person's self-image or self-concept (pp. 12-13).[3]

Given acceptance of these conditions by nurses, rules and standards of nursing practice can be developed for situations where patients are confronted with choices and decisions with respect to self-care or dependent-care or about choices to engage in the exercise or development of self-care agency or dependent-care agency. Nurses should view the six conditions as applicable to their own choices, as well as to patient choices.

Since persons have action tendencies toward that which they appraise as good (liked), a consideration of what is good is essential. "Good (as opposed to bad) implies full approval or commendation of someone or something in the respect under consideration, such as . . . excellence of condition, beneficial properties (p. 387). . . ."[4] Lonergan (pp. 596-602)[5] suggests three levels of the good or desirable. The first or elementary level is where what is good is object of desire. At this level, the good is particular and is coupled with its opposite bad. For example, "It is good that my dentist will see me today, for my tooth continues to ache." Lonergan suggests that the second level of good is the good of order in which recurring desires and aversions of members of social groups through intelligent control and insights into concrete situations result in arrangements for human living, including an "intelligible pattern of human relationships" in the family and in other social institutions. The good of order is dynamic, leading individuals to consider how their own actions are conditioned by existent arrangements, including patterns of relationships, and how their own actions to fulfill desires conditions the fulfillment of desires of others. The good of order is viewed as an aspect of human intersubjectivity. The third level of the good is that of value or worth "as the possible object of rational choices." Whatever is desired becomes a value when it is placed within some intelligible hierarchy as a possible object of choice within a situation of action.

The levels or aspects of the good as identified by Lonergan become important in practical endeavors such as self-care and nursing when unfamiliar possible courses of action to change situations are identified and are objects of choice. Persons become concerned with reasons for their action and begin a process of reflection by closely examining what could be done and investigating their motives for choosing courses of action. Desirability and usefulness of a course of action for goal achievement are considered, as is the fit or lack of fit of a course of action in the accepted order of things, for example, in the family or the health care system and the location of the course of action and the goal sought within each person's value hierarchy (pp. 610-611).[5] Insights about good as the object of desire, the good of order, and good as value or worth add another dimension toward respecting the practical intelligence of men, women, and children and to their choices of what to do and what not to do before initiating concrete courses of action to change their life situations.

SITUATIONS OF ACTION AND PHASES OF ACTION

The concept of nursing system and the self-care deficit theory of nursing presented in Chapter 3 reflect a deliberate action frame of reference and nursing's features as practical endeavor. Nurses act deliberately to produce systems of nursing for persons who have health-related action deficits for knowing and continually meeting their own or their dependents' therapeutic self-care demands. Nurses must become able to envision the wholeness of situations within which their patients engage or should engage in self-care or have it performed for them.

Context of action

Care systems for self or dependents articulate with and are subsystems of larger systems of personal daily living, which are parts of still larger systems of family or group living. These larger systems are understood by nurses as the context within which persons make judgments, choices, and decisions about self-care and dependent-care and follow particular courses of action.

This was clearly understood by a woman who on being told about her health problem and a recommended regimen of care responded with "If I do all these things there will be no time to lead my own life."

Nurses, too, must understand the context of their own actions when they work with patients in their homes, in clinics, or in resident care agencies such as hospitals or nursing homes. Nurses must have clear views of action systems of nursing care they produce that articulate (1) with other health care systems within health care agency contexts or the context of patients' homes, and (2) with systems for financing nursing and other forms of care required by nurses' patients.

Parsons (pp. 8n-9n)[6] introduced the term *unit act* to refer to the smallest distinct unit of doing something that made sense (was meaningful) within a larger action system (a compound act). For example, pushing an electrical switch to the on position is a unit act within the larger action system of illuminating an area of a room where a person has made the decision to sit and read. The elements of a unit act are identified in Fig. 4-1. In a later text, Parsons (pp. 44-45)[7] expands the term to "unit of action" to fit in problems of motivation.

The concept unit act is an important one for nurses, as well as other heal.h care workers, because each of their prescriptions for care may need to be broken down into series of unit acts so that patients can understand care prescriptions, choose to follow them, and proceed to follow them.

Phases of action

In attempts to continue to develop insights about deliberate action, the position is taken that actions to deliberately attain a goal are performed in phases. This applies to single units of action, as well as to related units, which together form systems of action. *Phase* is used to mean the appearance or emergence of different forms of human behavior as persons perform actions and series of actions in sequences (processes) to attain a goal or achieve a partial result. Two phases of deliberate action within concrete situations of action are identified in Fig. 4-2. Phase one includes investigative (estimative) type operations, proceeds to reflective understanding and judgment about the situation, including how a situation can be changed, and concludes with a decision about the ends to be sought and the means to be used. Phase two proceeds from the decision about what will be done and the design for doing it to the production of action sequences through which the end is reached, and the goal attained or not attained. Phase two also includes actions through which production is planned and controlled (including evaluation).

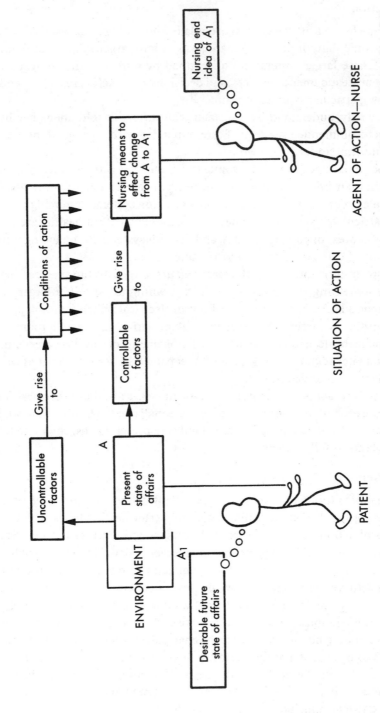

Fig. 4-1 Persons' elements of the unit act applied in a general way to nursing. *(From Nursing Development Conference Group, Orem DE, editor: Concept formalization in nursing: process and product, ed 2, Boston, 1979, Little, Brown & Co.)*

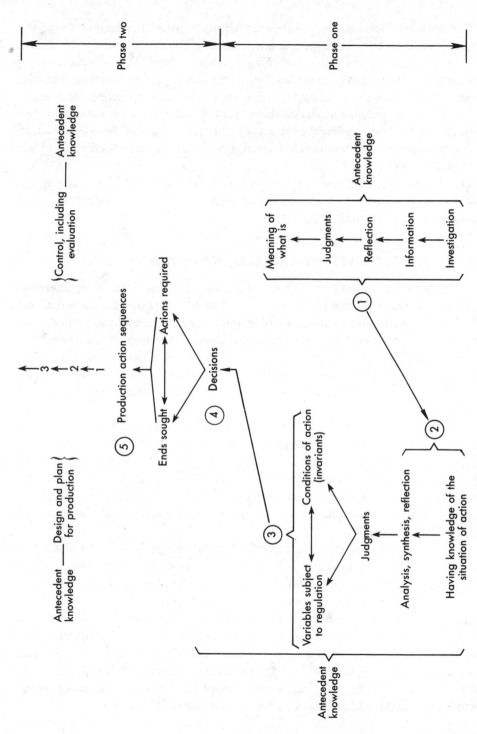

Fig. 4-2 Phases of deliberate action showing operations, results, and requirements for types of antecedent knowledge.

The Nursing Development Conference Group separated reflection about the course of action to be followed and decision making about what will be done from phase one, identifying them as constituting a separate phase. This schema involves three phases of action: the investigative, transitional, and production. Fig. 4-2 illustrates that persons who engage in deliberate action within concrete situations of action require antecedent knowledge about types of conditions, circumstances, and events that may occur in particular situations of action and about the types of action systems to be produced. More detailed descriptions of the phases of deliberate action are presented in Chapter 7.

The foregoing expositions of practical endeavor and deliberate action are presented in this chapter as a basis for understanding the characteristics of the practical science of nursing.

NAMING PRACTICE FIELDS AS FIELDS OF INQUIRY

A number of terms are used to refer to professional fields such as engineering, medicine, and nursing from the perspective of their accumulated, structured, and validated knowledge and their modes of inquiry. The terms include applied field, applied science, practice discipline, practical science, and science. Nurses have been reluctant not only to take a position about the proper object of nursing but also to take a position about naming nursing as a field of knowledge and inquiry. Nurses have used all of the terms just expressed, but few have expressed rationales for their use or attached meaning to particular terms.

In the previous edition of this textbook, both the terms *practice discipline* and *practical science* were used. In this edition, nursing as a field of inquiry and knowledge is referred to consistently as *practical science,* with theoretically practical components, and more practically oriented (practically practical) components. The reason for change is that knowledge about practical science must be used to develop a useful and valid concept of a practice discipline. The terms discipline, practice discipline, and applied field are described.

The term *discipline* means a branch or field of knowledge exhibiting a distinctive outlook and style of thinking, as well as distinctive organized ideas and concepts, methods of inquiry, and modes of understanding data. Disciplines of knowledge with their modes of inquiry are developed and advanced through the work of scholars, theorists, and researchers in the field who communicate their insights and the results of their investigations. The term *practice* in the context of practice discipline means that the ways of knowing and the organized facts, ideas, and concepts associated with the investigations of members of a discipline relate to elements of their practice field and serve to: (1) explain and describe elements of the practice field, and (2) bring together and organize knowledge in a way that prepares for action.

The term *applied field* is used more frequently than the term *practice discipline* to refer to the knowledge specific to professions and occupations. *Applied field* signifies that persons who engage in, for example, the practice of engineering or medicine or nursing extract from developed disciplines of knowledge, especially the natural sciences, ideas, laws, and theories that are useful to them in the resolution and solution of recurring problems in their practice fields. The term *applied field* minimizes the complexity of practice fields. The term is too narrow to be descriptive of all the constituent kinds of knowledge that constitute well-developed practice disciplines.

PRACTICAL SCIENCES

The term practical science is used by philosophers and philosophers of science within a philosophic system of moderate realism. Its referent is to modes of inquiry and fields of knowledge associated with the practical order of things, things that are doable. Wallace (pp. 273-293)[8] states that practical sciences are concerned with "principles and causes of things to be done." Practical science is contrasted with "theoretical science" concerned with things that are "knowable" and with "demonstrable knowledge" of the subject of investigation. Wallace[8] and Maritain (pp. 311-316, pp. 458-459)[9] state that practical science has theoretical or speculative parts, as well as parts that give direction to what to do or what not to do in distinct situations.

Three commonly recognized groups of practical science are identified by Wallace[8]: (1) ethnics or moral science concerned with human action in terms of its "being human or moral," (2) the health sciences (e.g., medicine and nursing), and (3) the sciences that deal with forces and objects from a production point of view (e.g., engineering).

The parts of practical sciences

Practical sciences include speculatively practical knowledge and practically practical knowledge.[9] Speculatively practical knowledge brings unity and meaning to the universe of action (action domain) of a practice field and to its elements. The theories and conceptual elements of the self-care deficit theory of nursing are speculative in mode. They describe and explain elements and relations within nursing practice situations, including principles and causes of their existence. The expressed theory of nursing system, which subsumes the theory of self-care deficit and the theory of self-care, is an example of how the practical science, nursing, constructs one subject (nursing system) "precisely as capable of being produced" while remaining in the speculative mode.

The second kind of knowledge, practically practical knowledge,[9] is more particularized, dealing with the details of cases, but always within the universal conceptualizations of the practice field, including its domain, elements, and types of results sought. This kind of knowledge is practical in that it is preparatory for action and includes rules and standards of practice and compositive in that it brings together knowledge necessary for taking action and organizes it according to actions and results. This form of knowledge is movement closer to concrete practice situations. Experience has a primary role in establishing what is needed for action, and practitioners within the profession have major roles in development of this kind of knowledge.

Practically practical knowledge in nursing science includes, for example, sets of care measures designed to meet a type of self-care requisite particularized for individuals of the same chronologic age, gender, and developmental state living under specified environmental conditions. Another example is rules for selection and use of methods of helping in relation to certain values of self-care agency and the nature and extent of types of self-care limitations.

Theoretical (speculative) nursing science has many of the features of science, unqualified by the adjective practical. In its development, methods of inquiry are used to investigate and analyze features of nursing practice situations and nursing cases. Investigators develop insights about perceived features and relations among them. They formulate insights as concepts. Expressed concepts of features and relations among them that are validated in concrete practice situations are the beginnings of descriptions and explanations of nursing's practice domain. Formulated and expressed concepts that are related can be synthesized or unified to form structures of related concepts. Syntheses can be expressed as static unions that express properties of persons, for example, therapeutic self-care demand, or as dynamic processes, as in the theory of nursing system where nurse and patient properties are conceptualized as necessarily interactive if a synthesis is to occur.

A third kind of knowledge is found within the structure of practice fields. Every practical science includes a number of *applied sciences*. Applied sciences are existent sciences that are put to use or are pursued to achieve some end outside the domain of the science. In practice fields, applied sciences are developed at points of articulation between theoretical or practical problems of a practice field and theoretical formulations of the science that is being applied. The formulations are selected because they are useful in resolving or solving types of problems in the practice fields. Examples of applied sciences include climateophysiology, medical microbiology, and surgical anatomy. The potential applied nursing sciences can be identified but are not developed.

Nursing as knowledge essential for use in achieving nursing results in social groups would be constituted within this framework from two types of practical nursing sciences and from a set of applied sciences. Nurses, unlike other professionals, rarely use the term *science* with respect to their own discipline. Nurses, however, appear willing to accept the idea of medical sciences and engineering sciences. Science is systematic empirical inquiry. It is concerned with affording meaning to concrete matters of fact. Myriads of facts have been and continue to be amassed within real situations of nursing practice. But facts do not make a science. Neither do the results of research, the fit of which into the structure of a science is unspecified. Developing the ideas and concepts, the laws, and the theories that describe and explain the elements of nursing's practice field is essential in making explicit the structure of nursing as a practical science and a set of applied sciences and in opening systematic avenues for research.

Stages of development

Science is activity with respect to entities to be understood not in their individuality in time-place localizations, but in their universality. Doing science is basically intellectual activity. Workers in science function as scholars, theorists, researchers, and, in the practical sciences, as developers of technologies and techniques for effecting change in concrete situations. Development of technologies and techniques is critical in practice fields since practitioners must move from intellectual conceptions of selected orders or correlations to be brought about to the effecting of those orders or correlations in concrete situations of practice. Technologies and techniques to effect change must be discovered, their validity and reliability under ranges of specified conditions established, and their undesirable effects if any set forth.

Workers in a science function with respect to whatever is presently known about their field or areas within their field of knowledge and inquiry that constitute their domain of activity.

Five stages

Five stages of development of the practical science nursing are identified (Fig. 4-3). Each stage is understood as a development of different kinds of knowledge within the domain and boundaries of nursing established by nursing's identified proper object. This as previously expressed is understood as a person's subjectivity to health associated deficits for engagement in self-care or dependent-care. Development is understood as movement from states of lesser to states of greater complexity with the emergence of detail with higher and higher levels of integration of existent and emerging structures and features.

The stages are identified as follows:
- Stage of description with descriptive explanation of properties of persons, movement, and change, and products of human action that are characteristic of nursing practice situations. Results of this stage are in the form of concepts; theories; and laws about persons, properties of persons, about movement or change in properties of persons or their operations, and about what is produced.
- A subsequent and linked stage of discernment and verification of variations in the qualitative and quantitative features of *person properties* concomitant with specific

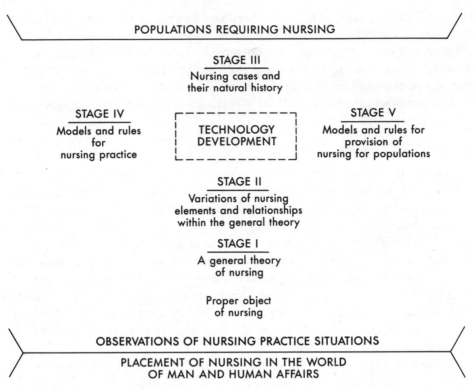

Fig. 4-3 Stages of understanding nursing.

values of factors, such as age and health state, known to condition human functioning, human development, and personal health and well-being of members of social groups. Results of this stage are conceptual relationships based on concomitant variation or correlations of features or values of person properties with factors that condition them. This stage demands the use of qualitative and quantitative measurement.

• Stage of description of instances where persons require and receive nursing — nursing cases. Descriptions include persons in space-time localizations, properties of persons, factors actively conditioning the values of patient and nurse properties, motion or change in properties of persons or in their operations in time-specific sequences. Also included are operational problems of nurses in providing nursing and problems of patients in accepting and receiving nursing, as well as the social and interpersonal features specific to the case. Cases are categorized according to one or more organizing principle, for example, who does the work of self-care — patient, nurse, dependent-care agent, or some combination thereof. Cases can be described by nurses to emphasize a particular feature of a case or some combination of features.

- Stage of synthesis of nursing practice models and the formulation of rules of practice for situations where the unit of a nurse's service is an individual, a dependent-care unit, a residence unit including families or other types of multiperson units. Nursing practice models are designs for nursing action based on perceived or hypothesized structures of (1) persons in relationships or (2) patient properties or components thereof, which vary within an established range. The values of patient properties give rise to particular requirements for nurse-patient interaction, use of a specific way or a combination of ways of helping, or for specialized nursing diagnostic or regulatory (treatment) measures. Practice models identify conditions that allow for positive movement or change in patient properties including probabilities for regression, nursing results that can accrue from nurses' maintenance of interpersonal unity with patients and their significant others, and through use of specific diagnostic and regulatory care measures. Nursing practice models are of two types: (1) nursing system models or total design models that lay out the features, the structure, and nursing action involved in the production of a nursing system within specific parameters, and (2) partial design models that lay out the features, the structure, and the nursing action demanded to establish units of design or parts of some combination of units of design (see Chapter 5).

  Rules of nursing practice associated with nursing practice models express principles to guide nurses within situations where persons and their properties vary within the range described in the model.
- Stage of description of populations requiring nursing to identify the incidence of types of nursing cases as a base for making inference about (1) kind and amount of nursing required by time periods for particular types of cases, (2) kinds of nursing results that should be sought by types of case, and (3) qualifications of nurses that reflect capabilities to provide nursing for types of cases that describe the population and the number of nurses with specific qualifications required. Item 3 would include the numbers and qualifications of nurses able to provide nursing consultation to patients and to other nurses. Changes in populations are reflected by factors that actively condition patient and nurse properties (basic conditioning factors), for example, the distribution of the population by age combined with the reason for being under health care, and with health care system factors, such as the use of particular medical diagnostic or treatment modalities that give rise to specific types of self-care requisites. Description is followed by synthesis of models for providing nursing to populations served.

  Developments of stages 3 and 4 contribute to the work of stage-5 development. Stages 4 and 5 yield not only rules for nursing, but also standards of nursing. Developments in stages 1 and 2 are necessary for definitive developments in stages 3, 4, and 5. The work of the Nursing Development Conference Group supports the statement that work with nursing cases and development of practice models may proceed along with or precede specific stage 1 and stage 2 developments.

Technologies

In addition to the developments expressed, there is a continuing need in nursing and other practice fields for the development, formalization, and validation of technologies essential for effective nursing practice. A *technology* is defined as an application of scientific knowledge to the practical purposes to be achieved in a field. In related fields, for example, nursing and medicine, a technology developed in one field may be used by persons in a related field. For example, some technologies for measuring cardiac and circulatory functioning are used by physicians and nurses; other measuring technologies, however, are used by medical specialists and specialized technicians. At times, technologies may be developed and be used productively without a rationale of why they work.

Nurses develop technologies in the course of their practice of nursing without recording them or verbally communicating them to other nurses for further development and validation. Nursing technologies include those related to human interaction and communication, as well as to the observational, diagnostic, and regulatory operations of nursing practice. The following listing of types of technologies required for nursing practice was developed in 1969 and appeared in a modified form in the first edition of this book. One technology for research on technologies is included in the listing (pp. 2-6).[10] This listing is an edited version of the original listing.

1. Technologies or processes through which interpersonal, intergroup relations are brought into existence and maintained as long as such relations are essential for achievement of nursing and nursing-related goals in specific types of practice situations.
2. Technologies of human assistance through which help or service is rendered by one person to another. The reasons for the requirements for help and for the matters about which persons need help determine the characteristics of assisting processes.
3. Technologies of individual personal care, which is self-administered by adults and administered by them to infants and children. When such care has as its goal positive health and when it has a base in scientifically derived knowledge it is referred to as *therapeutic self-care.*
4. Technologies for appraising, changing, and controlling human integrated functioning, with emphasis on physiologic or psychological modes of functioning in health and disease. These are technologies based in medical science.
5. Technologies to bond persons together in therapeutic relations (relations from which flow positively therapeutic results), which contribute to the maintenance of personal integrity and development, despite disease and disability.
6. Technologies for bringing about and controlling the position and movement of persons in their physical environments.

7. Research methods and techniques necessary for the initial and continuing formalization of the named practice technologies, their validation, and establishment of their validity and reliability for use under specified conditions and circumstances. Rules would be expressed for conditions of use in nursing practice situations.

The work of development and formalization of technologies and techniques of nursing practice is not adequately attended to by nurses and nursing practitioners. Whenever a practice technology is developed, it should be formalized to the degree possible at the time and validated through use and through research and rules for use under conditions encountered in nursing practice and should be formulated, expressed, and communicated within the profession.

Developments

The self-care deficit theory of nursing, with its constituent theories of self-care, self-care deficit, and nursing system, provides a way of looking at and investigating what nurses do and what nurses should do in social groups. It provides concepts, theories, and propositions for continued developments of the practical science of nursing. Concepts and theories descriptively explanatory of the elements, factors that condition the elements, and the products of and the outcome of nursing presented in Chapter 3 are stage 1 developments. The secondary or substantive structure of self-care, therapeutic self-care demand, self-care agency, and nursing agency described in subsequent chapters provide the foundations for stage 2 developments. Developments in stages 2 through 5 are critically important to provide generic nursing students with adequate textual references about the practical science of nursing.

Developments in all stages are underway, with contributions from teachers of generic undergraduate nursing students, registered nurses and nursing assistants, nursing practitioners in specialty areas of nursing, nursing researchers, nursing scholars, and theorists. Some developments are scattered, awaiting the efforts of scholars of self-care deficit nursing theory to organize specific developments and research findings within the structure provided by the theory. It is important to accept that nurses who embark on scientific development of nursing in one or more of its aspects have some degree of accumulated empirical knowledge of nursing within its broader context of health care, of scholarly achievement in sciences foundational to nursing and in the liberal arts and humanities, and of interest in scientific approaches to development of nursing as a practical science and as a set of applied sciences.

Persons who contribute to continuing development of nursing as a practical science (1) see the wholeness of nursing for one or more subpopulations as revealed by nursing's proper object and by a valid, adequate general theory of nursing; (2) have developing understanding of the characteristics of practical sciences, including the demand on nursing scientists to engage in analysis and synthesis dealing with complex masses of empirical data, to conceptualize recurring features of nursing situations, to theorize, to validate concepts and propositions of theories, and to develop measuring devices; and (3) have insights into nursing practice problems whose resolution and solution depend on the availability of structures of validated knowledge that combine nursing concepts and elements of nursing theories with facts and points of theory from already developed sciences or disciplines of knowledge (beginning development of applied nursing sciences).

Nurses who desire to contribute to nursing's continuing development as a practical science and a set of applied sciences seek understanding of the characteristics of these types of sciences, as well as the suggested stages of development of nursing science. As previously indicated, developments in stages 1 and 2 depend on nurses' experiential knowledge of nursing. This includes knowledge of nursing cases that is often incomplete. This dependence is well documented in the 1968 work of the Nursing Development Conference Group (pp. 141-145)[11] in which analyses of case material about persons nursed by members of the Group provided the basis for exploring the realities conceptualized in the patient property self-care agency and in "development of techniques for collection and analyses of data about self-care agency."

This work exemplifies how a stage 3 development (description of nursing cases) led to the continuing development and validation of the concept self-care agency, stage 2 development, and to development of an exploratory framework for assessment of self-care agency in persons suffering from ongoing disease processes, a stage 4 development. The 1968 explanatory framework for assessment of self-care agency of persons suffering from ongoing disease processes who are under the care of physicians was constituted from six articulated parts shown in Figs. 4-4 and 4-5. The figures were developed during the process of sorting data from one nursing case. The foci of assessment for the parts of the framework represented in the figure are restated below. The letters used are the same as the letters in Figs. 4-4 and 4-5.

- **A,** The person
- **A.1,** Self-image
- **A.2,** Care of self-image, factors affecting care of self-image
- **B,** The person's self-care system
- **B.1,** Action limitations with a basis in disease processes for which the person is under care (C), from physician's regimen of medical care (D), from other disease processes, from age
- **B.2,** Therapeutic self-care demand
- **C,** Disease processes and results and effects of same for which the person is under care. Establish and relate to **B.1** [and **B.2**]
- **D,** Physician'(s) regimen of medical care. Establish and relate to **B.1** and **B.2**

This early framework for assessment of self-care agency of persons suffering from disease processes and under medical care in concrete situations of nursing practice has

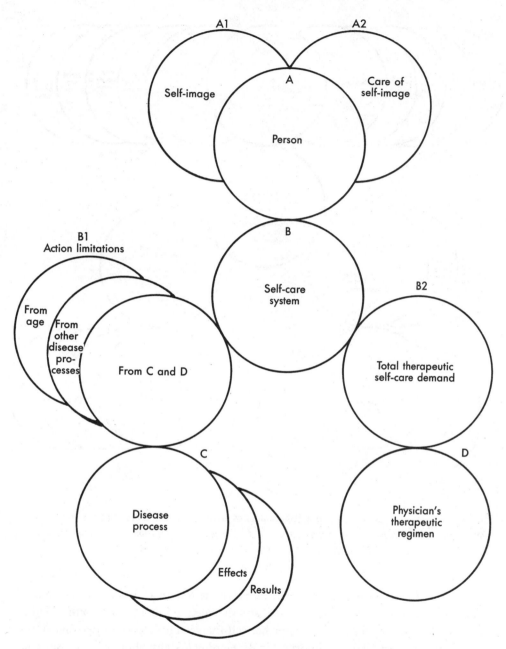

Fig. 4-4 A 1968 framework to assess self-care agency in the presence of disease. (*From Nursing Development Conference Group, Orem DE, editor: Concept formalization in nursing: process and product, ed 2, Boston, 1979, Little, Brown & Co.*)

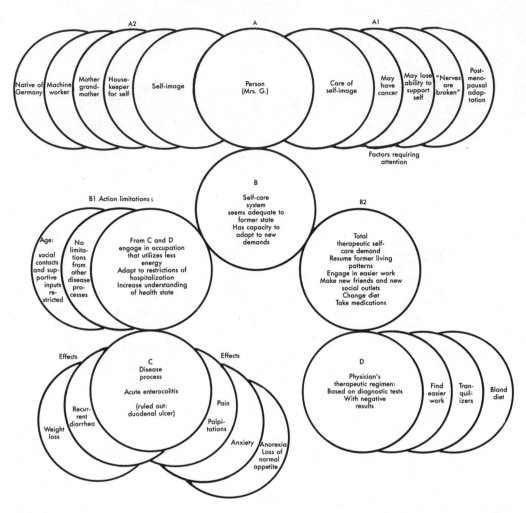

Fig. 4-5 Example of assessment of self-care agency using the 1968 framework. (*From Nursing Development Conference Group, Orem DE, editor: Concept formalization in nursing: process and product, ed 2, Boston, 1979, Little, Brown & Co.*)

as its central focus the person who is the nurse's patient with a "developed self-image," an ongoing task for "care of self-image," and the need to identify factors that require attention in the person's care of his or her self-image. This focus on persons and on their images of themselves is important in developing insights about what persons will and will not do in coming to know and in meeting their therapeutic self-care demands and in the exercise or development of their self-care agency in concrete situations of nursing practice.

Summary

Fig. 4-3 summarizes suggested stages of development of self-care deficit nursing theory within a frame of practical science. The figure includes features of the prescience phase of nursing's development as a field of knowledge and inquiry.

The stages of development of self-care deficit nursing theory and developments within various stages have characteristics of a normative model of nursing, reflecting what nurses ought to know and what they ought to bring about. The historical model of nursing was deficient because it represented nurse role in terms of tasks to be learned and performed, it did not define the domain and boundaries of nursing, it underplayed the role of the professional nurse with respect to nursing's contribution to health care, and it did not contribute to nurses' development of honest regard for themselves as therapeutically trained persons. The five suggested stages of development of the practical science nursing reflect but deviate to some degree from the traditional stages represented for the development of sciences, namely (1) the stage of natural history, which is largely descriptive of what is the case; (2) the stage of normative thinking, which is what ought to be the case; (3) the stage of science proper, which is the stage of explanation and validation of hypotheses; and (4) the stage of application.

The nursing profession should be concerned not only with nurses and their practice of nursing but also with the practical science of nursing. This science can only be developed and formalized through the activity of nurses with the talents and interests of nursing scholars, theorists, researchers, and developers who at the same time may be nursing practitioners or teachers of nursing or who work closely with practitioners (Fig. 4-6).

KNOWING NURSING'S DOMAIN

Nurses who are effective practitioners of nursing recognize when persons are in need of nursing, but they may not be able to express with clarity the bases for their recognition of need. Inability to express what nurses do when they nurse and why they do what they do characterized many graduates of nursing programs in the United States into the last quarter of the twentieth century.

Nursing developed and continued to manifest the characteristics of a task-oriented occupation rather than a profession with a focus on human beings with discernible requirements for nursing.

As the need to make nursing available to more and more people was recognized in the beginning period of modern nursing, attention became focused on the *action domain of nursing practice*. Components of the action domain of the nurse often were expressed (1) as *recurring tasks* that were performed by nurses according to standardized procedures, that is, routine courses of action and specifications for task

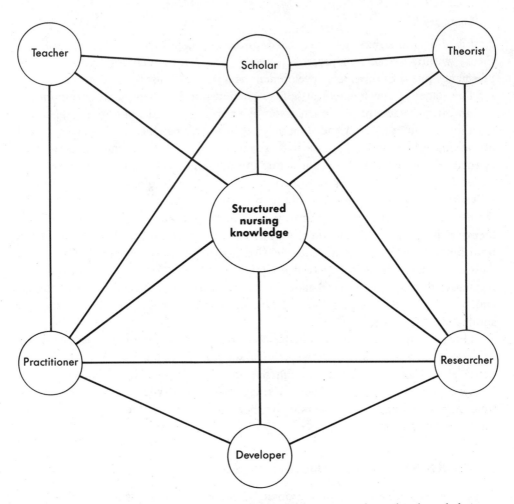

Fig. 4-6 Professional roles and role relationships with structured nursing knowledge as a common element.

performance, and (2) as rules to which nurses should adhere. Nursing as *taught* in nursing schools and programs became task-oriented rather than person-oriented. It was up to the individual nursing student and nurse to seek understanding of the personal and interpersonal aspects of nursing and incorporate these into practice.

This historical emphasis on *tasks and procedures* within the *action domain of nursing practice* seems to have stilled or overruled nurses' interest in the questions: What gives rise to human requirements for nursing? Why can people benefit from nursing? Nurses' failure to attend to these questions resulted in an absence of agreement among nurses about what nursing is and is not. As a result the question of *what tasks nurses should perform* continues to arise whenever boundary questions between nursing and medicine or nursing and some other field of practice arise. For example, the lack of clarity about the practice domain of nurse practitioners is essentially a boundary problem, the solving of which requires insights about how human requirements for nursing differ from human requirements for medical care. As long as a majority of nurses are willing to define boundary problems in terms of tasks and procedures, nursing cannot be properly moved to fulfill its human and social mission. Tasks separated from the human and environmental factors, conditions, and circumstances that specify why and when and by whom they should be performed *provide no basis for understanding nursing as care or art or as knowledge that grounds the nurse's art.*

As the twentieth century ends, social conditions in the United States should cause nurses to recall the social conditions in Europe and America during the nineteenth century. The physically and mentally sick and the poor and destitute are still with us in hospitals and other care facilities, in their homes, and on the streets. The chronically ill as well as the acutely ill, the aged and the aging, and the young with impaired structural or functional integrity can benefit from many forms of care including nursing. The "trained nurse" of the nineteenth and early twentieth centuries made a difference in society. Perhaps more interest on the part of nurses in why people need and can benefit from nursing would help nurses to better focus their attention and orient their actions so that they can produce more enduring effects and results for persons under their care. Some nurses have thrown off the tasks showered on them from other practice fields and are in a position to advance nursing as a practice field. Nurses who do this are addressing the human and social problems that are associated with needs of people for nursing.

REFERENCES

1. Arnold MB: Patterns of action: Emotion and personality. In Neurological and physiological aspects, vol II. New York, 1960. Columbia University Press, p. 198.
2. Kotarbinski T: Praxiology, an introduction to the sciences of efficient action, (trans. Olgierd Wojtasiewicz), Pergamon Press, 1965, New York, pp. 47-48.
3. Orem DE: Motivating self-care—the reality, persons as self-care agents. Conference papers Hospitals in the Community—A Vision, The Wesley Hospital, Auchenflower, 4066, Queensland, Australia, 1988, pp. 12-13.
4. Webster's dictionary of synonyms, ed 1, Springfield, Mass, 1951, GB Merriman Publishers.
5. Lonergan BJF: Insight. A study of human understanding, New York, 1958, Philosophical Library, pp. 596-602.
6. Parsons T: The structure of social action, New York, 1937, McGraw-Hill Book Co., pp. 44-45.
7. Parsons T: The social system, New York, 1951, The Free Press, pp. 8-9n.
8. Wallace WA: Essay XIII: Being scientific is a practice discipline. From a realist point of view, essay on philosophy of science, ed 2, Lanham, Md, 1988, University Press of America, p. 275.
9. Maritain J: The speculative order and the practical order. The degrees of knowledge, translated from the 4th French edition, under the supervision of Gerald B Phelan, New York, 1959, Charles Scribner's Sons.
10. Orem DE: The levels of nursing education and practice, Alumnae Magazine of the Johns Hopkins Hospital School of Nursing, 68:2-6, 1969.
11. Nursing Development Conference Group, Orem DE, editor: Concept formalization in nursing: process and product, ed 2, Boston, 1979, Little, Brown, and Co.

SELECTED READINGS

Allison SE: A framework for nursing action in a nurse conducted diabetic management clinic, J Nurs Admin 3:53-60, 1973.

Denyes MJ: Orem's model used for health promotion: directions for research, Adv Nurs Sci 11:13-21, 1988.

Dodd MJ: Patterns of self-care in cancer patients receiving radiation therapy, Oncol Nurs Forum 11:23-27, 1984.

Evers GCM: Appraisal of self-care agency, A.S.A.—scale, Assen/Maastricht, The Netherlands, 1989, Van Gorcum & Co.

Fawcett J: Orem's self-care framework (with an annotated bibliography). In Conceptual models of nursing, ed 2, Philadelphia, 1989, FA Davis, pp. 205-261.

Frey MA, and Denyes MJ: Health and illness self-care in adolescents with IDDM: a test of Orem's theory, Adv Nurs Sci 12:67-75, 1989.

Gast HL, et al: Self-care agency: conceptualizations and operationalizations, Adv Nurs Sci 12:26-38, 1989.

Gulick EE: Parsimony and model confirmation of the ADL self-care scale for multiple sclerosis persons, Nurs Res 36:278-283, 1989.

Hammonds TA: Self-care practices of Navajo Indians. In Riehl-Sisca J, editor: The science and art of self-care, Norwalk, 1985, Appleton-Century-Crofts, pp. 171-195.

Orem DE, and Taylor SG: Orem's general theory of nursing, In Winstead-Fry P, editor: Case studies in nursing theory, New York, 1986, National League for Nursing, pp. 54-71.

CHAPTER 5

The function of design in nursing practice

Nurses are admonished to develop plans for nursing care in concrete practice situations, but over the years scant attention has been given to comprehensive design as a function of the professionally educated nurse engaged in nursing practice. **Design** is recognized in professional fields as prior to and as an essential basis for development of detailed plans for using formulated methods to achieve goals. Design (p. 622),[1] like plan, denotes a proposed way of making or doing something. Design, however, sets forth the disposition of individual elements and details of elements through careful ordering and calculation and suggests a definite pattern for the work to be done. Design implies reference to the achievement of order and the elimination of friction or lack of harmony among the distinct parts or elements of a complex whole. Design also designates attention to integrity of the parts as well as the order, harmony, and integrity of the whole that is to be produced.

The elements of the self-care deficit theory of nursing and their designated relationships identifies or points to concrete conditions and factors that become parts to be dealt with in the production of nursing. Through working with these parts and understanding them and the relationships among them in concrete nursing situations, nurses and nursing students become able to design and produce nursing. Nursing is not a naturally existent entity. It is something constructed and produced by nurses. It is made in time and over time in some place(s) by one or more persons for another person or persons. Simon[2] refers to structured validated knowledge about what is constructed or made as "sciences of the artificial."

VARIATIONS IN DESIGN IN PRACTICE FIELDS

Nurses provide help or care in the form of nursing for persons of different ages, in different stages of development, in different health states, and in different time-place localizations. Those who can be helped through nursing become the center of any design for nursing. Men, women, and children who are patients of nurses are unitary beings with singular ways of living and singular life histories. Their behaviors may be disorderly or abberant; spontaneous and unpredictable; or they may behave with accountability and responsibility. All are subject to conditions and conditioning, but it is the individual man, woman, or child who provides that which can be affected (conditioned) (p.50).[3]

The self-care deficit theory of nursing, with its focus on the realities of men, women and children, their properties that are nursing-relevant, and on motion or change that occurs in nursing practice situations, points to elements and features of concrete situations of nursing practice with which nurses must deal. These elements and features must be known in detail by nurses, known in their relations to the essential work of producing systems of nursing care for individuals or units comprised of individuals. Designing systems of nursing rests on nurses' knowledge (1) of the work to be done and (2) the realities to be dealt with in doing the work. Effective nursing rests on creative design but design that conforms to what is needed and what can be done in practice situations at this time(s), in this place.

Direct personal health services such as nursing are directed to the health and well-being of individuals singly or in groups. Systems of nursing care or systems of medical care are constituted from action sequences, series of events over time to which persons who are nurses' or physicians' patients contribute according to their capabilities. Results of direct personal health care are understood in terms of changes in human or environmental features. Results of health care do not take on existence apart from persons in environments. Nor can the work of designing nursing for a particular individual or group occur in a time period that differs from the time period when systems of nursing care are being produced. In fields such as architecture and engineering, design is complete as are plans and specifications before construction is begun. In both types of fields, however, professionals must know the work to be done and the concrete realities to be dealt with in designing and doing the work.

Areas of nursing design

Any exercise in explicating the design function in nursing practice demands recognition that through performance of this function nurses form units of design, which, when ordered to one another and finally arranged in a creative, orderly, harmonious fashion, constitute patterns for the production of nursing systems toward attainment of nursing results. Design activity begins before production and before planning for production, although there may be the appearance of simultaneity. Understanding the design function in nursing requires acceptance that units must be designed one by one and that the nature of the work of designing of one unit differs from the work of designing other units. Nurses must know the realities to be dealt with in designing each unit; they must also know that different units of design may deal with the same concrete entities and use the same data.

When formed, units of design may exist only within nurses as images of selected elements and features of nursing practice situations in relationship one to another and together constituting a unitary structure. Units of design may be recorded in writing or they can be communicated verbally. Units of design represent *results* of those aspects of the work of doing nursing that must be in process or completed before the helping or taking care of aspects of nursing begin. The totality of a design for a system of nursing may emerge immediately with minimal information or it may emerge over time.

Six design units are suggested for consideration. Their identification and acceptance rest on a number of assumptions, including the following:

- Nursing has societal, interpersonal, and technologic aspects.
- The self-care deficit theory of nursing, through the substantive structure of its conceptual elements, points to the realities that nurses deal with in nursing practice situations.
- Nursing design is accomplished through analysis and synthesis of concrete elements of nursing practice situations bringing them into orderly relationship to form structural units the elements of which can be creatively brought together to constitute a pattern to guide the production of systems of nursing toward attainment of nursing goals.

The six design units are identified as follows (see Fig. 5-1):

A. Delineation within the contract or agreement to receive nursing, nursing's area of jurisdiction in the health care of persons for whom nursing is sought, and an outlining of the health care goals to which nursing will contribute
B. Establishment of the main features and relationships of a socially legitimate and functional unit of individuals who are person elements of nursing practice situations
C. Identification of the usual or current components of self-care or dependent-care systems being produced by or for persons who are nurses' patients whenever this information is nursing relevant as a base for judging adequacy of care and approaches to change when change is required
D. a Establishment of the components of therapeutic self-care demands of persons under nursing care necessary for continuing regulation of their functioning and development, keeping the components in conformity with (1) changes in the number and kinds of self-care requisites and changes in the values at which each should be met, and (2) factors that condition the means that can be validly and reliably used to meet self-care requisites; and
D. b Establishment of the resources needed to meet the components of patients' therapeutic self-care demands
E. Establishment of the degree to which persons' who as nurses' patients (1) can responsibly exercise their developed and operational self-care capabilities without harm to self; and (2) continue to develop, improve, or increase their self-care capabilities. Degree would be established in relation to components of the therapeutic self-care demand and the frequency of meeting components.
F. Establishment of the design(s) for the production of a system(s) of nursing with definitions of and differentiation of nurse roles, patient roles, and roles of

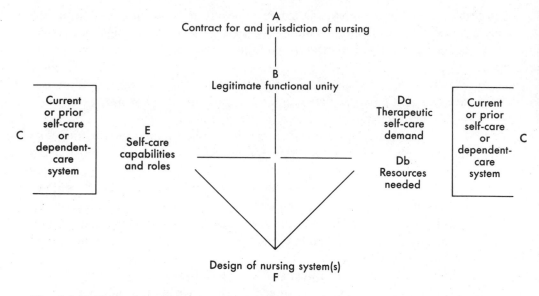

Fig. 5-1 Design units, nursing practice situations.

participating others with specification of methods of assistance to be used, the nursing results to be sought, and factors the presence of which would indicate the need for change in the design of the nursing system or a transfer from a nursing system to a self-care or a dependent-care system. Roles are expressed in terms of actions to be performed in order to know and meet patients' therapeutic self-care demands and to protect or to regulate the exercise or development of self-care capabilities or dependent-care capabilities.

Through the work of development of the six design units nurses establish the patterns and boundaries and specifications within which they proceed through nursing to overcome or compensate for the action limitations of their patients for knowing and meeting their therapeutic self-care demands and for protecting and regulating patients' exercise or development of their capabilities to engage in self-care within the framework of their self-management capabilities.

Design units serve different purposes. Design unit A sets limits on what nurses do; for example, nursing's area of jurisdiction in a health care situation may range from nurses providing help in knowing and meeting certain identified components of a person's therapeutic self-care demand to nurses' continuous care of persons in comatose states. Design unit B describes the person elements of the operational unit involved in the provision of nursing. Design unit C provides information about the qualitative and quantitative features of current or past self-care or dependent-care systems as one basis of measuring adequacy and determining the need for and possibilities for bringing about change. Design unit D develops the characteristics of and the details for the work of meeting the self-care requisites of patients and the resources needed. Design unit E sets limits for what patients can and probably should do in knowing and meeting their own therapeutic self-care demands and in their regulation of the exercise or development of self-care capabilities. Design unit F provides the pattern for the production of a system of nursing through establishment of role responsibilities and relationships.

As previously indicated, the development of design units proceeds along with the production of help and care. Nursing design units with their elements enable nurses to seek understanding of their need, not only for conceptualizations of elements but also for images of the details, features, and relationships of all the elements that give form and pattern to the work of nursing. Nurses who accept the foregoing suggestions about the function of nursing design must work through the fit of this function into their already formulated conceptualizations of nursing process. Nursing students who learn how to develop nursing design units and also learn the process operations of nursing practice (investigative and diagnostic, prescriptive, and productive) will be less confused and will understand how design units relate to nursing process.

To the degree that values of their elements remain stable, design units provide the standards and rules nurses need to meet and follow to overcome or compensate for self-care limitations of patients in knowing and meeting their own therapeutic self-care demands and in regulating the exercise or development of their self-care capabilities (or dependent-care capabilities). The process operations of nursing are considered in Chapter 9.

ELEMENTS OF DESIGN UNITS

Nursing design in the concreteness of nursing practice situations has its foundation in the contract or the agreement between parties to provide and receive nursing. The first suggested unit of design is concerned with laying out of nursing's area of jurisdiction within the context of the health care and the family or broader social situation of persons seeking nursing. The parts of this and other design units are presented in outline form. The parts of units are expressed as types of information required and the kinds of judgments to be made and statements about how nurses use the resulting information and judgments.

Design unit A: contract for and jurisdiction of nursing

The development of design unit A establishes for nurses who is to be nursed and the person's position(s) in the structure of a family or a residence group and in the health care system, the names of the contracting parties, general framework for cooperation and coordination of action and functions of communication, and the fit of nursing into the broader systems of health care of persons seeking nursing. It ensures the legality of the nursing situation. If nurses are to have this kind of a foundational framework for their nursing endeavors, the following elements of investigation and judgment are suggested.

A.1   Persons(s) to be nursed by name, age, and gender, position in family, residence; single or married, if single, name and residence of next of kin, if married, name and residence of spouse

A.2   Reasons for seeking nursing at this time

A.3   Prior care givers: self, dependent-care agent, nurse

A.4   Time of request for nursing

A.5a Projected character of requirements for nursing in terms of extent and whether periodic or continuous

A.5b Projected time duration of requirements for nursing

A.6   Location(s) for receiving nursing

A.7   Parties to the agreement or contract for nursing
   a. Adult person(s) who require nursing or next of kin or spouse by name; or adult legally responsible for a dependent person, adult or child, who requires nursing by name
   b. Health care agency by name or nurse in private or group practice of nursing by name(s)

A.8   Position in the health care system
   Under active medical care from physician(s) by name
   Under medical supervision from physician(s) by name
   Under care of other health professionals by name and field

A.9   Reason(s) for being in the health care system

A.10 Health care goals being sought; nursing's fit as contributory to goal achievement

A.11 Impact of reasons for person(s) being in the health care system on their families or friends; obvious requirement for concern for, attention to, or provision of guidance and counseling for families and friends

A.12 Establishment of the authority and responsibility of nurses in accord with nursing's area of jurisdiction

A.13 Number and qualifications of nurses needed and the kinds of resources required

A.14 Method of financing nursing

   Design unit A requires for its development information generally obtained when persons are admitted to residence health care agencies or institutions or placed on patient rosters of home health care agencies or clinics. However, nurses must obtain some information from patients, their relatives, or from their physicians. The elements of design unit A established in each concrete situation of nursing practice must be held in mind by nurses throughout the nursing period.

Design unit B: a legitimate and functional unity

Identifying the persons and the relationship among them with respect to their functioning in the nursing practice situation is done initially and thereafter as frequently as necessary. This design unit establishes the persons to be associated with one another; establishes general requirements for communication, coordination of action, and cooperation; fosters persons acting with an operative, dynamic sense of duty; and establishes the characterizing developmental and functional features of the person(s) to be nursed. It ensures the nursing legitimacy of the situation of nursing practice. The following are the suggested elements established and ordered to one another.

B.1a Capabilities of persons who are nurses' patients for self-management in a customary or a changed environment

B.1b Self-management limitations associated with age and developmental stage, health state factors, health care system factors, environmental features

B.2a Degree to which persons who are nurses' patients have been providing their own self-care, degree to which assistance with self-care has been provided and by whom, or have been provided care within a dependent care system

B.2b Existent limitation for engagement in self-care by type of self-care operation — estimative, decision making, productive

B.3 Projections about probable emergence of types of self-care limitations or worsening of existent ones or overcoming existent ones

B.4 Degree to which members of families or friends will be involved with the nurses' patients and their needs for association and communication with nurses

B.5 Existent and required capabilities and areas of nursing responsibility of nurses who are operational participants in the nursing situation during specified time periods with specification of areas of independence and interdependence and modes of communication

B.6 Need for nursing consultation

B.7 Interpersonal features of the nursing situations according to the general characteristics of the agreement or contract for nursing with general role specifications

B.8 Modes of communication and documentation relative to the kinds of events that demand immediate communication, for example, patient to nurse, nurse to patient, nurse to nurse, patient and nurse to physician, patient to family, nurse to family, family to nurse

B.9 Communication channels for nurses' patients who need assistance with respect to personal affairs and interests outside the domain of nursing

B.10 Modes for fostering an active, operative, dynamic sense of duty in all participants

Design unit B identifies the operational participants in the nursing situation, recognizes areas of independence and interdependence of functioning, designates modes and channels of communication, and identifies general areas of responsibility of participants.

Design unit C: self-care or dependent-care system components

Given nursing's area of jurisdiction in a health care situation, it may be necessary initially or at other times to know the components of patients' self-care or dependent-care systems. This information is necessary if nurses must know the adequacy of some or all components or if new components must be introduced.

C.1 Establish what the patient or dependent-care agents customarily do (care practices engaged in) to meet universal self-care requisites and the frequency of use of named care practices

C.2 Establish the developmental self-care requisites that are understood and the care measures used to meet them

C.3 Know obstacles that interfere with the methods of care that are regularly used to meet universal and developmental self-care requisites

C.4 Establish the presence or absence of types of care system components to meet health deviations self-care requisites, including what the patient experiences and discernible effects and results of particular components

C.5 Establish how self-care or dependent-care system components articulate with patients' and dependent-care agents' patterns of daily living

Design unit C is formed through recounting by a patient or dependent-care agent of what is being or has been done to meet patients' self-care requisites with some degree of stability or what has been recently introduced. Nurses also observe what patients and dependent-care agents do.

Design unit D: therapeutic self-care demand

Design unit D establishes the amount and kind of action that is essential-to-desirable to control factors (keep them within norms compatible with human life, health, development, and well-being) that contribute to the regulation of human functioning and development. For example, meeting the universal self-care requisite "maintain a sufficient intake of food" provides for an intake of food (the factor being controlled) that is in accord with established norms for quality and quantity of food required according to (1) age and developmental stage and state of an individual; (2) conditions and circumstances under which the person lives, for example, an active or sedentary life, hot or cold climates; and (3) health states characterized by certain disorders.

Design unit D is developed through investigation, data analysis, synthesis of data, and judgments about qualitative and quantitative values at which self-care requisites should be met, along with specifications about frequency and timing. Values of requisites are particularized for individuals, means are selected for meeting requisites, and work of meeting each particularized self-care requisite is outlined in the form of sets of care measures to be performed and resources required.

Details about self-care, self-care requisites, and therapeutic self-care demands are given in Chapter 6. Here only elements of the design unit are set forth.

D.1a   Establish from authoritative sources values at which each universal self-care requisite should be met for individuals of the patients' age and gender, developmental stage and state, and environmental conditions under which persons live.

Know the values at which universal self-care requisites have been or are being met for the patient.

Know existent or predicted conditions and circumstances that indicate need for change from recommended norms or from values at which universal requisites have been or are being met.

Calculate the qualitative and quantitative values at which each universal self-care requisite should be met.

D.1b   Establish from authoritative sources and from experiential knowledge valid and reliable means for meeting each requisite, for example, means for food intake for a three month old infant with a cleft palate.

Know existent conditions and circumstances that interfere with use of the usual valid and reliable means for meeting each requisite, for example, the inability of a patient to swallow as related to maintaining an adequate intake of food.

Know conditions internal to patients as well as external conditions and circumstances that constitute obstacles to or interferences with meeting each requisite, the nature of the interference, tested ways for surmounting the interference; and estimating if, how, and to what degree the effects of the obstacle can be controlled, for example, the effects of emphysema on maintaining an adequate intake of air.

Establish for each universal self-care requisite the means that will be used to meet each universal self-care requisite at values particularized for patients and establish the sets of care measures, which, if effectively performed, should attain these goals of meeting each requisite.

Identify for each universal self-care requisite the resources needed to meet each requisite using the selected means, identifying resources in relation to each set of care measures.

D.2   Establish the developmental type of self-care requisites that nurses' patients have been or are meeting.

Know developments that are in process in patients and the environmental conditions that will promote physical, psychological, cognitive, and social developments; know developments that should be brought about because of existent or emerging conditions and circumstances, for example, need for rehabilitation of the self-concept because of the presence of disabling conditions.

Know existent conditions and circumstances that interfere with or are obstacles to development, and the degree to which they are controllable through use of valid and reliable means.

Identify developmental self-care requisites associated with patients' age and gender, stage of development, and health state; establish the environmental conditions and other means through which they can be met and the resources required.

D.3   Establish the health deviation type self-care requisite associated with patients' states of health and their system of medical care that patients have been or are meeting.

Identify specific features of the health states of patients and the diagnostic and treatment modalities used in their medical care with knowledge as to how they are being experienced by patients and the impact on patients. Express existent and emerging health deviation self-care requisites, including the qualitative and quantitative values at which they should be met, including changes in values of universal self-care requisites.

Identify the sets of care measures to be performed given particular health-deviation self-care requisites, selected means for meeting them, and the resources required.

D.4   Establish the order that should exist between and among the sets of care measures through which universal, developmental, and health-deviations self-care requisites are to be met.

Structure sets of care measures in relation to time and place of performance, energy demands of performance, economy of use of resources, and other factors such as duration of time required for performance.

Identify essentiality and contributions of sets of care measures to the continuing regulation of patients' functioning and development.

Design unit D, the calculation of patients' therapeutic self-care demands establishes one of the patient properties identified in the self-care deficit theory of nursing. It specifies the self-care to be produced by or for patients.

Design unit E: patients' self-care roles

The outcome of design unit E is the establishment of what patients' can do, should do, or should not do in the interest of their own health and well-being while under nursing care to meet specific particularized self-care requisites, to protect their power of self-care agency, and to continue to develop capabilities to know and meet their own therapeutic self-care demands.

E.1   Know the components of patients' therapeutic self-care demands that they (a) have been or are meeting and can continue to meet without assistance and (b) have been or are meeting and can continue to meet with guidance and support.

Know emerging internal or external conditions and factors that will interfere with one or both of the foregoing and their probable time of occurrence.

E.2   Know the components of patients' therapeutic self-care demands that they cannot or should not meet (for reasons of health and well-being) at this time and for some projected time duration.

E.3   Know the changes that patients should make in their customary systems of self-care with respect to identified and evaluated components in order to bring them in accord with their current, calculated therapeutic self-care demands, including the fit of new or changed self-care components into their patterns of daily living.

E.4   Know the new or adjusted self-care operations (estimative, critical judgment and decision making, and production) that patients or their dependent-care agents must learn to perform and the facilitating powers to be developed if required changes in self-care or dependent-care systems are to be brought about.

E.5   Know patients' or dependent-care agents' capacities for learning and for making required adjustments.

E.6   Know the psychological and physiologic limitations of dependent-care agents.

Design unit E furthers the establishment of the goals to be sought for and by patients and establishes the foundations for design unit F.

Design unit F: design of the nursing system(s)

This unit involves nurses in the creation of designs for unifying nurse action, patient action, and action of participating others to achieve results and goals experienced in terms of (a) knowing and meeting patients' therapeutic self-care demands continuously in time, (b) protecting developed and developing powers of patients to manage themselves and to engage in self-care, and (c) regulating patients' exercise or development of self-care capabilities. The following elements of design are identified.

F.1   Initial and continuing establishment by nurses of their roles in the immediate and subsequent meeting of the therapeutic self-care demands of patients and their use of methods of assistance that conform to patients' self-management capabilities, their stages of development, their levels of available energy, their needs for safety and protection, their overt limitations for engagement in self-care, and their fears and concerns.

Provide for communication of information about and coordination of role responsibilities of nurses who contribute to the immediate achievement of nursing results during the twenty-four hours of the day or whenever one nurse is replaced by another.

F.2   Nurses' initial and continuing establishment and adjustment of patient roles and roles of participating others in meeting of patients' therapeutic self-care demands in accord with patients' developed and developing and operational capabilities for engagement in self-care, the exercise of which is unrestricted by health state or health-care system factors.

F.3   Nurses' and patients' or participating others' designation of areas of functioning requiring coordination of action and cooperation and use of designated methods of communication if the productive work of meeting patients' therapeutic self-care demands is to be accomplished effectively and economically.

F.4   Nurses' and patients' or participating others' initial and continuing establishment of their respective role functions in protecting the self-management and self-care capabilities of patients and in regulating the exercise or development of patients' self-care capabilities.

F.5   Nurses' continuing establishment of their own professional responsibility for conduct of the provision of nursing with recognition of interdependence of patients and participating others, as well as the independence of each as a legitimate participant in the nursing situation.

F.6   Establish conditions that should foster effective functioning and bring about the order and the dynamic sense of duty on part of all—nurses, patients, participating others.

Design unit F sets the specifications for who will do what toward achievement of nursing goals.

VARIATIONS IN NURSING SYSTEMS DESIGN

Variance in nursing system design is described first in relation to nursing's area of jurisdiction in health care situations where nursing is being sought or provided. Then variance is related to role responsibility differences for nurses, patients, and participating others in nursing practice situations.

Variance in areas of jurisdiction

Nurses' governing or leadership role in nursing practice situations is determined by nursing's area of jurisdiction in specific health care situations. This role is established by the contract or agreement to provide nursing and to be nursed. This formalizes the reason for seeking nursing and defines the authority of and the responsibilities to be fulfilled by nurses. If an agreement is unfulfilled or improperly fulfilled through failure of health care agencies to ensure the presence of nurses who know what nursing is needed, who design systems to ensure the production of nursing, and who produce it, then agencies may be suspected of contract nonfulfillment. If nurses in situations do not exercise their nursing authority and fulfill their nursing responsibilities they are suspected of malpractice.

Areas of nursing jurisdiction should be expressed in terms of nursing with designation of the following:

• Total to limited responsibility of nurses for the safety and protection of nurses' patients according to their stable or changing self-management capabilities and their self-care limitations in their situations of daily living;

• Total to limited responsibility for continuous knowing and meeting of patients' therapeutic self-care demands by overcoming or compensating for patients' self-care limitations;

- Areas of responsibility for assisting nurses' patients to protect their developed self-care capabilities and their self-management capabilities;
- Areas of responsibility to assist patients to regulate (1) exercise of developed and operational capabilities to engage in self-care and (2) development of new capabilities for self-care or making adjustments in existent ones;
- Areas of responsibility for the design of dependent-care systems and the development of dependent-care agents.

Design units A and B are concerned with identifying and laying out the details of nursing's area of jurisdiction and the governing role of nurses in defining and attaining nursing goals within nursing's area of jurisdiction in health care situations.

Establishing nursing's area of jurisdiction sets forth nursing's situational boundaries and should identify points and areas of articulation with medical and other health care systems, as well as self-care and dependent-care systems, that are operational and will continue to be operational as patients are nursed. It also establishes the matters to be communicated and lines of communication.

Role variance

As identified in the preceding section, the extent of the governing or leadership role of nurses in practice situations is defined by nursing's area of jurisdiction in health care situations. The governing role of nurses extends to all facets of developing nursing situations. It includes the design function as developed in preceding sections. It includes continuous efforts to bring about and maintain association, integration, and interaction among participants in the nursing situation. The governing role also extends to ensuring production of nursing and attainment of nursing goals for patients. The governing role of nurses includes the actual production of continuous nursing whenever the health states of patients are in continuous flux, the therapeutic self-care demand is complex and in continuous change, and the life or integrity of patients is in jeopardy.

Nurses' decisions within the design function about their own roles in the continuing production of systems of nursing are made in relation to decisions about patient roles and roles of participating others in their designs for nursing systems. Nursing system design (design unit F) involves the making of judgments and decisions about methods of helping that are valid in relation to patients' limitations for engaging in self-care and reasons for or causes of these limitations. Each method of helping described in Chapter 2 casts helpers and those helped into distinct roles. Self-care limitations of patients and their developed and operational self-care abilities provide one basis for nurses' decision about methods of helping that are valid for use in the situation and in so doing cast patients in specific roles in relation to the production of care that is needed by them.

Five general roles of adolescent or adult patients appropriate in the designs of systems of nursing are identified. Roles as expressed reflect the operations to be performed.

- No active role as observer or operator whenever there is absence of sensory consciousness in patients
- Active role as participant observer and contributor of nursing relevant information about self and environmental features
- Active role as a participant operator in meeting components of his or her existent or emerging therapeutic self-care demand
- Active role as a participant investigator in calculating components of his or her therapeutic self-care demand
- Passive to active role as learner in understanding self-care requisites and mastering use of specific means to meet them

These roles, except for the first, can be combined. For example, the second and fourth roles can be fulfilled by persons with limitations of movement. Roles two, three, four, and five may be combined according to capabilities of patients and the need for role performance at particular times throughout the period of nursing.

When nurses' patients are infants or children, they should first be considered in terms of their needs to be taken care of and to be cared for in their uniqueness as individuals. Infants and children should be accepted as experiencing, as seeking to know what is around them, and as able to tolerate certain approaches to them but not others. Infants and children should be considered as active participants and be helped to participate in accord with their developmental states in systems of nursing designed for them.

The number of nurses brought into the design of nursing systems in addition to nurses with the governing and leadership role should vary according to (1) the degree of complexity and stability of patients' therapeutic self-care demands; (2) the stability of health states of patients with resultant effects on their therapeutic self-care demands and their self-management and self-care capabilities and limitations; (3) the essential contribution of nursing to the health and well-being of persons to be nursed. Nurses with vocational or broad, technical-type preparation for nursing are valuable in stable nursing situations. Nurses with deep technical-type preparation and experience are valuable in the production of nursing where intricate technologies are needed to meet self-care requisites of patients. The relationship of these nurses to nurses in the governing or leadership role must be well developed and maintained, and their contributions to the production of nursing for patients over time should be well defined. In some settings, vocationally trained attendants or aids provide care. In settings where attendants and aids are used, nurses may or may not fill governing or leadership roles. In situations where there are no nurses, attendant service, not nursing, takes place.

Other participants in nursing practice situations whose roles should be identified in nursing system designs include members of patients' families or friends who contribute to meeting selected components of patients' therapeutic self-care demands whenever their roles are consistent over time. Also members of families or friends of patients may fill the "sitter" role. Sitters stay with patients to ensure their protection if they are not capable of self-management in their environments, secure nursing help for them as needed, and assure patients that they are not alone.

VALIDITY OF NURSING SYSTEMS DESIGNS

Nursing systems designs are valid whenever the design for what is to be produced conforms with what is and what should be. Validity demands the identification of what is to be produced, the goals to be attained through its production, and the numbers and qualifications of persons by time periods who can produce the designed nursing system. Validity also demands that any designed system meet criteria for effectiveness and economy of time and resources. Specialists in nursing system design (1) know in detail the self-care capabilities and limitations and the therapeutic self-care demands of persons with special health and developmental problems and (2) have participated in developing effective systems for producing nursing that attain nursing goals and results.

Designs for nursing systems are valid only for that period during which elements of design units A, B, D, and E maintain the values initially used by nurses in governing and leadership roles to create the design of a nursing system(s) for particular patients. The initial product of design unit F may be for a series of nursing systems designs to be followed sequentially whenever nurses can predict changes in elements of design units A, B, D, and E in some time frame.

ARTICULATIONS OF NURSING SYSTEMS

Known predictable areas of articulations of nursing systems with other systems of care must be incorporated into designs for them. Sometimes this can be accomplished before the actual production of care; at other times, articulations must be designed during production. If there are self-care or dependent-care systems in operation at the time nursing is to be provided, nurses must make judgments and decide which is to be viewed as the major system and which is to be considered the subsystem of care. For example, if a person living at home has help from nurses relative to designated components of a therapeutic self-care demand, the meeting of which are beyond the person's functional competencies, then it is realistic to consider the major system to be the person's ongoing self-care system. The same consideration would hold when nurses contribute a subsystem of nursing to an ongoing dependent-care system for adults or children. On the other hand, nursing is the major system when patients or participating others have defined but limited roles in the production of continuous care of the patient.

Designing and developing articulation of subsystems of action with main systems of action demand timing of performance of care measures with the same goal orientations by persons in different roles. They also demand current information about the effects of performance of care activities to attain one set of goals on care activities directed to attain another set of goals. For example, a person in his home may be responsible for all aspects of self-care, including those related to continuous control of a condition of diabetes mellitus and impaired cardiac functioning with help from nurses whose area of jurisdiction is defined in terms of meeting self-care requisites associated with or arising from a leg ulcer and vascular surgery on the same lower extremity. The nurse within this area of jurisdiction must not only know the components of the person's self-care system as related to diabetes and cardiac functioning but also obtain information to judge adequacy of control. The nurse within this defined area of nursing jurisdiction must coordinate nursing efforts with those of the patients' vascular surgeon. However, the nurse's responsibility also extends to advising and counseling the patient about other self-care requisites that are inadequately met. This may include advising him to contact his internist or cardiologist.

Nursing systems design can become very complex and require frequent redesign. Nurses must develop habits of mental imagery, allowing them to see whole systems of nursing in terms of parts, function of parts, and articulations among them. Timing and designing articulations with other health services is of great importance when nurses' patients are undergoing extensive medical diagnosis or specialized therapies that place them in contact with a variety of health care workers and often require them to move from one place to another. Under these conditions, control of fatigue and special protection from hazards should be built into the patients' therapeutic self-care demands.

REFERENCES

1. Webster's dictionary of synonyms, ed 1, Springfield, Mass, 1951, GB Merriman Publishers, p. 622.
2. Simon HA: Sciences of the artificial, Cambridge, 1969, MIT Press.
3. Weiss P: You, I and the others, Carbondale and Edwardsville, Ill, 1980, Southern Illinois University Press, p. 50.

SELECTED READINGS

Backscheider JE: Self-care requirements, self-care capabilities and nursing systems in the diabetic nurse management clinic, Am J Public Health, 64:1138-1146, 1974.
Garrett AP: A nursing system design for a patient with myocardial infarction. In Riehl-Sisca J, editor: The science and art of self-care, Norwalk, 1985, Appleton-Century-Crofts, pp. 142-160.
Merton RK: On theoretical sociology, New York, 1963, Macmillan Co., pp. 39-45.
Nursing Development Conference Group: A general concept of nursing system. In Orem DE editor: Concept formalization in nursing: process and product, Boston, 1979, Little, Brown and Co., pp. 105-127.
Sorokin P: Familistic, contractual, and compulsory relationships and systems of interaction (groups). In Social and cultural dynamics, revised and abridged in one volume, Boston, 1957, Porter Sargent Publisher, pp. 436-452.

CHAPTER 6

Self-care, self-care requisites, therapeutic self-care demand

Self-care is action of mature and maturing persons who have developed the capabilities to take care of themselves in their environmental situations. Persons who engage in self-care have the requisite action capabilities — the agency or power to act deliberately to regulate factors that affect their own functioning and development.

SELF-CARE

In the term *self-care*, the word *self* is used in the sense of one's *whole being*. Self-care carries the dual connotation of "for oneself" and "given by oneself." The provider of self-care is referred to as a *self-care agent*. The provider of infant care, child care, or dependent adult care is referred to by the general term *dependent-care agent*. The term *agent* is used in the sense of *the person taking action*. **Self-care** is the practice of activities that individuals initiate and perform on their own behalf in maintaining life, health, and well-being. Normally, adults voluntarily care for themselves. Infants, children, the aged, the ill, and the disabled require complete care or assistance with self-care activities. Fig. 6-1 illustrates the concept of self-care and dependent-care agents.

Infants and children require care from others because they are in the early stages of development physically, psychologically, and psychosocially. The aged person requires total care or assistance whenever declining physical and mental abilities limit the selection or performance of self-care actions. The ill or disabled person requires partial or total care from others (or assistance in the form of teaching or guidance) depending on his or her health state and immediate or future requirements for self-care. Self-care is an adult's continuous contribution to his or her own continued existence, health, and well-being. Care of others is an adult's contribution to the health and well-being of dependent members of the adult's social group.

Self-care has purpose. It is action that has pattern and sequence and, when performed effectively, contributes in specific ways to human structural integrity, human functioning, and human development.

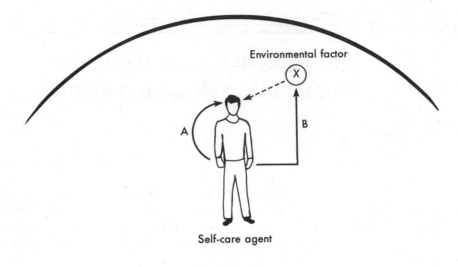

Environmental factor

Self-care agent

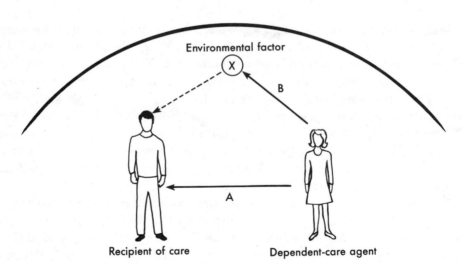

Environmental factor

Recipient of care   Dependent-care agent

Fig. 6-1 Self-care and dependent-care agents (A, care directed to self or to another who is the recipient of care; B, care directed to the regulation of environmental factors; X, environmental factor).

Formalization of the concept self-care

I expressed my formulated insight that maturing and mature individuals do take care of themselves on a day-to-day basis and that they are subject to health associated limitations for doing this in my 1965 descriptive definition of nursing, in my formalization of nursing's proper object, and in the definition of self-care that appears in the first paragraph of the preceding section. Through my efforts and those of the Nursing Development Conference Group the concept self-care was formalized in 1969.

The work of formalization is described in the first and second editions of *Concept formalization in nursing: process and product*. This work included investigation of the working definition of self-care to determine if the concept was useful in handling data from concrete nursing practice situations. Early stages of the process of formalization involved formulation, expression, and acceptance of a set of initial premises and three sets of propositions, generalizations about self-care.

Initial premises and propositions

Because self-care occupies a pivotal position in the self-care deficit theory of nursing, premises and propositions about self-care, as they appear in the first and second editions of *Concept formalization in nursing: process and product*, are reproduced with minor revisions.

Premises

In 1965, I developed two premises about self-care, which the Nursing Development Conference Group revised and accepted in 1969 (p.132).[1]

1. Self-care is conduct. It is ego-processed. It is learned activity, learned through interpersonal relations and communications.
2. Adult persons have the right and responsibility to care for themselves to maintain rational life and health; they may have such responsibility for other persons.
   a. Infant and child care, care of the aged, and care of adolescents include the giving, assisting with, or supervising the self-care of another.
   b. Social assistance will be needed by adult persons whenever they are unable to obtain needed resources and maintain conditions necessary for the preservation of life and promotion of health for themselves or for their dependents; such assistance may be needed for the accomplishment or the supervision of self-care.

The identification of self-care as conduct "reflects the essence of the concept: self-care is behavior, it exists in reality situations," p. 134.

Propositions

The propositions I developed in 1965, which were studied, revised, added to, and accepted by the Nursing Development Conference Group in 1967, are organized in three sets (p. 133).[1]

SOME PROPOSITIONS ABOUT SELF-CARE

Set One — Conditioning Factors
1. Self-care conduct is affected by self-concept and by the level of maturity of the individual.
2. Self-care conduct is affected by culturally derived goals and practices.

3. Self-care conduct is affected by the scientifically derived health knowledge possessed by a person.
4. Self-care conduct is affected by placement in the family constellation.
5. Self-care conduct is affected by membership in social groups exclusive of the family, for example, friendship and work groups.
6. Adults may or may not choose to engage themselves in specific self-care actions.
7. Lack of scientifically derived knowledge about self-care, disorders of health and malfunctioning, lack of self-care skills, and inadequate habits of self-care limit what a person can do with respect to his own self-care or in assisting another person in such matters.

Set Two — Self-Care in Health and Disease

1. Self-care contributes to and is necessary for a person's integrity as a psychophysiologic organism with a rational life.
2. Each person must perform or have performed for him each day a minimum of activities directed to, or performed for the sake of, himself in order to continue his existence as an organism with a rational life. If health is to be maintained and improved, he must perform additional activities. In the event of disease, injury, or mental or physical malfunctioning he must perform other activities to sustain life or improve health.
3. Self-care directed to the maintenance and promotion of health requires a scientifically derived fund of knowledge about self-care goals and practices as well as related skills and habits.
4. Disease, injury, and mental or physical malfunctioning may limit what a person can do for himself, since such states may limit his ability to reason, to make decisions, and to engage in activity to accomplish self-care goals. Disease, injury, and mal- functionings may involve structural changes as well as functional changes, which may necessitate the use of specialized self-care measures, some of which may be medically prescribed.

Set Three — Behavioral and Resource Demands of Self-Care

1. Self-care requires general knowledge of self-care goals and practices as well as specific knowledge about self, including health state, and about the physical and social environment. It also requires internalization of insights and sanctions and motivation. Acquiring specific knowledge involves making observations and judgments and leads to understanding of present self-care requirements as well as the self-care deficit; it may require contact and interactions with workers in the health services.
2. Self-care includes seeking and participating in medical care prescribed by the physician in the event of deviations or departures from health, and periodic scientific evaluations of health states.
3. Self-care requires internally oriented activities directed to the control of behavior; self-care also requires externally oriented behavior directed to the control of the environment, to establishing contact and communication with others, and to the securing and utilization of resources.
4. Self-care requires the use of resources that may include living in a healthful or a therapeutic physical and social environment; consumption of water, food, and drugs;

application of physical agents and drugs to external surfaces and to those internal surfaces that communicate with the exterior; introduction of drugs into the body tissues to supply substances that the body is not producing; use of artificial devices to control the position of the body or its parts, or to aid in movement; use of prosthetic devices to facilitate functioning . . . pp. 133-134.

This early work with respect to self-care led to the continued development of the substantive structure of the concept and to the formulation expression of the theory of self-care discussed in Chapter 3.

Self-care requisites are formulated and expressed insights about actions that are known to be necessary or hypothesized to have validity in the regulation of aspects of human functioning and development. Formulated self-care requisites name two elements. One element is the factor to be controlled or in some way managed to keep aspects of individuals' human functioning and development within norms compatible with life, health, and personal well-being. The second element is a specification of the nature of the action to be performed. The two types of elements are readily identified in this self-care requisite: Maintain food intake at a quality and quantity sufficient to keep human functioning and human development within norms compatible with life, health, and personal well-being in relation to existent human and environmental conditions and circumstances.

Self-care requisites thus are understood as expressions of action to be performed by or for individuals in the interest of controlling human and environmental factors that affect human functioning and human development. Self-care requisites are expressions of purposes to be attained, results desired from deliberate engagement in self-care. They are the reasons for doing actions that constitute self-care.

SELF-CARE REQUISITES

Three types of self-care requisites are identified: universal, developmental, and health-deviation. They rest on the following assumptions:
- Human beings, by nature, have common needs for the intake of materials (air, water, foods) and for bringing about and maintaining living conditions that support life processes, the formation and maintenance of structural integrity, and the maintenance and promotion of functional integrity.
- Human development, from intrauterine life to adult maturation, requires the formation and maintenance of conditions that promote known developmental processes at each period of the life cycle.
- Genetic and constitutional defects and deviations from normal structural and functional integrity and well-being bring about requirements for (1) their prevention and (2) regulatory action to control their extension and to control and mitigate their effects.

Self-care requisites are generalizations about the purposes that individuals should have when they engage in self-care. Conceptualized self-care requisites that have been validated by their successful use in aiding individuals to manage their health and well-being become elements of the general culture or remain within the domains of the health care professions. Self-care requisites must be known before they can serve as the purposes of self-care. Universal self-care requisites should become known by all educable adults. Ideally, this also holds for developmental self-care requisites. For both types of requisites, however, reliable knowledge is not always effectively selected and adequately organized for public dissemination. Health-deviation self-care requisites usually become known by those who have genetic or constitutional defects or health deviations or whose family members or associates have such defects or health deviations.

When self-care requisites are viewed as formulated and expressed generalizations about the purposes of self-care, the ways and means through which these purposes can be attained is an important consideration in understanding self-care as human action. For example, an adult who is judged by herself and her physician to be edematous and in a state of fluid and electrolyte imbalance has, as one object of self-care, this prescribed health-deviation self-care requisite: to maintain fluid intake at no more than 1000 ml during each 24-hour period. This is an adjustment of the universal self-care requisite to maintain a sufficient intake of water. The actions to achieve this purpose must be known and be within the capabilities of the person with the self-care requisite (or another person who can act for the individual).

In addition to making judgments and decisions about the kinds of fluids to be ingested and the distribution of amounts over the 24 hours of the day, there are action sequences for procuring the fluids, preparing them as necessary for ingestion, measuring them into appropriate utensils, drinking them, and accounting for the fluids taken at particular times and for the entire 24-hour period. Throughout each 24-hour period there would be actions for self-restraint, self-orientation, and maintenance of awareness of the purpose of self-care. Acceptance of oneself as being in need of this kind of care (or at least willingness to attain the purpose of care) is also required.

The operations required to maintain fluid intake within a specified maximum may be thought of as a segment of a person's daily self-care. Since self-care directed to achieve a particular object is necessarily a series of actions performed in some sequence, self-care is properly referred to as an action system or a dynamic process. It is helpful for nurses and other care providers to conceptualize all self-care actions performed in sequence as constituting an individual's self-care system. Actions directed to meet particular, individual self-care requisites can be conceptualized as constituting subsystems of the total self-care system. The ways and means for meeting particular self-care requisites can be described in terms of (1) general method and (2) required operations or actions. In the example outlined in Table 6-1 the general method is drinking, the natural method used by human beings after infancy to

Table 6-1   Elements of an action system to meet a particularized self-care requisite

Particularized self-care requisite	General method	Sets of required operations
Maintain fluid intake at no more than 1000 ml every 24 h	Ingestion by mouth, drinking from a container	Seek and validate knowledge of the requisite, its meaning, its duration, and projected effects Prepare self, materials, and the environmental setting Consume measured fluids and account for the amounts consumed Monitor self for evidence of effects — desired or adverse Communicate results of monitoring to the prescribing physician

consume substances in a liquid state. The sets of operations in Table 6-1 identify the kinds of actions to be taken to achieve partial results toward accomplishing one particular self-care purpose, using a specified method.

Required operations vary with general method. If the general method selected for use in the example in Table 6-1 was injection of fluids into a vein (intravenous administration of fluids), the types of operations required would conform in a general way to the sets named in Table 6-1 but the specific actions would differ. When the general method and required operations for achieving a type or range of purposes have been identified, tested, and integrated into an explicit system of action, the result is a formulated process that becomes part of the technologic knowledge of particular practice disciplines, for example, the intravenous administration of fluids. Nurses develop capabilities to (1) identify the self-care requisites of their patients, (2) select or confirm the general methods through which each identified requisite can and will be met, and (3) identify the actions to be taken in meeting each specific self-care requisite. Nurses should also develop their powers to identify and conceptualize not only specific self-care requisites, but also the total demand for self-care action. The self-care actions to be performed for some duration in order to meet known self-care requisites by using valid methods and related sets of operations or actions is termed the *therapeutic self-care demand*. An individual's self-care demand cannot be known until it is calculated. One result of effective nursing in some nursing situations is that patients become able to calculate their own therapeutic self-care demands, even persons who, because of limited movement, may not be able to execute some of the actions within the demand.

A therapeutic self-care demand is a humanly constructed entity, with an objective basis in information that describes an individual structurally, functionally, and developmentally. It is based on the theory that self-care is a human regulatory function and in facts and theories from the human and environmental sciences. Formulating a therapeutic self-care demand requires investigating and understanding what self-care requisites exist and judging what can and what should be done to meet them. A therapeutic self-care demand is essentially a prescription for continuous self-care action through which identified self-care requisites can be met with stipulated degrees of effectiveness. Each person has requisites for self-care; to the degree that these are known and the ways for meeting them understood, individuals will experience demands for action to care for themselves (or dependent family members). Self-care is deliberate action that is practical in orientation. Performing a self-care measure involves making a choice. This is so even with routine practice such as those related to food selection or personal hygiene. Unless self-care activities have become habitual practices, there is a need for reflection about what should be done and how it will be done. Knowledge of human functioning, one's present condition and circumstances, and known care measures provide a basis for such reflection. Some techniques for care in health and in illness are a part of the general culture. Others become known to individuals and families because of specialized education or practical experience in using the techniques. There is often a lag between developed techniques and their use. Available resources may affect the use of self-care techniques. Interests and motives are also determining factors. Individuals and families may adapt themselves to chronic ill health rather than learn about therapeutic care measures.

Self-care and care of dependents may be well intentioned but not therapeutic. It is necessary to determine the therapeutic value of practices prescribed by the general culture and even by health professionals. A single self-care practice or a whole system of self-care is therapeutic to the degree that it actually contributes to the achievement of the following results: (1) support of life processes and promotion of normal functioning; (2) maintenance of normal growth, development, and maturation; (3) prevention, control, or cure of disease processes and injuries; (4) prevention of or compensation for disability; and (5) promotion of well-being. Some of these results are required by all persons on a continuing basis during all stages of the life cycle, but others are required only in the event of disease or injury.

Self-care is a practical response to an experienced demand to attend to oneself. The demands may originate in the individual, for example, a person experiencing a lack of energy or intense emotional reactions, or from knowledge that a care measure should be performed because it is health-promoting. Demands may originate from others, for example, the directives of parents to children or health workers to clients and patients or neighbors and friends. The demand as experienced is a stimulus to which the person responds in some manner. Demands may be met or ignored. Awareness of the demand may remain even when the demand has been ignored. A person may identify the presence of a tumor and know he or she should seek medical assistance, but does not and yet worries about having cancer. When persons know that what they are experiencing is significant to life or health, they feel a heavy responsibility toward themselves.

The self-care demands that all people experience and the demands experienced when there is illness, injury, or disability have two aspects: the purpose of requisite self-care and its nature. Self-care considered as a practical response requires answers to two questions: What is the nature of the demand? What will constitute a therapeutic response to the demand?

Self-care requisites are expressions of the kinds of purposive self-care that individuals require. They should be expressed in terms of action, for example, "maintain a sufficient intake of water." Three types of self-care requisites are identified and discussed here. Each type represents a category of deliberate actions to be taken by or for individuals because of their functional and developmental needs as human beings. Persons seeking understanding of self-care and self-care requisites will search for further descriptions and explanations.

- Universal self-care requisites are common to all human beings during all stages of the life cycle, adjusted to age, developmental state, and environmental and other factors. They are associated with life processes, with the maintenance of the integrity of human structure and functioning, and with general well-being.
- Developmental self-care requisites are associated with human developmental processes and with conditions and events occurring during various stages of the life cycle (e.g., prematurity, pregnancy) and events that can adversely affect development.
- Health-deviation self-care requisites are associated with genetic and constitutional defects and human structural and functional deviations and with their effects and with medical diagnostic and treatment measures.

When these three types of requisites are effectively met, they are productive of human and environmental conditions that (1) support life processes, (2) maintain human structures and human functioning within a normal range, (3) support development in accord with the human potential, (4) prevent injury and pathologic states, (5) contribute to the regulation or control of the effects of injury and pathology, (6) contribute to the cure or regulation of pathologic processes, and (7) promote general well-being. From the perspective of preventive health care, effectively meeting universal and developmental self-care requisites in healthy individuals is ideally in the nature of primary prevention of disease and ill health. Meeting health-deviation requisites may aid in the control of pathology in its early stages (secondary prevention) and in the prevention of defect and disability (tertiary prevention). Effectively meeting the universal and developmental self-care requisites is essential when there is pathology in order to maintain human structure and functioning and to promote development and thereby contribute to rehabilitation. Rehabilitation focuses on developmental self-care requisites associated with conditions resulting from pathology, medical diagnoses or treatment procedures, or the results of inadequate nursing or dependent care.

Universal self-care requisites

Eight self-care requisites common to all human beings are suggested.
1. The maintenance of a sufficient intake of air.
2. The maintenance of a sufficient intake of water.
3. The maintenance of a sufficient intake of food.*
4. The provision of care associated with elimination processes and excrements.
5. The maintenance of a balance between activity and rest.
6. The maintenance of a balance between solitude and social interaction.
7. The prevention of hazards to human life, human functioning, and human well-being.
8. The promotion of human functioning and development within social groups in accord with human potential, known human limitations, and the human desire to be normal. *Normalcy* is used in the sense of that which is essentially human and that which is in accord with the genetic and constitutional characteristics and talents of individuals.

These eight requisites represent the kinds of human actions that bring about the internal and external conditions that maintain human structure and functioning, which in turn support human development and maturation. When it is effectively provided, self-care or dependent care organized around universal self-care requisites fosters positive health and well-being. The box on page 127 presents general actions for meeting these eight requisites. The results of meeting each of them contribute in different ways to health and well-being.

The maintenance of sufficient intakes of air, water, and food provides individuals with the materials required for metabolism and energy production. The provision of effective care associated with elimination processes and excrements should ensure the integrity of these processes and their regulation, as well as effective control of the materials eliminated. The maintenance of a balance between activity and rest controls voluntary energy expenditure; regulates environmental stimuli; and provides variety, outlets for interests and talents, and the sense of well-being that comes from both. The maintenance of a balance between solitude and social interaction provides conditions essential for developmental processes in which knowledge is acquired, values and expectations are formed, and a measure of security and fulfillment is achieved. Solitude reduces the number of social stimuli and demands for social interaction and provides conditions conducive to reflection; social contacts provide opportunities for

---

* Constituents of foods that human beings need are referred to as nutrients. These include proteins and the amino acids of which they are composed, fats and fatty acids, carbohydrates, minerals, and vitamins. Water is also a constituent of many foods.

General sets of actions for meeting the eight universal self-care requisites

1. Maintenance of sufficient intakes of air, water, food
   a. Taking in that quantity required for normal functioning with adjustments for internal and external factors that can affect the requirement or, under conditions of scarcity, adjusting consumption to bring the most advantageous return to integrated functioning
   b. Preserving the integrity of associated anatomic structures and physiologic processes
   c. Enjoying the pleasurable experiences of breathing, drinking, and eating without abuses
2. Provision of care associated with eliminative processes and excrements
   a. Bringing about and maintaining internal and external conditions necessary for the regulation of eliminative processes
   b. Managing the processes of elimination (including protection of the structures and processes involved) and disposal of excrements
   c. Providing subsequent hygienic care of body surfaces and parts
   d. Caring for the environment as needed to maintain sanitary conditions
3. Maintenance of a balance between activity and rest
   a. Selecting activities that stimulate, engage, and keep in balance physical movement, affective responses, intellectual effort, and social interaction
   b. Recognizing and attending to manifestations of needs for rest and activity
   c. Using personal capabilities, interests, and values as well as culturally prescribed norms as bases for development of a rest-activity pattern
4. Maintenance of a balance between solitude and social interaction
   a. Maintaining that quality and balance necessary for the development of personal autonomy and enduring social relations that foster effective functioning of individuals
   b. Fostering bonds of affection, love, and friendship; effectively managing impulses to use others for selfish purposes, disregarding their individuality, integrity, and rights
   c. Providing conditions of social warmth and closeness essential for continuing development and adjustment
   d. Promoting both individual autonomy and group membership
5. Prevention of hazards to life, functioning, and well-being
   a. Being alert to types of hazards that are likely to occur
   b. Taking action to prevent events that may lead to the development of hazardous situations
   c. Removing or protecting oneself from hazardous situations when a hazard cannot be eliminated
   d. Controlling hazardous situations to eliminate danger to life or well-being
6. Promotion of normalcy
   a. Developing and maintaining a realistic self-concept
   b. Taking action to foster specific human developments
   c. Taking action to maintain and promote the integrity of one's human structure and functioning
   d. Identifying and attending to deviations from one's structural and functional norms

the interchange of ideas, acculturation and socialization, and the achievement of the human potential. Social interaction is also essential to obtain the material resources essential to life, growth, and development.

Prevention of hazards to life, functioning, and well-being contributes to the maintenance of human integrity and, therefore, to the effective promotion of human functioning and development. The promotion of human functioning and development (promotion of normalcy), in turn, prevents the development of conditions that constitute internal hazards to human life and to human functioning and development. It also promotes conditions that lead individuals to feeling and knowing their individuality and wholeness, to cognitional objectivity, and to freedom and responsibility as human beings.

One aspect of the development of areas of knowledge about the self-care requisites is the explication of relationships among them. For example, the requisites *prevention of hazards* and *promotion of normalcy* must be related to each of the other six requisites, as illustrated in Fig. 6-2, in relation to maintenance of a sufficient intake of air, water, and food. Care givers can inquire as to how requisites for prevention of hazards and promotion of normalcy articulate with the other six requisites by seeking answers to questions in the following series.

Three questions for investigation are suggested for the requisites maintenance of sufficient intakes of air, water, and food.

- What is a sufficient intake of air, water, and food under known or hypothesized internal and external conditions? For example, should water and food intake be adjusted under conditions of heat stress, and if so, how?
- What hazards, if any, may be associated with meeting each of these requisites for the intake of materials? How can identified hazards, such as the presence of

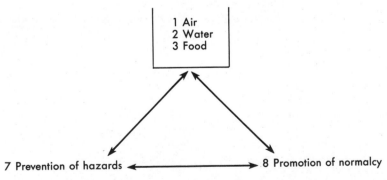

Maintenance of a sufficient intake of:

1 Air
2 Water
3 Food

7 Prevention of hazards   8 Promotion of normalcy

Fig. 6-2 Interrelations of some of the universal self-care requisites.

noxious substances in inspired air, water, or food and food intakes that are not sufficient, be eliminated or controlled?

- In meeting these three requisites for material intakes, can normal functioning and development be promoted, and if so, how (e.g., the institution and maintenance of patterns of food consumption based on a knowledge of the nutrients in consumed food, not just on habits and preferences)?

To be effective the provision of care associated with elimination processes and excrements requires answers to the following:

- What are the elimination patterns of individuals? Are current patterns congruent with former patterns?
- What care practices or care measures are associated with acts of elimination and the disposal of excrements?
- Do the identified elimination patterns or the care practices (or lack of them) in and of themselves constitute hazards?
- What hazards, if any, are associated with preparation for or engagement in elimination under the individual's internal and external conditions?
- What constitutes the norm for elimination for an individual? If elimination patterns are presently outside the norm, how can normal functioning be brought about?
- What care practices related to acts of elimination and disposal of excrements would benefit individuals and the social group?

The provider of care in relation to maintaining a balance between activity and rest and a balance between solitude and social interaction would need to answer the following questions:

- What constitutes a balance between rest and activity and between solitude and social interaction under prevailing internal and external conditions?
- What kinds and degrees of rest and activity or solitude and social interaction constitute a hazard under existing conditions?
- What kinds and degrees of rest and activity or solitude and social interaction can be expected to maintain human structure and promote human functioning and development in relation to the human potential and its limits and at the same time be in compliance with the interests, desires, and talents of the individual?

Care givers would need to answer the following questions with respect to the association between prevention of hazards and promotion of normal human functioning and development:

- What hazards to human life, functioning, and development exist in the individual's environment?
- What will happen to an individual if a hazard is not eliminated or controlled?
- What patterns of action should individuals develop and exercise in order to become aware of or prevent or control hazards?

- What individual interests, values, and actions with respect to known hazards are causing conditions that impair human structure and functioning or are obstacles to normal human functioning and development?

Four questions may guide inquiry about requisites for maintenance of normalcy.

- What internal or external factors are suggestive of or positive indicators of specific requisites for the promotion of normalcy with respect to (1) individualization and personalization and (2) human functioning described psychologically, cognitively, or biologically?
- Can these requisites be phrased in a way that can be understood and serve as a guide in the selection of care measures?
- What courses of action would be effective and possible under existent or predicted conditions?
- Are individuals involved in regimens to attain some personalized or group goals that are hazardous to personal well-being, health, or life?

Meeting the universal self-care requisites through self-care or dependent care is an integral part of the daily living of individuals and their social groups, but it tends to become separated from the fabric of human life when certain conditions predominate. These conditions include (1) contamination of air, water, and food with noxious materials; (2) scarcity of food and water; (3) conditions that adversely affect the work, recreational, educational, and religious activities and the daily living patterns of human groups; and (4) illness, defects, specific pathology, and disability of social group members. Under such conditions individuals as well as the social group as a whole will focus attention on these self-care requisites and may act to bring about conditions under which they can be effectively met.

Each of the eight universal self-care requisites from either a qualitative (kind) or a quantitative (amount) perspective or both becomes differentiated for individuals or groups in relation to differences in age, gender, developmental state, health state, sociocultural orientation, and resources. The varieties of practice within social groups and the range of practices used by individuals reflect not only long-term adjustment to environmental conditions but also the kind and amount of knowledge that has been acquired, is transmitted, and is put to use with respect to these universal requisites for care.

Developmental self-care requisites

Initially these requisites were subsumed under the universal self-care requirements. They have since been separated out to emphasize their importance and because of their number and diversity. Developmental self-care requisites are either specialized expressions of universal self-care requisites that have been particularized for developmental processes or they are new requisites derived from a condition (e.g., pregnancy) or associated with an event (e.g., loss of a spouse or parent).

There are two types of developmental self-care requisites; type 2 has two subtypes.

1. Bringing about and maintaining conditions that support life processes and promote the processes of development, that is, human progress toward higher levels of the organization of human structures and toward maturation during:
   a. The intrauterine stages of life and the process of birth
   b. The neonatal stage of life when (1) born at term or prematurely and (2) born with normal birth weight or low birth weight
   c. Infancy
   d. The developmental stages of childhood, including adolescence and entry into adulthood
   e. The developmental stages of adulthood
   f. Pregnancy in either childhood or adulthood
2. Provision of care associated with effects of conditions that can adversely affect human development.
   Subtype 2.1: Provision of care to prevent the occurrence of deleterious effects of such conditions.
   Subtype 2.2: Provision of care to mitigate or overcome existent deleterious effects of such conditions.
   Conditions include:
   a. Educational deprivation
   b. Problems of social adaptation
   c. Failures of healthy individuation
   d. Loss of relatives, friends, associates
   e. Loss of possessions, loss of occupational security
   f. Abrupt change of residence to an unfamiliar environment
   g. Status-associated problems
   h. Poor health or disability
   i. Oppressive living conditions
   j. Terminal illness and impending death

The first category of developmental self-care requisites articulates with each of the eight universal self-care requisites. The requisites in this category when effectively met should contribute to the prevention of developmental disorders and promote development in accord with the human potential.

The types of problems named in the second category do not constitute an exhaustive list. In some nursing situations, the kinds of problems named may be a central focus of care; in other situations, the results of the problems are considered a qualification on action within the particular situation. For example, the developmental problem of "failure of healthy individuation" may provide a central, organizing focus for nursing action in some child nursing situations. On the other hand, the arrested cognitive development of an adult, associated with "educational deprivation," may be accepted as a qualification on action since it is not likely to change during the duration of a nursing situation. Nurses will move to help patients learn and develop personally, regardless of their stage of cognitive development, but the methods used will be selected in light of the stage of operational knowing the patient has achieved. The following excerpt from descriptive materials about one member of an adult ambulatory population exemplifies this nursing approach.[2]

> Mr. M. is a 66-year-old diabetic who has never been to school, who thinks very concretely, who cannot read, who can distinguish colors but not name them, and who has fairly good motor ability. Recently he was asked to begin testing his urine at home and the nurse began teaching him. Content had to be broken into small units and presented slowly. After two sessions Mr. M. did learn to test his urine and repeated demonstrations by him at subsequent clinic visits indicate that he continues to do it accurately. As a result the clinic staff can be certain that they have accurate information about test results. Mr. M. is extremely pleased at having learned to do this and views this as an important *self-development*. During his last clinic visit he said to me, "You know, I've had this diabetes 4 years now and nobody ever did as much for me till I got tied up to this nurse. She done more for me in this time and now I know more than I did before" (p. 789).

Health-deviation self-care requisites

These self-care requisites exist for persons who are ill or injured, have specific forms of pathology including defects and disabilities, and who are under medical diagnosis and treatment. Obvious changes in human structure (edematous extremities, tumors), in physical functioning (difficult breathing, limited movement of a joint), or in behavior and habits of daily living (extreme irritability in relations with others, sudden changes in mood, loss of interest in life) focus a person's attention on himself or herself. These changes may raise questions. What is wrong? Why is this happening? What should I do? Family members and friends may also ask the same questions when they observe these obvious deviations from health. Changes that occur subtly and gradually are not detected as quickly as those that appear suddenly and dramatically. In instances where inability to focus attention or attend to oneself is part of the disease process (for example, a cerebral accident), manifestations of the disease may be noted first by family members or co-workers. When a change in health state brings about total or almost total dependence on others for the needs to sustain life or well-being, the person moves from the position of *selfcare-agent* to that of *receiver of care*. Parents also experience a similar change in position when a child's health deviation demands care that exceeds their capacities as *child care agents*. Evidence of health deviations leads to demands for determining what should be done to restore normalcy. In modern society, this would be expressed as a demand for medical diagnosis and treatment. Seeking and participating in medical care for health deviations are self-care actions.

Health deviations may bring about feelings of illness or of not being able to function normally. These feelings, which are related directly or indirectly to the nature of the health deviation, will influence what the person may choose to do.

Disease processes may also be functional in individuals and may not be accompanied by feelings of illness. The localized or generalized nature of the effects of disease or injury are related to feelings of illness. For example, a person with a simple fracture may feel well despite some discomfort, but a person with a "cold" may feel quite ill. In either situation, a disease or injury is something to be lived with and lived through, since disease and injury have some duration over time. The duration varies with the nature of the disease or injury. Some diseases terminate only with death, whereas others are brought under control by biologic processes with or without human intervention using medically derived measures. The characteristics of health deviations as conditions extending over time determine the kinds of care demands that individuals experience as they live with the effects of pathologic conditions and live through their duration.

Disease or injury affects not only specific structures and physiologic or psychological mechanisms but also integrated human functioning. When integrated functioning is seriously affected (severe mental retardation, comatose states, autism), the individual's developing or developed powers of agency are seriously impaired either permanently or temporarily. Conditions that limit physical mobility, even when such limitations are severe, may be less disruptive of integrated human functioning than emotional and mental disorders. Extreme limitations of physical mobility or sensory deprivation as in total blindness may lead to emotional and mental problems, which, if unresolved, can interfere with human integrated functioning. Whenever health deviations result in disfigurement or disability, there is a demand for specialized medical and nursing assistance to prevent further deviations in human functioning.

Self-care requisites arise not only from disease, injury, disfigurement, and disability but also from medical care measures prescribed or performed by physicians. Medical care measures may modify structure (surgical removal of organs) or require behavioral modification (control of fluid intake). Pain, discomfort, and frustration resulting from medical care also create requisites for self-care to bring relief. Some medical care measures introduce hazards into a person's life situation. For example, the possibility of dependence on prescribed drugs or the risks attendant on anesthesia and major surgical intervention are real problems. The use of these measures necessitates the use of protective care measures. The specific techniques of medical diagnosis and treatment used will produce particular self-care requisites. Nurses must know and be alert to these results and requisites.

This analysis of health-deviation self-care has shown that in abnormal states of health, self-care requisites arise from both the disease state and the measures used in its diagnosis or treatment. Understanding these types of self-care requisites requires a foundation of knowledge in medical science and medical technology. Modern medical advances require nurses to be well grounded in pathology and in various medical technologies if they are to assist effectively individuals with health-deviation self-care. If persons with health deviations are to become competent in managing a system of health-deviation self-care, they must also be able to apply relevant medical knowledge to their own care.

There are six categories of health-deviation self-care requisites:

1. Seeking and securing appropriate medical assistance in the event of exposure to specific physical or biologic agents or environmental conditions associated with human pathologic events and states, or when there is evidence of genetic, physiologic, or psychologic conditions known to produce or be associated with human pathology
2. Being aware of and attending to the effects and results of pathologic conditions and states, including effects on development
3. Effectively carrying out medically prescribed diagnostic, therapeutic, and rehabilitative measures directed to preventing specific types of pathology, to the pathology itself, to the regulation of human integrated functioning, to the correction of deformities or abnormalities, or to compensation for disabilities
4. Being aware of and attending to or regulating the discomforting or deleterious effects of medical care measures performed or prescribed by the physician, including effects on development
5. Modifying the self-concept (and self-image) in accepting oneself as being in a particular state of health and in need of specific forms of health care
6. Learning to live with the effects of pathologic conditions and states and the effects of medical diagnostic and treatment measures in a life-style that promotes continued personal development

---

Exercise to assist in learning to obtain information about dependent-care systems for children and adults

1. Select a friend who is the responsible adult or one of the responsible adults providing continuing care for a child in the family. Make sure the person is willing to answer questions about giving care.
   a. Ask the person to tell you about how he or she cares for the child. Tell the person that you are interested in the components of care as they are understood by persons who involved in giving care. Ask the person to proceed by telling you what he or she does.
   b. Record what the person tells you, attending to the person's focus (1) on care to meet the universal developmental, and health deviation self-care requisites and (2) on what is said about the child's role in care.
   c. Ask questions if necessary to get a description of the care provided.
   d. As a conclusion, ask the person how he or she feels about being in the role of care giver.
2. Follow the same procedure for a person providing care for an adult member of a family or a household.

THERAPEUTIC SELF-CARE DEMAND

The symbol or name therapeutic self-care demand was introduced by the Nursing Development Conference Group in 1970. Before the formalization of the concept, the terms *action demand* and *self-care demand* were used to refer to the amount and kind of self-care that persons should perform or have performed for them within a time frame.

The concept and the reality

The conceptualization of therapeutic self-care demand is modeled on **deliberate action**. The self-care requisite component of the concept (Fig. 6-3) are purposes or goals to be achieved. Methods or technologies are means through which self-care requisites can be met. The courses of action related to each requisite indicate the kinds and sequences of actions to be performed in using a selected method or technology to meet a particularized self-care requisite (see Table 6-1). In concrete situations where persons take care of themselves or in dependent-care or in nursing situations, therapeutic self-care demand is a time-specific calculation of the sets of actions judged to have validity and reliability in controlling factors that affect human functioning and development. The calculation is based on data about individuals and their life situations. Control or various degrees of regulation of factors, means keeping factors at values which are within the range that is compatible with human life, human development, health, and well-being.

In all practice situations, the factor to be controlled or in some way regulated must be understood in its relationship to the functioning and the development of men, women, and children in the interests of life, health, and well-being. Factors may be intrinsic or extrinsic to persons. Pain experienced by infants, children, or adults is an example of an intrinsic factor; environmental hazards are extrinsic to persons. Both

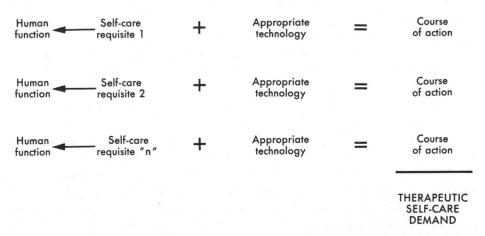

Fig. 6-3 Structural and action elements of components of therapeutic self-care demands.

intrinsic and extrinsic factors should be understood when possible in terms of their characteristics and the history of their presence and development. For example, a parent who abuses a child is a hazard to the life, health, and well-being of the child; but the abusive behavior of the parent has specific characteristics and a history of development, both of which must be known to select the valid and reliable means to protect the child. The intrinsic factor of pain must be investigated to determine how, when, and for how long the pain is experienced; its association with specific types of events; and its history.

Factors that demand regulatory action and are expressed as self-care requisites are associated with the age and gender of individuals, their developmental and health states, their environments, and their patterns of living. These distinguishing features of men, women, and children, along with other features are called basic conditioning factors within the context of the self-care deficit theory of nursing.

Basic conditioning factors and therapeutic self-care demand

Factors internal or external to individuals that affect their abilities to engage in self-care or affect the kind and amount of self-care required are named basic conditioning factors. These factors were identified and have been worked with since 1958. They were named in the early 1970s by the Nursing Development Conference Group. The original listing included the first eight factors or types of factors identified below. Factors 9 and 10 have since been added.

1. Age
2. Gender
3. Developmental state
4. Health state
5. Sociocultural orientation
6. Health care system factors; for example, medical diagnostic, and treatment modalities
7. Family system factors
8. Pattern of living including activities regularly engaged in
9. Environmental factors
10. Resource availability and adequacy

The list is not complete and should be amended whenever a new factor is identified.

The named factors condition therapeutic self-care demands in a number of ways. Some such as age, gender, and developmental state, as well as physical environmental factors, affect the value at which a universal or developmental self-care requisite should be met. For example, the age and developmental state of an infant affect the amount, composition, and state of food given at a single feeding. The factors health state and health care system factors condition the therapeutic self-care demand through (1) the emergence of new self-care requisites, for example, a requisite to control or manage the experiencing of pain; or (2) the requirement of changes in values at which the universal or developmental requisites would normally be met.

Age, gender, and developmental state also condition the means (methods, technologies, techniques) that can be used to meet universal and developmental self-care requisites.

Health state factors and health care system factors sometimes bring about human conditions that interfere with, constitute obstacles to, meeting universal or developmental type requisites, for example, an infant's or adult's inability to swallow. Such obstacles must be overcome to meet requisites. This often necessitates the use of technologies designed for this purpose. The use of gastric tubes and gastrostomy tubes for feeding individuals who cannot take food by mouth and swallow are well-known examples.

Nurses should take an objective approach to investigation of the conditioning effects of age and gender, physical aspects of development, health state, health care system factors, and environmental factors on component parts of the therapeutic self-care demands of their patients. Nurses can help patients take an objective approach to identifying the conditioning effects of such factors as nurses and patients work to calculate patients' therapeutic self-care demands. As part of such investigations, nurses should recognize the importance of patients' subjective information about self-care requisites they are aware of that are based on what they are experiencing, for example, the requisite for control or management of nausea or anxiety.

The basic conditioning factors patterns of living, sociocultural orientations, family system factors, and social environmental factors affect the therapeutic self-care demands of individuals, largely by limiting what self-care requisites and means for meeting them will be accepted and admitted as constituent components of persons' therapeutic self-care demands. For example, whenever persons' patterns of living involve habitual use of tobacco, *the self-care requisite to keep the lungs and body free of tar and other harmful substances* is an actual requisite and the *means to meet it is to stop smoking* with use of all the *care measures* needed to achieve this freedom from harmful substances. However, habitual smokers, for example, may not be able to admit the means and necessary care measures into their therapeutic self-care demands.

Sociocultural orientations of persons to health and health care, the care measures prescribed by their culture, and the care measures families will and will not accept all condition what will or will not be admitted into therapeutic self-care demands of family members. For example, the sociocultural orientations of some individuals determines the kind of protein-containing food that they will eat. Such factors require subjective approaches if nurses are to develop insights about them in concrete practice situations. It may not be enough for nurses to understand features of a common culture of a social group. They may need to know culture elements internalized by individuals and by members of families into their self-concepts and value systems.

Resource availability and adequacy affect primarily the selection of means to meet self-care requisites and the associated care measures. For example, the availability of protein-containing food and its cost determine what individuals can do about meeting the universal requisite to maintain food intake sufficient for persons living under specified conditions. Resource availability, by affecting the way in which a requisite is particularized for an individual, and the means available to meet a requisite affect the required series of care measures to be performed with respect to resource use.

Calculation of the therapeutic self-care demand

Calculation in this context is understood as an investigative process with elements of hypothetico-deductive reasoning. Engagement in the process is a search for answers to the question: What series and sequences of actions regulatory of human functioning and development should this individual perform (or have performed by another) within specified time frames in the interests of life, health, and well-being? The process results in the production of nursing design unit D identified in Chapter 5.

In concrete situations, calculating an individual's therapeutic self-care demand proceeds component by component. A component, a unit of a therapeutic self-care demand, becomes known from the following operations:

1. Identification, formulation, and expression of a single self-care requisite in its relation to some aspect(s) of human functioning and development. This includes particularizing the values and frequency with which it should be met.
2. Identification of the presence of human and environmental conditions that are (1) enabling for meeting the requisite or (2) not enabling and constitute obstacles to or interference with meeting it.
3. Determination of the methods or technologies that are known or hypothesized to have validity and reliability in meeting the requisite under prevailing human and environmental conditions and circumstances.
4. Laying out the sets and sequences of actions to be performed when a particular method or technology or some combination of them are selected for use as the means through which the particularized requisite will be met under existent and emerging conditions and circumstances.

The result of this process, as related to a single self-care requisite, is the laying out of the structural features of one component of a person's therapeutic self-care demand (operations 1 through 3) that determine the action features or elements of the demand (operation).

The baseline or foundation of a person's therapeutic self-care demand(s) is constituted from universal self-care requisites and developmental self-care requisites particularized for the person by age, gender, developmental stage, pattern of living, and environmental conditions and circumstances. These self-care requisites have their foundations in the nature of human beings, some features of which are common to other living things and not in the factors that condition them. Therapeutic self-care demands of persons whose states of health are within established norms for their age and developmental states have universal and developmental components. Universal components include those that are disease preventive in nature, such as requisites for immunizations for specific diseases.

For persons who are ill, injured, or suffering from specific medically diagnosed health deviations, the universal and developmental self-care requisites as particularized for persons of their age, gender and developmental state, patterns of living, and environmental conditions serve as reference points for adjustments necessitated by health state factors and health care system factors such as a prescribed medical treatment.

In laying out the structural features of specific components of individuals' therapeutic self-care demands, nurses work first to identify and formalize requisites that are essential for the maintenance of life processes (for example, the maintenance of a sufficient intake of air that meets physiologic needs) to those that prevent personal harm or injury or health deterioration, to those that maintain health or promote movement to a higher level of human functioning, to those that contribute to a state of human well-being under existent conditions and circumstances.

Scholarly work to organize existent and validated knowledge about universal, developmental, and health-deviation-type self-care requisites is needed for nursing purposes. Some work has been done by teachers in programs of nursing education and by researchers. One comprehensive contribution was made through the University of Michigan project, Development of Criterion Measures of Nursing Care, which focused on adults hospitalized for health conditions treated medically or surgically. Nurses developed the criterion measures for all the universal-type self-care requisites and for selected health-deviation-type self-care requisites.

The identification and formulation and expression of health-deviation-type self-care requisites must be learned by every nurse and nursing student. The process may begin with a physician's medical order for a patient under nursing care. A medical order, such as cleanse and dress surgically made incisions in left leg twice a day, is a prescription of a method for meeting a self-care requisite that is unexpressed, namely, to promote wound healing in relation to the human function of maintenance of skin integrity. In other instances nurses must move from symptoms that patients are experiencing or signs of health disorders to identification, formulation, and expression of self-care requisites and to selection of means for meeting them. In some instances nurses or nurses and patients together select the means; in other instances the need for a means to meet a requisite may require referral to the physician.

Health-deviation-type self-care requisites, like universal and developmental requisites, have their origins in the anatomic and functional features of human beings. Health state considered as a basic conditioning factor for persons' therapeutic self-care demands is viewed as an expressed formulation of an assessment of whether or not the anatomic features and the functioning of individuals is within or outside established norms for individuals of particular ages in particular developmental stages.

The methods or technologies that are valid in meeting health-deviation-type self-care requisites have their foundations in common-sense approaches, in the medical sciences, or in nursing. The methods or technologies to meet universal and developmental self-care requisites have their primary foundations in the human sciences, including the fields of human development and human behavior.

The baseline, scientifically determined values at which universal- and developmental-type self-care requisites should be met for individuals by age, gender, and development state should be mastered by every nursing student. This knowledge is antecedent to practice with reference to calculating therapeutic self-care demands of individuals.

When persons are acutely ill, injured, or suffering from specific disorders of health, nurses in calculating therapeutic self-care demands focus on health state as the active basic conditioning factors and seek answers to two questions: Is this or that feature of a person's health state interfering with or is an obstacle to the meeting of universal or developmental type self-care requisites? What health deviation self-care requisites are associated with specific features of a person's disordered state of health and with medically prescribed measures for diagnosis and treatment?

The activity element of each component of a therapeutic self-care demand may include three types of actions: (1) those directed to the person performing or for whom the care measure is performed, (2) those directed to required resources, and (3) those that meet the self-care requisite. Persons must accept themselves as being in need of the functional or developmental regulation expressed by the requisite and in need of the means for meeting it, must secure and prepare materials and equipment required, must prepare self as required, and then proceed to perform the actions through which the self-care requisite is met. The developed activity element of each component of a therapeutic self-care demand is the procedure for meeting a particularized requisite.

The calculation of the therapeutic self-care demands requires antecedent knowledge of human structure and functioning, human growth and development, family life, occupational life, and preventive health care. It also requires current and historical information about particular individuals and groups. There is also a need for up-to-date information about valid and reliable processes or technologies for (1) identifying the presence and effects of factors that affect the values of self-care requisites or limit the methods that can be used for meeting requisites and (2) meeting specific care requisites. Methods for meeting self-care requisites should be examined and understood within the cultural context of social groups and within the total care systems of social group members. Some self-care or child care measures in use within social groups may be effective and therapeutic; but health care professionals who are outsiders may perceive these measures as harmful, take steps to change them, and thereby harm individual social group members.

The adult gradually comes to have some understanding of his or her own self-care demands through an accumulation of day-to-day experiences, and parents often come to understand the care demands of their children in this fashion. Persons who are care agents for socially dependent individuals should be able to calculate the current and projected self-care demands on those under their care. Adolescents and adults ideally develop knowledge and skills that will enable them to calculate their own self-care demands in relation to developmental processes, to events in the life cycle, and to a range of environmental conditions that affect human functioning, human development, and general well-being. The recognition of some adverse condition in the environment or in the individual or group usually results in the need to look at the totality of the self-care requisites and to identify the methods and the courses of action that will bring a therapeutic return. Nursing professionals require highly developed specialized skills in calculating the therapeutic self-care demands for persons and groups within their defined domains of nursing practice.

Design of the therapeutic self-care demand

Calculation of a therapeutic self-care demand has a focus on components. The design of a therapeutic self-care demand has a focus on essential to ideal relationships among components. **Action** components must be related in time and place frames of reference for the 24 hours of the person's day. Factors to be considered include the need to maintain a time-specific relationship between certain particularized requisite, for example, the relationship between food intake and insulin administration in persons with diabetes mellitus. Other factors include organizations of components to ensure economy of time and effort and proper articulation with other activities of personal and family life.

Adjustment in design is needed each time new self-care requisites emerge or existent ones change significantly. Design requires knowledge of existent developed components of therapeutic self-care demands and their functional relatedness or independence from one another. Self-care can be burdensome and at times overwhelming for individuals. A good design of the therapeutic self-care demand can lessen stress from performance to meet it.

Variations in therapeutic self-care demands

Types of variations relate to composition, complexity, and stability. The therapeutic self-care demand varies according to the self-care requisites from which it is made. At least two variations occur, which can be identified in relation to preventive health care:
1. A primary prevention self-care demand
   a. Universal self-care requisites
   b. Developmental self-care requisites (type 1 and type 2.1)
2. A secondary or tertiary prevention self-care demand
   a. Health-deviation self-care requisites or developmental self-care requisites (type 2.2)
   b. Universal self-care requisites
   c. Developmental self-care requisites (type 1 and type 2.1)

From the perspective of preventive health care (sometimes referred to as preventive medicine), the therapeutic self-care demand sets forth the kinds of continuing health care that (all things being equal) will prevent disease or its extension, maintain health or promote a more desirable health state, and positively contribute to the individual's human development. Meeting one's therapeutic self-care demand (or that of another) is engaging in preventive health care, which includes seeking and actively participating in the care provided by health professionals.

Calculating and meeting the therapeutic self-care demands of individuals are not adequately attended to by nurses in some nursing situations. Meeting universal self-care requisites and developmental requisites is often neglected, even in institutions where patients are supposed to receive and are charged for nursing. The use of the general comprehensive theory of nursing described in Chapter 3 should be an aid to nursing students and nurses for understanding the importance of the knowledge and skills organized around the therapeutic self-care demands of patients.

The mix of types of self-care requisites in a therapeutic self-care demand indicates the complexity of individuals' continuous care requirements and is an index of the kinds of knowledge and the range of skills required by persons who can act to meet the demands. Individual deficits in self-care or care of dependents may arise from the composition and complexity of the therapeutic self-care demands, as well as from the health or developmental states of care recipients. Nurses need to have the diagnostic skill of identifying the self-care deficits of adult patients in meeting their current or projected therapeutic self-care demands. A related diagnostic skill is that of determining the infant or child care or dependent adult care competencies of responsible adults who seek for nursing socially dependent family members. The range of therapeutic self-care demands of individuals who can benefit from nursing (a nursing population) and the range of self-care (or dependent-care) deficits of these individuals are indications of the kind and amount of nursing required. Care demands and deficits are also indicators of the kinds of abilities that would qualify nurses for practice.

Therapeutic self-care demands also vary in relation to the stability of their components. Some demands are stable over days, weeks, or months; others have no stability since their components are in constant flux. When therapeutic self-care demands of individuals are unstable and complex, the continuous presence and activity of highly skilled, experienced nurses in the governing or leadership role are required to protect the life, health, and well-being of persons under nursing care.

SELF-CARE THEORY REVIEW

The theory of self-care expresses the view that human beings are persons who have attained some degree of self-possession. This is the only view of human beings that is compatible with the expressed insights about self-care as a human regulatory function.

Within the theory of self-care, person and environment are identified as a unity characterized by human-environmental interchanges and by the impact of one on the other. Person-environment constitutes a functional type of unity with a concrete existence. It is in our thought processes that we consider individuals as apart from their environments. Thinking patient-environment is a sophisticated mode of thought developed by nursing practitioners who learn to include themselves within their patients' environments.

In nursing practice situations the theory of self-care guides nurses in the calculation of their patients' therapeutic self-care demand, in designing systems of nursing or dependent care to ensure that self-care requisites will be met, and in performing or guiding actions through which the components of the care demand are met.

The theory of self-care also guides nurses to make critical observations in their first contacts with patients to determine evidence that a self-care or a dependent-care system is in process. If there is no system of care in operation, meeting care requisites of the patient immediately becomes a part of nursing care. If there is a system of self-care or dependent care in operation, nurse and patient or nurse and dependent-care agent together will reach some temporary agreement about who will now perform the care measures that together constitute the ongoing care system. After initial or definitive nursing diagnosis, temporary agreements may be confirmed or changed. Continuing self-care is essential for life, health, and personal well-being. Nurses must understand its nature and ensure its continuous provision when persons come under nursing care.

REFERENCES

1. Nursing Development Conference Group, Orem, DE, editor: Concept formalization in nursing: process and product, Boston, 1979, Little, Brown & Co., p. 132-134.
2. Backscheider, JE: The use of self as the essence of clinical supervision in ambulatory patient care, *Nurs Clin North Am*, Philadelphia, 1971, p. 789, WB Saunders.

SELECTED READINGS

Harris L and Associates, Inc.: Healthy lifestyles/unhealthy lifestyles, a national research report of behavior, knowledge, motivations and opinions concerning individual health practice, New York, 1984, Gartland Publishing.

Nursing Development Conference Group: Nursing system variables and cerebrovascular accidents. In Orem DE, editor: Concept formalization in nursing: process and product, ed 2, Boston, 1979, Little, Brown and Co., pp. 249-272.

Orem DE, and Taylor SG: Case study in Orem's general theory of nursing. In Winstead-Fry P, editor: Case studies in nursing theory, New York, 1986, National League for Nursing, pp. 59-68.

School of Nursing, University of Missouri-Columbia: Clinical and culural dimensions around the world. Papers and abstracts presented at the First International Self-Care Deficit Nursing Theory Conference, Kansas City, Missouri, October 15-18, 1989, Columbia, Missouri, 1989, School of Nursing, University of Missouri-Columbia, the Curators of the University of Missouri.

Aukamp VA: Self-care practices of pregnant women, 21 page addendum

Griffin JB: Operationalizing Orem in the cultural assessment of child bearing, pp. 127-146 (Korean mothers and USA fathers).

Hanucharurnkul S: Social support, self-care, and quality of life in cancer patients receiving radiotherapy, pp. 187-212.

Harris JL: Self-care actions of chronic schizophrenics associated with meeting solitude and social interaction requisites, pp. 165-183.

Riley CP: Effect of a pulmonary rehabilitation program on self-care of patients with chronic obstructive pulmonary disease, pp. 89-102.

Utz, SW, et al: Perceptions of health status and body image in persons with mitral valave prolapse, pp. 157-160.

Youniss J: Parents and peers in social development, a Sullivan-Piaget perspective, Chicago, 1980, University of Chicago Press.

CHAPTER 7

Self-care agency and dependent-care agency

Self-care agency and **dependent-care agency** refer to human capabilities of individuals to perform actions to take care of themselves and others. Nurses must understand the actions that constitute self-care and dependent-care, as well as the capabilities that are enabling for performing these kinds of actions.

Being able to perform competently one kind of goal-oriented action does not indicate that persons have ability to perform other, different kinds of actions. For example, a competent accountant may not have developed capabilities for construction work, for meal preparation, and for some components of self-care. Powers of persons to engage in particular kinds of goal-achieving action is referred to as agency. Developed powers of agency of adults extend over a range and that range should include self-care and dependent-care.

Conceptualization of agency depends on prior conceptualizations of voluntary, deliberate goal-achieving actions and action sequences.

SELF-CARE AGENCY, A HUMAN POWER

Self-care agency is the *complex acquired ability* to meet one's continuing requirements for *care* that regulates life processes, maintains or promotes integrity of human structure and functioning and human development, and promotes well-being. Self-care agency of individuals varies over a range with respect to its development from childhood through old age. It varies with health state; with factors that influence educability; and with life experiences as they are enabling for learning, for exposure to cultural influences, and for use of resources in daily living. Self-care agency of individuals at this time or that time is conditioned by factors that affect its *development* and its *operability*. Its *adequacy* is measured against the component parts of the therapeutic self-care demand, that is, the demand on individuals to engage in self-care (Fig. 7-1).

Self-care is human endeavor, learned behavior, that has the characteristics of deliberate action (see Chapter 4). Self-care is produced as individuals engage in action to care for themselves by influencing internal and external factors to regulate their own internal functioning and development. Self-care actions engaged in over time are

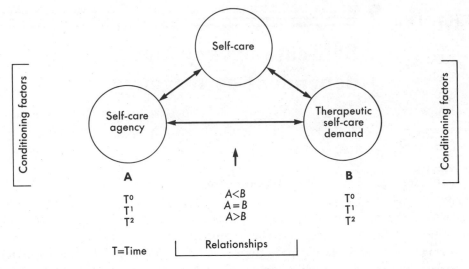

Fig. 7-1 Adequacy values of self-care agency as related to therapeutic self-care demand may vary over time.

performed by persons in their environmental settings and within the context of their patterns of daily living. Sometimes the meeting of one's requirements for self-care rules out engagement in preferred activities. At other times, self-care is interspersed with the other activities of daily life and is not a major focus of attention. The human ability named *self-care agency*, the ability for engaging in self-care, develops in the course of day-to-day living through the spontaneous process of learning. Its development is aided by intellectual curiosity, by instruction and supervision from others, and by experience in performing self-care measures. It has been conceptualized as a unit because of the specific practical endeavor, self-care, to which it is directed. Self-care has form and content. The form of self-care is that of deliberate action and its phases. The content derives from the purposes to which it is directed, the self-care requisites, and the courses of action that are effective in meeting them.

The ability to engage in self-care is also conceptualized as having form and content. Self-care agency is conceptualized as taking the form of a set of human abilities for deliberate action: the ability to attend to specific things (this includes the ability to exclude other things) and to understand their characteristics and the meaning of the characteristics; the ability to apprehend the need to change or regulate the things observed; the ability to acquire knowledge of appropriate courses of action for regulation; the ability to decide what to do; and the ability to act to achieve change or regulation. The content of self-care agency derives from its proper object, meeting self-care requisites, whatever those requisites are at specific moments.

Self-care agency can be examined in relation to individual capacities, including their skill repertoires and the kinds of knowledge they have and use, for engaging in a range of practical endeavors. Individual abilities can be described in terms of *development, operability,* and *adequacy* (p. 205).[1] The **development** and **operability** of self-care agency can be affected by genetic and constitutional factors as well as by culture, life experiences, and health state. Development and operability are identified in terms of the kinds of self-care operations individuals can consistently and effectively perform. The adequacy of self-care agency is measured in terms of the relationship of the number and kinds of operations that persons can engage in and the operations required to calculate and meet an existing or projected therapeutic self-care demand. Determining the adequacy of self-care agency is essential if judgments about the presence or absence of self-care deficits are to be made.

The art of nursing includes making a comprehensive determination of the reasons why people can be helped through nursing. An important aspect of this determination is diagnosing the abilities of an individual to engage in self-care (or dependent care) now or in the future and appraising these abilities in relation to the person's therapeutic self-care demand. Unless self-care agency is accurately diagnosed, nurses have no rational basis for (1) making judgments about existing or projected self-care deficits and the reasons for their existence, (2) selecting valid and reliable methods of helping, or (3) prescribing and designing nursing systems.

Self-care is performed largely out of habit, but individuals who have not thought about their self-care role may need to be helped to look at themselves as self-care agents in order to understand the values to which their habits commit them and to appraise the adequacy of their self-care abilities. Examining one's self-care habits, appraising the benefits derived from one's self-care as practiced, recognizing needs for change, and becoming knowledgeable about new self-care requisites are important for maintaining the adequacy of the individual's self-care agency. New self-care requisites resulting from changes in internal or external conditions necessitate additional knowledge, adjustments in some types of developed skills (for example, perceptual skill), and examination of one's willingness to pursue particular courses of self-care action. Persons with specific types and values of self-care requisites are important as subjects for exploratory research about the creation, use, and effectiveness of self-care practices.

Self-care agency (or dependent-care agency) is defined by qualities ascribed to individuals. If nursing is to take place, nurses must have the abilities to view their patients as self-care and dependent-care agents and to diagnose patients' abilities for engagement in continuous and effective care. To do this, nurses must be able to accept individuals, families, and groups as being in specific stages of development and particular states of health and well-being. What persons can do with respect to practical affairs (including self-care) varies with age and developmental state, as well as with health state. Nurses must understand the limits of the biologic features of human beings (e.g., blood vessels), but they must also strive to understand the human capacities for self-care and self-management.

SELF-CARE AGENCY CONCEPTUALIZED

The formalization of the concept self-care agency occurred between 1958 and 1970. Initial insights about the human property named self-care agency were expressed as capabilities and limitations of individuals for engagement in self-care. Gradually, the name *self-care agency* came into use. The formalization of the structure of the concept was facilitated by the formulation of propositions about self-care agency to express current understandings. The propositions expressed critical judgments about the patient property self-care agency based on insights derived from experiences in concrete nursing practice situations or results of analyses of nursing case materials. The model for this movement is experience, understanding, critical reflection, and critical judgment. Early insights about self-care agency are expressed in the following eight propositions (p. 183).[1]

1. Self-care agency is a complex, acquired human characteristic or quality.
2. Self-care agency is the power of an individual to engage in the operations essential for self-care.
3. The exercise by an individual of the power that is named self-care agency results in a system of actions directed to reality conditions in self or environment in order to regulate them; or its exercise results in a design and plan for such a system of action.
4. Self-care agency can be conceptualized as an action repertoire of an individual.
5. Self-care agency can be characterized in terms of abilities and limitations of an individual for engagement in self-care.
6. Conditions and factors in the environment of an individual affect the development of and the exercise of self-care agency.
7. Persons are subject to time sequential needs for the exercise of self-care agency.
8. Self-care agency is an estimative capability and a productive capability for self-care.

The structure of the concept was formalized as a three-part structure:

1. A broad conceptual structure constituted from capabilities for performing estimative, transitional, and productive self-care operations
2. A set of power components enabling for performance of self-care operations
3. Five sets of foundational capabilities and dispositions articulating with the power components in their relationships to operational capabilities

Historically, the movement of conceptualization was from the broad conceptual structure, to the foundational capabilities and disposition, and finally to the enabling power components. The structural features of the concept self-care agency are described in the historical sequence of development.

Broad conceptual elements: capabilities for self-care operations

The broad structure of the concept self-care agency is understood in relation to and modeled on operations specific to the phases of deliberate action, namely, estimative operations, transitional operations of reflection, critical judgment, and decision making, and production operations through which the purposes specified by self-care requisites and calculated as a therapeutic self-care demand are achieved. Thus, self-care agency is understood as developed capabilities of individuals to engage in the named self-care operations in order to know and meet their requirements for self-care within time and place frames of references. Fig. 7-2 illustrates the property self-care agency and its broad conceptualized structure.

An identification of suboperations of the estimative, transitional, and production operations of self-care was developed to provide insight into the three operational capabilities. In describing the suboperations, the terms *self-care requisites* and *therapeutic self-care demand* are not named. They are implicit in the descriptive statements. The estimative, transitional, and productive operations and their results are identified in sequential relationships (pp. 192-193).[1]

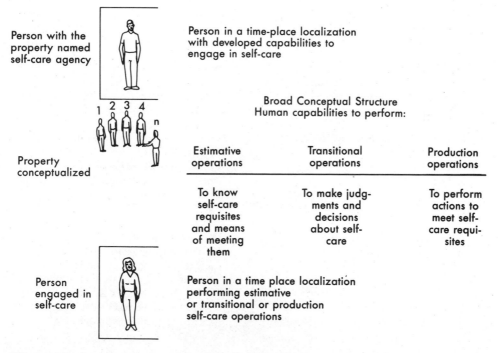

Fig. 7-2 The broad conceptual structures of self-care agency.

SELF-CARE OPERATIONS AND RESULTS

Operations	Results
Estimative Type	
1. Investigation of internal and external conditions and factors significant for self-care	Empirical knowledge of self and environment
2. Investigation of the meaning of characterized conditions and factors and their regulation	Experiential knowing (based in part on acquired technical knowledge) of the meaning of the existent conditions and factors for life, health, and well-being
3. Investigation of the question: How can existent conditions and factors be regulated (i.e., changed or maintained)?	Technical knowledge of what can be regulated and the means available for effecting regulation
Transitional Type	
4. Reflection to determine which course of self-care should be followed	An affirming judgment that one course of self-care is preferred, or that a series of courses is preferred, or that none should be pursued
5. Deciding what to do with respect to self-care	A decision to engage in or not engage in specific regulatory self-care operations
Productive Type	
6. Preparation of self, materials, or environmental settings for the performance of a regulatory-type self-care operation	Conditions of readiness for performing self-care operations for regulatory purposes
7a. Performance of productive self-care operations with specific regulatory purposes within a time period	Knowledge that regulatory measures are in process or are completed

7b. Determining presence of and monitoring, during performance, conditions known to affect effectiveness of performance and results	Information that conditions and factors affecting performance and results
	  a. Are or are not present
	  b. Are or are not under control if present

8. Monitoring for evidence of effects and results
  a. Desired
  b. Untoward
	Information about events indicating that regulation is
	  a. Being achieved
	  b. Not being achieved
	Knowledge of untoward results
	  a. Absence of
	  b. Presence of

9. Reflection to determine evidence of and adequacy of regulatory results	An affirming judgment as related to specific self-care regulatory operations
	  a. Self-care should continue
	  b. Self-care should be discontinued
	    (1) To be resumed at a specific time
	    (2) Not to be resumed as related to the operations in question

Operations	Results

10a. Decision about regulatory operations
    a. Continue action
    b. Close action
    c. Cease action but resume at a spe-
       cific time
10b. Decision about estimative operations
    a. Continue to use results obtained
       from estimative operations (current
       data base)
    b. Begin a new series of estimative
       operations

The capabilities to engage in the named operations is understood as self-care agency. Actual engagement of persons in the operations within time and place frames of reference is self-care.

Some human foundations of self-care agency

Another stage in the formalization of the concept self-care agency dealt with the question: Are there common human foundations for engagement in deliberate action including self-care?

Understandings of group members about self-care agency were advanced by Louise Hartnett Rauckhorst's 1968 development of a conceptualization of voluntary human action involving motor activity (pp. 135-141).[1] Two complementary models were structured to make explicit the physiologic and psychological features of deliberate action. The psychological model of action included three articulated frames: a central veridical frame focused on persons in physical environments; a sociocultural frame focused on persons in social environments with given roles and role expectations; and a personal frame of reference focused on personal values, self-as-felt and known, ideal self, and long-range goal orientations. The physiologic model of action associates higher mental processes with sensory and motor neurologic functioning in the execution of internally and externally oriented actions. These models provided one foundation for the development of the secondary or substantive structure of the theoretical concept self-care agency and for its continued formalization and validation. Hartnett's models do not negate the fact that it is the person who acts. They express the complexity of deliberate human action and point the way toward expression of the foundational capabilities, dispositions, and orientations of individuals relevant to ability and willingness for performing self-care operations, as well as other forms of deliberate action.

The step of explicating the human foundations of self-care agency was formalized by Joan E. Backscheider in 1970 and 1971 in the form of a survey list of general capabilities essential for engagement in self-care. The survey list included "physical, mental, motivational, emotional, and orientative capabilities" and resulted from

Backscheider's work in a nursing clinic for ambulatory adults with diabetes mellitus. Her three-pronged approach to nursing diagnosis was expressed in a 1971 article published in 1974 (pp. 1138-1146).[2] The approach included:

- Inquiry to determine regulatory goals to be achieved through self-care and the care measures to be used
- Analyses of the foregoing to determine the estimative and the production-type self-care operations that would need to be performed to achieve the regulatory goals
- Inquiry to determine ability of patients to perform the action components of the estimative and production self-care operations

The first element of the approach results in information, judgments, and decisions about components of patients' therapeutic self-care demands. The second element involves analysis of what should be done as well as *if–then* type of reasoning — if patients are to perform x,y,z care measures associated with components of their therapeutic self-care demands, they must have X',Y',Z' developed and operative action capabilities. The third approach involves assessment of patients' action capabilities to determine the presence or absence of requisite capabilities.

Bachscheider's survey list revised in 1979 as five sets of capabilities and dispositions is shown in Table 7-1. The sets identified as *Selected Basic Capabilities* are foundational not only for engagement in self-care but also for other forms of activity. For example, persons with conditions that negatively affect sensation and perception are limited in performing estimative-type operations regardless of the nature of the action. The set of *Knowing and Doing Capabilities* is constituted from those that affect knowing and reasoning and the making of right judgments and decisions in life situations and includes the learned skills that affect communication, as well as investigative and production-type operations. The set *Dispositions Affecting Goals Sought* expresses conditions that affect persons' willingness to look at themselves and accept themselves as self-care agents, to accept themselves as in need of particular self-care measures, or to be able to perform certain self-care measures. The members of the set *Significant Orientative Capabilities and Dispositions* are determinants of persons' interest and willingness to engage in self-care, to be concerned about health, or to be able to engage in self-care.

Whenever persons under nursing care need to perform new and additional self-care measures, to adjust or change presently performed measures, or to resume self-care after a period of being taken care of, nurses' assessment of patients' foundational capabilities and dispositions as suggested in the survey list is an essential aspect of nursing practice. The sciences and disciplines of anatomy, physiology, psychology, cognitive development and functioning, psychopathology, and social psychology are some of the fields basic to understanding the capabilities and dispositions included in the survey list.

Table 7-1 Human capabilities and dispositions foundational for self-care agency

Conditioning Factors and States	Selected Basic Capabilities — I	Selected Basic Capabilities — II	Capabilities and dispositions — Knowing and Doing Capabilities	Dispositions Affecting Goals Sought	Significant Orientative Capabilities and Dispositions
Genetic and constitutional factors	Sensation, Proprioception, Exteroception	Attention	Rational agency	Self-understanding, Self-awareness	Orientations to: Time, Health, Other persons, Events, objects
Arousal state	Learning	Perception	Operational knowing	Self-image, Self-value	Priority system or value hierarchy: Moral, Economic, Aesthetic, Material, Social
Social organization	Exercise or work	Memory	Learned skills: Reading, Counting, Writing, Verbal, Perceptual, Manual, Reasoning	Self-acceptance, Self-concern, Acceptance of bodily functions, Willingness to meet needs of self	Interest and concerns, Habits, Ability to work with the body and its parts
Culture	Regulation of the position and movement of the body and its parts	Central regulation of motivational emotional processes	Self-consistency in knowing and doing	Future directedness	Ability to manage self and personal affairs
Experience					

From Nursing Development Conference Group, Orem DE, editor: Concept formalization in nursing: process and product, ed 2. Boston, 1979, Little, Brown & Co., p. 212.

The survey list should be developed through use; it is not a complete or even an adequate development of human capabilities and dispositions foundational to self-care and other forms of action.

Power components enabling for self-care operations

In continuing investigation of the substantive structure of the concept self-care agency, the need to identify human capabilities that were empowering for engagement in the operations of self-care became evident. The reasoning process moved from the characteristics of self-care operations, as identified in the listing of *Self-care Operations and Results*, to a visualization of the human capabilities needed for their performance. Estimative self-care operations are operations of inquiry that seek both empirical and technical knowledge for purposes of knowing and understanding what is, what can, and what should be brought about with respect to taking care of self. The transitional operations of reflecting, judging, and deciding with respect to self-care matters are grounded in what individuals know about the self-care situation, their experiences and the knowledge about self-care requisites and measures for meeting them, as well as their values and their willingness. Productive operations are doing operations to achieve practical results demanding preparation for and performance of self-care measures, monitoring performance as well as their effects and results, and making judgments and decisions about subsequent actions.

It was concluded that the human powers enabling for performing self-care operations would be of a nature intermediate between human functioning and human dispositions as described in the survey list and the estimative, transitional, and production-type self-care operations. Ten power components necessary for having the capabilities to engage in self-care operations, were formulated and expressed (see accompanying box). The capabilities are expressed as a single series and not in relation to the estimative, transitional, and productive operations. Fig. 7-3 depicts the substantive components of the concept *self-care agency*.

The power components have been used both in nursing practice and in research since their publication in 1979. They need refinement and continued development with respect to their own structure and to their articulation with self-care operations and foundational capabilities and dispositions.

PERSONS AS SELF-CARE AGENTS

As individuals engage in self-care, they exercise their developed and operational abilities to manage themselves in their time-place localizations. They determine what self-care is required, make decisions about what self-care requisites they will meet and how they will meet them, perform the required activities, and determine their effects and results.

Self-care on a day-to-day basis is interspersed among other kinds of activities or

Power components of self-care agency (pp. 195-196)[1]

1. Ability to maintain attention and exercise requisite vigilance with respect to self as self-care agent and internal and external conditions and factors significant for self-care
2. Controlled use of available physical energy that is sufficient for the initiation and continuation of self-care operations
3. Ability to control the position of the body and its parts in the execution of the movements required for the initiation and completion of self-care operations
4. Ability to reason within a self-care frame of reference
5. Motivation (i.e., goal orientations for self-care that are in accord with its characteristics and its meaning for life, health, and well-being)
6. Ability to make decisions about care of self and to operationalize these decisions
7. Ability to acquire technical knowledge about self-care from authoritative sources, to retain it, and to operationalize it
8. A repertoire of cognitive, perceptual, manipulative, communication, and interpersonal skills adapted to the performance of self-care operations
9. Ability to order discrete self-care actions or action systems into relationships with prior and subsequent actions toward the final achievement of regulatory goals of self-care
10. Ability to consistently perform self-care operations, integrating them with relevant aspects of personal, family, and community living

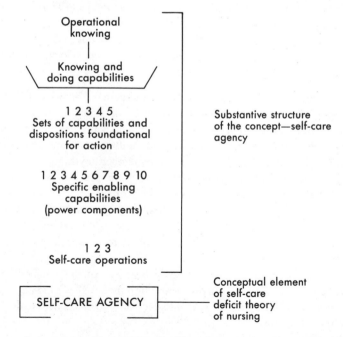

Fig. 7-3 Substantive conceptual structure of self-care agency showing one set of foundational capabilities and dispositions and operational knowing as a member of the set.

it is an aspect of another activity, for example, lifting or carrying a heavy object in a manner that prevents back injury or muscle strain. When persons are well, self-care is not a major concern; interests and activities are centered around personal and family life, work, and special interests. Occasionally, individuals must make choices between self-care and other activities. Parents who care for a sick child or who give up needed sleep and relaxation because of a family crisis are common examples of choices involving self-care.

Self-care is affected not only by the individual's family position and roles but also by health state. During illness, usual activities, even usual self-care activities, are disrupted and new self-care requirements may take over a large portion of a day. This is illustrated in the following self-analysis and personally recorded experiences and activities of a nursing practitioner and teacher during an attack of influenza. The recordings begin on the third day of the illness.

Saturday: Felt miserable. I knew I should see a doctor but had no energy or desire to get myself there. The thought of going seemed too much to face. Also, since I know no physician and since it is Saturday, I know I don't have the energy to hunt for one. Consulted with Joyce, a neighbor. What I was really asking was for her to motivate me to do something since I knew I would not be able to do it alone. She looked up some names and suggested that I call from her apartment.

Called the first man who handled it by telephone. He told me to treat it symptomatically (which was what I had been doing) since it is unresponsive to antibiotics. I have taken aspirin for elevated temperature, cough medicine, and hot drinks and fluids.

Up until today I felt the need to sleep a lot. Today I am not so drowsy, but my attention span is short and I have to find ways to divert myself — frequent changes of reading material, light reading only, a little knitting.

Sunday: More energy today in spurts. Felt a need to be more active with different types of things, so I repotted plants and wrapped a package. I find myself annoyed because I can't read heavier things. I keep trying, but this just increases my frustration. Read the papers thoroughly. The *Times'* crossword puzzle is good intellectual stimulus because you can put it down and pick it up and you don't have to remember anything.

Slightly nauseated today, probably from coughing. Have to watch the "quality" of fluids. Can take juices and coke but not milk and coffee.

I am much more croupy this evening. Chest is congested. Had difficulty bringing up anything at first. In desperation I asked Joyce, who was going to the pharmacy, to bring me some tincture of benzoin [for a croup kettle]. It is good to have someone like Joyce. It makes this all seem more manageable.

Did a lot of paroxysmal coughing but finally began to cough up mucus. It is a somewhat frightening sensation. My initial reaction was to stop the coughing and not expectorate. But after doing that two or three times, I knew I had to bring it up. It's hard to do this effectively without too much distress.

Very irritable.

Monday: Soon after I got up, I took a check on the status of my symptoms. I felt better. My temperature was 98° for the first time since Thursday. I still did some paroxysmal coughing. I thought my chest felt clearer. My throat was still sore, and my ears were very stuffy. On the whole I felt I was somewhat better. I talked to two people on the phone (in process of cancelling my appointments for the day), both of whom were horrified at how I sounded. This was a shock to me since I decided that on the whole there was improvement. I realized that I could not determine whether I was objectively "still bad," but I would have to trust my own assessment of improvement.

I talked to two other persons (for the same reason), both of whom had recently had flu. Both communicated anxiety by relating my symptoms to their condition. One identified with the ear stuffiness, which in her case developed into otitis media. She suggested use of hot mineral oil drops. The other person said that it was urgent to drink two gallons of fluids a day, which I knew I could not do. After talking to each one, I had a very temporary reaction of feeling overwhelmed, of feeling aware of the importance of what each had said, but of being uncertain about it. I decided to try to increase my fluid intake somewhat and to observe the ear symptoms more closely.

I think my reaction to these contacts was to have my level of anxiety raised. On my own I had to devise a means of adapting and observing. If I had not been able to do this, I would have been left in a rather uncomfortable state.

My attention span is not much better today. I start but don't complete things. I need to be physically active but have limited energy.

My day has been characterized by intermittent naps and more frequent paroxysms of productive coughing. I continue to produce mucous plugs but feel better, and my chest feels clearer in between coughing spells.

One thing that is interesting is that with all this inactivity I have had no indication of muscle spasm in my back [due to muscle damage resulting from surgery]. I have only done my exercises twice since becoming ill [a set of exercises prescribed by the orthopedist]. On the recent trip to Georgia where I sat all day for two days, I very much felt the need for exercise. The level of my resistance to having to sit and to that experience may have made the exercise need greater. Sometimes at night after a long stretch of sleeping I awake with a feeling of being cramped, but my current need for physical and mental inactivity seems to override my need for physical movement. Friday I could not have done the exercises; today it felt good to do them. They were just enough.

Tuesday: Decided not to go to work today. My symptoms are gradually subsiding, and I would like to keep it that way. My energy comes in spurts, and I decided not to expend it in one long flame. I still have a stuffy ear, chest congestion, and paroxysmal coughing. I am losing creativity in dealing with them. They just exist now. My menstrual period began today, and I always have a little less energy the first day.

Eating is difficult, or more accurately, planning meals to eat. I just can't get interested in it. I have no idea how well-balanced my meals are. I eat if I become interested in food. I have taken too much prune juice. I have minor gastric disturbance and some diarrhea. I have no juice on hand except prune.

I decided to walk to the grocery store, which is one-half block away. I needed to do this to test how much strength had returned. I walked there and back with my groceries and then took a nap for an hour. I am glad I decided to stay home today.

I have begun to do some work — thinking-type. I organized the class I have to present tomorrow and am writing a report of interactions with a patient I have been seeing for four months on an outpatient basis. I feel good about getting the report written; the longer I avoided it, the longer it got. It is interesting and a good stimulation but I must stop now and go sit in a chair where I can lean back and rest.

As the nurse describes her experiences, self-care was the central focus of her daily living. Adjustment of other activities to available energy was in itself self-care action. Seeking medical care was an attempt to have a medically prescribed course of action to follow in the management of the symptoms of influenza. The nurse was able to manage her own care, but not without anxiety. She sought and received help from her friend. Unsolicited advice was perceived as relevant to a degree but also anxiety-producing. The difference in the objective and subjective assessments of "how sick" she was gives insight into the importance of understanding any illness as a continuum and of the need to look for change and evaluate change over time. The statement on Tuesday, the sixth day of the illness, that the symptoms "just exist now" may be evidence of human adaptation to existing conditions and the human tendency to accept and live with a situation once its novelty is lost or when there is a decrease in the intensity of stimuli.

DEVELOPMENT OF SELF-CARE AGENCY

Self-care is learned behavior. As children grow, foundational capabilities and dispositions for engagement in forms of deliberate action including self-care develop. They learn what to do and what not to do in gradually widening areas of human living. They develop behavioral repertoires for taking action when various combinations of conditions and circumstances prevail in themselves or in their environments. In many cultures, children learn how to protect themselves from accident and injury. They may be admonished to and learn to conform to cultural practices with respect to consumption of food and water, elimination, rest and sleep, solitude and social interaction, and to achieve normalcy within their social group. Such learning results in the development by children of the powers for action identified previously as *power components of self-care agency*. These power components develop in relation to performed operations through which specific decisions are made, purposes formulated, and productive actions generated.

Learning self-care

Learning to engage in and continuous engagement in self-care are human functions. The central requisites for self-care are learning and the use of knowledge in performing externally or internally oriented sequences of self-care actions. The *self-care agent,* the provider of self-care, is open to cultural elements in the nature of known self-care requisites and ways of meeting them. Some of these elements would be known requisites and measures of care that have been integrated into the general culture. Others would be elements that are medically prescribed for individuals or groups. *Medical* is used here in the sense of those systems of medicine that prevail within particular cultures and social groups.

The self-care provider or agent performs actions that have either an *internal* or *external orientation.* Whether a self-care action is internal or external in orientation can be determined by observation, by eliciting subjective data from the self-care agent, or both. The internally and externally oriented self-care actions listed here provide a general index of the validity of helping methods.* The four types of externally oriented self-care actions are: (1) knowledge-seeking action sequences, (2) assistance- and resource-seeking action sequences, (3) expressive interpersonal actions, and (4) action sequences to control external factors. The two types of internally oriented self-care actions are: (1) resource-using action sequences to control internal factors and (2) action sequences to control oneself (thoughts, feelings, orientation) and thereby regulate internal factors or one's external orientations (Fig. 7-4).

Understanding self-care as deliberate action with internal and external orienta- tions aids nurses in acquiring, developing, and perfecting skills needed for (1) securing valid and reliable information to describe the self-care systems of individuals, (2) analyzing information descriptive of self-care and dependent-care systems, and (3) making judgments about how individuals can and should be helped with respect to performing the self-care operations from which a therapeutic self-care demand is constituted. When the courses of action, or action sequences, of a therapeutic self-care demand are known, they can be identified and grouped according to their internal and external orientations.

Nurses must understand self-care actions classified according to their internal or external orientations with respect to their relationships to each of the five ways of helping. For example, the helping method of *doing for or acting for another* does not correlate with self-care actions directed to the control of thoughts, feelings, and orientations. On the other hand, the method does correlate with self-care actions in which resources are sought or used in controlling external or internal factors.

Ways of determining and meeting one's self-care needs are not inborn. Broadly speaking, the activities of self-care are learned according to the beliefs, habits, and practices that characterize the cultural way of life of the group to which the individual belongs. In some cultures, a sick person assumes that he or she has displeased the spirit of a dead ancestor and will ask a shaman (a medicine man) for help in appeasing the

---

* Five helping methods are described in Chapter 1. They are identified as acting for or doing for, supporting, guiding, providing a developmental environment, and teaching.

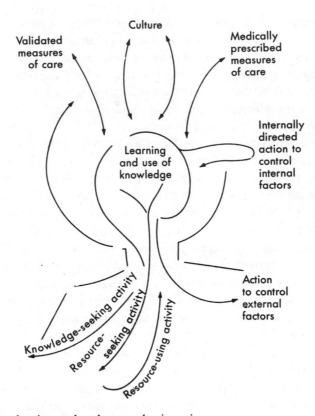

Fig. 7-4 Self-care has internal and external orientations.

spirit. In a scientifically advanced culture, people assume that sickness has some natural explanation, such as an infection, an indiscretion in eating or drinking, or the presence of a growth or tumor; and they will seek care from medical doctors. Keeping the body clean is a meaningless gesture in some cultures but an acceptable precaution in others. Even within scientifically advanced cultures, some groups may know more about health matters than other groups in the same society. In the more knowledgeable groups, care may be taken to meet nutritional and sanitary requirements when preparing food and to secure immunization and routine health checkups. In less knowledgeable groups, these precautions may be unknown or regarded indifferently or rejected.

The individual first learns of cultural standards within the family. Hence, there are many variations in self-care practices. The child learns from parents or guardians, who learned from their parents or guardians. While growing up, the child learns of additional and improved ways of self-care from other persons: teachers, classmates, neighbors, friends, and playmates. When health knowledge is widespread and applied, the preventive care measures that are carried out on a community basis—water purification, sewage disposal, and regulated practices in the processing of milk and other perishable foods—provide not only community service but also education and guidance on a broader community health basis. Individuals in each community must provide the leadership, daily effort, and financial and other resources required to start and maintain these services. If there is a breakdown in community services or if services are not provided, the burden of carrying out healthful practices falls upon individuals. For example, they may be required to boil or chlorinate water after a flood or engage in these practices routinely in areas where the water supply is not safe for internal use. Some environmental hazards, such as air pollution in large cities, are relatively uncontrolled, and persons living in such areas can do little to protect themselves except by stimulating community action, remaining indoors, or changing residence.

As indicated previously, self-care requires both learning and use of knowledge as well as enduring motivation and skill. The learning process includes the individual's gradual development of a repertoire of self-care practices and related skills. Ideally, children are helped to develop images of themselves as responsible self-care agents by gradually learning to perform care measures through which self-care requisites are met, for example, bathing, brushing teeth, looking to ensure that it is safe to cross a street, not touching hot objects. Self-care measures executed daily tend to become integrated into the fabric of daily living, and the purposes to be achieved through use of the measures (the self-care requisites being met) may not be kept in mind. Openness to oneself and to one's environment and to known and validated self-care requisites and cultural self-care practices are prerequisites for learning as well as for engaging in continuous and effective self-care.

The individualized factors of age, developmental state, and health generally determine the scope of self-care activities a person can perform. In addition, each adult's established pattern of responding to external and internal stimuli will affect decisions and other actions relative to self-care. Adult values and goals also affect the selection and performance of self-care actions in health or in illness. Self-care measures compatible with a person's goals and values are likely to be seen as beneficial. Their practice, however, depends on the person's judgment of whether he or she can perform the measures. The first step in the practice of self-care is answering these questions: Is it beneficial for me? Can I do it? Among adults, accepting oneself as being in particular functional and developmental states and having specific structural characteristics is another prerequisite for engaging in self-care that regulates human functional and developmental processes.*

---

* See Nursing Development Conference Group, pp. 280-282, for Melba Anger's, General ideal set of self-care actions, a model for use in working out the sets of care measures essential for meeting self-care requisites through the use of given technologies.

Understanding self-care as deliberate action

Deliberate action was described in Chapter 4. The following description of self-care as deliberate action should lead to further insights about deliberate action and about the development and exercise of self-care agency.

Distinguishing deliberate action

Self-care and care of dependents are forms of human activity referred to as deliberate action. This means that it is purposeful goal- or result-seeking activity. It also implies that the meaning of the result sought is identified before the action is taken. This can be done at various levels of understanding. For example, adults tend to care for themselves and their dependents to sustain, protect, and promote human functioning. If adults approach care with a background of scientific knowledge, they may see results in terms of integrated functioning, as in bringing about a new metabolic balance through the controlled intake of nutrients. A person may also formulate results in terms of what he or she hopes to experience, for example, to feel better or, as related to dental hygiene, to have a "fresh" mouth or, when under dental care for a pathologic condition of the gums, to stop bleeding. Deliberate action is essentially action to achieve a foreseen result that is preceded by investigation, reflection, and judgment to appraise the situation and by a thoughtful, deliberate choice of what should be done. An adequate concept of deliberate action includes ideas to describe circumstances leading to the decision about what should be done and events and circumstances necessary to bring about the result selected. Action is deliberate when it is based on an informed judgment about the outcome(s) being sought from acting in a particular way.

Deliberate action is distinguished from physiologically and psychologically "programed mechanisms" for responding to internal and external conditions. These are reflex activity (sneezing), instinctual urge (impulse to seek food), emotional reaction (sudden arousal of fear and movement to avoid a falling object), and feelings of pleasantness and unpleasantness (discomfort and the desire to change position after sitting for a long time). These activity patterns, however, often serve as forces motivating individuals to focus attention on present conditions and reflect on their meaning, consider the possible outcomes of various courses of action, formulate a judgment on the appropriate action, and then decide to take a concrete course of action. This can be illustrated by an analysis of the common example of individuals deliberately maintaining specific positions for medical or dental examinations or treatments despite discomfort or even pain. Knowledge of the results of moving and not moving affect the individual's decision to control position. Physiologic or psychological mechanisms and habits will affect how long individuals can exert control over their position. Deliberate action is always self-initiated, self-directed, and controlled in regard to presenting conditions and circumstances. Human development includes learning how to take deliberate action about the commonly encountered conditions of human existence and daily living within specific environments.

The structural elements of concrete action systems, including self-care, dependent care, and nursing systems, are discrete, that is, single actions. A discrete action (e.g., the lifting of one's hand) when taken out of its position within a sequence of actions (e.g., drinking a glass of water) may not convey the purpose and hence the meaning of the action within the particular sequence. As mentioned earlier, Talcott Parsons used the term *unit act* to refer to the smallest assembly of goal-oriented actions that make sense (i.e., convey meaning within a system of action) (pp. 44-45).[3] It is important for nurses to understand action sequences in terms of the discrete actions and unit acts from which they are constituted. For example, what kind and number of discrete actions must be performed to meet the self-care requisite "to maintain a sufficient intake of water" by taking the quantity of water by mouth that satisfies the criterion measures for being sufficient? Some examples of discrete actions include grasping a glass, holding a glass, and lifting a glass containing a known quantity of fluid.

Two examples of nurses' use of their understanding of action sequences required for meeting self-care requisites are given in articles by Backscheider (pp. 1138-1146)[2] and Pridham (pp. 237-246).[4] As previously described, Backscheider was concerned with the assessment of the self-care abilities of members of an adult, ambulatory nursing population to meet their particularized self-care requisites associated with the condition diabetes mellitus. To develop a standard against which to assess the action abilities of patients, Backscheider analyzed the action sequences involved in meeting care requisites common to the population. Pridham investigated the same nursing questions from a somewhat different perspective. Her concern was to explore and collect data as a basis for judging the self-care capabilities evidenced by a hospitalized child with diabetes mellitus who was under nursing care. The question to be answered was: What role can the child fulfill in her own self-care? Manifestation of and criteria for judging the psychological development of the child (and factors affecting it) in relation to her self-care role were one focus of the investigation. Both of these investigations clearly point to the relationship between the (1) *demand* on individuals to consistently and effectively perform particular self-care actions in some sequence, with proper adjustments to prevailing internal and external conditions, and (2) their self-care *action capabilities* at particular times in the life cycle under particular living circumstances.

Estimative and transitional operations

Persons who can produce effective self-care have knowledge of themselves and knowledge of environmental conditions. Before they can affirm the appropriate thing to do, they must gain knowledge of the courses of action open to them and of their effectiveness and desirability. Effective producers of self-care bring the first phase of self-care to closure by making a decision about the actions they will take and those they will avoid.

Providers of self-care require two kinds of knowledge: empirical knowledge of events and of internal and external conditions and antecedent knowledge that aids them in making observations, attaching meaning to their observations, and correlating the meaning of events and conditions with possible courses of action. Knowledge extends to (1) internal or external conditions relevant to health and well-being, for example, stiffness and pain in the joints of the hands or feet; (2) characteristics of the conditions, for example, the degree of stiffness related to the mobility of the joints or the degree of the constancy and severity of the pain; (3) the meaning of these conditions for health and well-being, for example, that the identified conditions indicate an improvement or worsening of a diagnosed joint disorder; and (4) the beneficial or harmful results that will come about by taking one course of action in preference to another, for example, consulting the physician, resuming a prescribed therapeutic regimen that has been neglected, or using the affected parts of the body. The qualitative and quantitative requirements for empirical and antecedent knowledge are related to the number and kinds of self-care requisites, methods for meeting them, external conditions, including the location and availability of resources, and other factors.

Under a daily living routine, self-care requisites follow a normal and consistent pattern. The decisions of an adult in regard to meeting self-care requisites are "programed" in the sense that experience A calls for deliberate action B. When a person is in ill health, however, the usual pattern of the therapeutic self-care demand changes. The ill person may experience new and more self-care requisites in a totally different time distribution, and more knowledge and effort may be needed to arrive at valid judgments about self-care. In fact, medical or nursing assistance may be necessary for the judgments to be valid.

Another self-care requisite may affect the decision making. For example, a need for food may occur at the same time that a person has received a medical order to take "no food" for some time. Making judgments and decisions about self-care must take into account time specifications and the precedence that meeting one self-care requisite takes over meeting other requisites. Environmental conditions are also relevant to making judgments and decisions about self-care. The number and nature of the inquiries the self-care provider makes about environmental conditions vary with the provider's familiarity with the surroundings. A person may be half awake yet have sufficient information to decide what he or she can and will do about being cold. In an unfamiliar place, a person may decide that being cold has advantages over changing air temperature or circulation.

Individuals must have some understanding of the meaning and value of self-care to make rational and reasonable self-care judgments and decisions. Level of maturity, knowledge, life experiences, habits of thought, and health state will all affect this understanding. Knowledge of self-care measures useful in meeting self-care requisites varies with life experiences. Opportunities for learning about self-care vary with families and communities. This learning process, which is continuous throughout life, is necessary for understanding self-care and being motivated to make decisions about it and to produce it for oneself and one's dependents.

Knowledge of the purposes and meaning of self-care provides the basis for appraising and attaching value to engaging in particular courses of self-care action. Factors internal to individuals may interfere with appraisal and with judgments and decisions, for example, extreme agitation, inexperience, or level of cognitive development. External factors, such as lack of resources or extreme social pressure, also affect judgments and decisions. Nurses should understand that at times self-care decisions may be based on the meaning care activities have for significant others. For example, a person decides to follow a particular course of self-care action because it will please the family. Regardless of motive, the decision to follow a particular course of self-care action determines whether an individual will take action to meet specific self-care requisites.

Knowing what conditions are relevant to health and well-being and why they are relevant at various stages of the life cycle is essential for effective engagement in the investigative, judgment-making, and decision-making activities of the first phase of self-care action. Judgments may be *rational* in that they are preceded by thought about what conditions exist and what can be done. Judgments may not be *reasonable*, however, in that they are not in accord with the existing therapeutic self-care demand and existing circumstances relating to health and well-being. Both scientific knowledge and common-sense knowledge are essential in the first phase of self-care. The investigations and the ensuing judgments and decisions made in the first phase give expression to the culture of individuals and to their self-images as self-care agents. Some individuals hesitate or refuse to investigate conditions that are significant for self-care. Other individuals are willing to explore what exists and what is possible but have difficulty in making judgments about what can and should be done, whereas others have difficulty in making the final decision about what to do. If the first phase of self-care action does not end with a decision, phase two will not ensue.

Production operations

Phase two begins with the decision about the course of action to be followed in relation to the specific demand or set of demands for self-care. The choice of what will or will not be done terminates the first phase of deliberate action. The choice made sets the goal for phase two because it specifies what kind of action will be taken. The questions raised by the self-care agent now include: How can I proceed in relation to my choice? What must I do? What resources do I need? Do I have them? Can I perform all the actions correctly and effectively at the time when they should be performed and for as long as they need to be performed? Will other duties interfere? How will I know if I am proceeding correctly? What rules will I follow? How will I know if I am getting the results I want? Who can help me if I need help?

The accomplishment of the various kinds of universal, developmental, and health-deviation self-care requires *expenditure of effort to satisfy the demands for care* as these demands are known and understood when action begins or as it proceeds. Effort will be demanded until specific results are achieved and as frequently as the result is required or until there is evidence that the effort is not productive. Effort is not random but deliberate. It is directed by the agent toward the result desired by following some standard technique or procedure or by adjusting action to the factors in the situation that can be changed or controlled. Attention is focused on the action performed and on evidence to be used in judging if the action is correct and if the desired result is or has been achieved. Deliberate effort should cease when the self-care agent knows that the desired result has been achieved. Effort may be withheld or changed if there is evidence that the result is not being achieved or that some other result is preferable. Expenditure of effort in self-care may not be pleasurable, and it may eliminate opportunities for other activities.

The essential condition for the expenditure of effort to meet self-care demands in specific situations at specific times is the ability to initiate and persevere in self-care to achieve desired results. This results from (1) having specific and requisite knowledge and skills, for example, knowing how to obtain dental care, how to make an appointment, and how to describe the problem; (2) being sufficiently motivated to initiate and continue efforts until results are achieved; for example, the desire to avoid loss of teeth may motivate a regimen of dental hygiene for months or years; (3) being committed to meeting particular demands for care to the degree that forgetting is eliminated or minimized and proper priority is afforded to measures of care; for example, thoughtful performance and a routine for performing prescribed dental care; (4) being able to execute the movements required; and (5) having energy and a sense of well-being sufficient to initiate and sustain self-care effort; for example, in severe illness or disability a person may be unable to care for teeth and gums. Being able to initiate and sustain self-care effort to achieve the desired result is related to the kinds of self-care required, to external conditions, and to internal factors that affect the ability to perform deliberate actions.

Individuals may be able to initiate and persevere in self-care action to meet universal requirements if they follow routine practices but may be unable at a particular time to change old practices or to add new practices. Becoming able may involve changing one's ideas about health and illness, developing new skills, and becoming committed to new ways of proceeding. This may be very difficult for some individuals despite their knowledge that the changes should be made. Engagement in health-deviation self-care may be more difficult since abilities are specified both by the demands for care arising from the health deviation and by the medical therapy prescribed. As previously stated, specific knowledge and skills that have a base in medical science and technology are required for health-deviation self-care. Changes in medical technology have produced sometimes complicated demands for management of self-care. For example, in some kinds of drug therapy the individual may have to divide pills, take a different dose on specified days, or follow one series of doses for five days. Development of readiness to engage in health-deviation self-care may require specialized assistance. Perseverance in self-care may require assistance in the form of support and guidance.

Having some understanding of the meaning and value of self-care is fundamental to engaging in it. Some factors affecting understanding and meaning were described under the first phase of self-care. Knowledge of self-care demands and the measures to meet them is essential. Knowledge must be applied not only in the initiation of action but also throughout the performance. Knowledge must be applied to guide the performance of specific tasks and to make the practical judgments required about what to do next. Lack of skill in task performance, failure to validate judgments, or inability to make judgments will adversely affect the accomplishment of self-care. Factors in the external environment, for example, availability of resources, may affect either the initiation or the continuation of self-care action.

Initiation of and perseverance in action to meet self-care demands demonstrate the individual's power of agency in this form of deliberate action. Any action limitation decreases powers of agency and may give rise to a need for assistance. Action limitations related to the individual's health state constitute the reasons why people need nursing.

SELF-CARE AGENCY, PRACTICAL CONSIDERATIONS

Nurses, other health workers, and the public must understand that self-care is work requiring energy expenditure, time, and resources. It cannot be done without the requisite enabling human capabilities and without knowledge of what should be done. Persons' calculated therapeutic self-care demands express the kind and amount of work to be done. Persons' capabilities to engage in self-care at particular times and places identify their abilities to do the work of self-care.

As previously mentioned, self-care agency, conceptualized as a complex of human capabilities particularized for one kind of action or work, named self-care can be investigated in relation to its development, operability, and adequacy.

Self-care agency, developed and developing

The presence or absence of the capability named self-care agency when concretely considered is related to the stage of development of individuals, including their development of self-direction with respect to goal selection and their physical, cognitive, and psychosocial development. Self-care agency reveals itself as the developed or developing capability to engage in the *investigative and decision-making phase of self-care* (phase one) and the capability to engage in the *production phase of self-care* (phase two). There may be an unequal development of capabilities for phase one and phase two operations due to the states of development of individuals. For example, children learn to perform and do perform some measures of self-care before learning the related investigative operations. This does not rule out young children's determinations that they want or don't want to perform this or that self-care measure. Children also make decisions that they want to learn how to perform certain care measures so that they can be the care agent with respect to aspects of required, prescribed, medical treatment measures, for example, giving themselves medication by injection. Some adults whose cognitive development has been arrested because of lack of schooling or other factors may have greater capability for becoming proficient in performing operations of the productive phase of self-care than for investigative operations.

Self-care agency can be identified as *present* when it is *developed* or is *developing*. Development is associated with certain situations that call for self-care action and with care measures to attain certain ends or goals. In other words, self-care agency at particular times reveals itself in the performance by individuals of learned sequences of self-care actions to meet foreseen goals and that its appraisal requires investigations of what individuals do and do not do consistently in self-care. Self-care agency is considered *absent* when capabilities for performing operations for both phases of self-care are undeveloped. This holds for infants even though their *inherent capacities for action* and *impulses to action* are operative, for example, the action impulses and the inherent action capacities exhibited in the feeding behaviors of infants. Arnold describes the feeding behaviors of infants as implying "wanting, appraising, liking, and disliking," as well as recognition that "no more is wanted," and "an impulse to stop" (pp. 54-55).[5]

Capacities for self-care that are developed and could be made operative by individuals are sometimes not exercised. This may be through deliberate choice, by forgetting, or because factors of time or place or the availability of required resources did not allow for performance of self-care operations. Such situations must be differentiated from situations where the capability for self-care is developed but cannot be made operational *at all* or to *some degree* because of structural or functional conditions associated with specific pathologies, states of illness, injury, and disability.

The degrees of development of self-care agency of individuals in concrete situations of daily living and in nursing practice situations can be identified for persons of various ages within the following five developmental categories (p. 205).[1]
1. Undeveloped
2. Developing
3. Developed but not stabilized
    a.   in need of continued development
    b.   in process of continued development

      c.   in need of redevelopment
      d.   in process of redevelopment
   4. Developed and stabilized
      a.   in need of redevelopment
      b.   in process of redevelopment
      c.   redeveloped and stabilized
   5. Developed but declining

The development or redevelopment of self-care agency by individuals throughout their life cycles should be understood as associated with the human desire to know, the power to learn, and movement to higher and more complex stages of personal development.

Self-care agency, operability, and adequacy

Questions about the operability and adequacy of self-care agency of individuals assume some degree of its development. It is recognized that self-care agency, whatever its degree of development at particular times under some human conditions and circumstances, cannot be exercised at all or only to a limited degree. Health states of individuals or specific effects of a health disorder or injury can adversely affect their performance of self-care operations and the operability of their foundational capabilities and dispositions for self-care. At particular times, persons can be so adversely conditioned by human and environmental factors that their self-care agency is not operative or only partly operative for some time.

The adequacy of self-care agency is critical in nursing practice situations. Lack of adequacy and the health or health-related reasons for lack of adequacy of self-care agency of persons seeking nursing determine the legitimacy of nursing practice situations. Critical judgments of nurses about the adequacy of patients' self-care agency presume knowledge of patients' calculated therapeutic self-care demands or components of them and the capabilities required for meeting them and making needed adjustments. Nurses must also know the degree of development and operability of persons' developed powers of self-care agency in making final judgments about adequacy and the reasons for the adequacy or the degree in inadequacy of self-care agency of individuals under nursing care.

Self-care limitations

Persons who engage in self-care are knowing about themselves, their functional states, and the care that they need. They want to know. They appraise, investigate, and make judgments and decisions. They engage in result-achieving courses of action and are able to manage themselves in their environments. Self-care abilities are expressions of what persons have learned to do and can do in the investigative and decision-making phase of self-care and in its production phase under presenting human and environmental conditions. Self-care limitations are expressions of that which restricts individuals from providing the amount and kind of self-care that they need under existent and changing conditions and circumstances.

Self-care limitations are expressed in terms of restricting influences on the operations of self-care. Three kinds of limitations are identified: restrictions of knowing, restrictions on judgments and decision making, and restrictions on result-achieving actions in either the investigative or production phases of self-care.

Limitations of knowing about one's own functioning, about needed self-care, and about the operations through which self-care is accomplished are associated with individuals' past experiences and with what is being experienced in the present. Some conditions and factors associated with limitations of knowing are identified in three sets.

Set one

- Changed modes of functioning that are new and are not understood; lack of fit between what one has experienced and what one is experiencing
- New unrecognized requirements for self-care associated with changed functional states
- New self-care requisites that are parts of a prescribed regimen of health care that are not understood
- Lack of knowledge essential for performing the operations needed to meet specific self-care requisites using specified methods and measures of care

Set two

- Impairments of sensory functioning, of perception, and of memory that interfere with the acquisition of empirical knowledge or recall of knowledge
- Disturbances of human integrated functioning that adversely affect empirical consciousness, cognitive functioning, and rationality associated, for example, with (1) organic conditions that are productive of toxic states, (2) mental and emotional illness, (3) brain disorders, and (4) effects of material substances such as prescribed or unprescribed drugs

Set three

- Dispositions and orientations that result in perceptions, meanings, and appraisals of situations that are not in accord with reality
- Movement away from action to acquire new and essential knowledge
- Modes of cognitive functioning that affect mental operations associated with knowing when action is to be taken, adjusting action to existent or emerging conditions and knowing when to stop action, and with organizing sets of actions into meaningful sequences toward result achievement

The three sets of limitations of knowing differ in kind; therefore, persons with such limitations require different kinds of help with respect to self-care. The first set expresses absence or lack of required knowledge. The second set expresses limitations for knowing environmental conditions and for knowing self and environment. The third set expresses psychic and cognitional limitations for developing insights about situations, for seeking to acquire knowledge, and for the knowing that is basic to doing in result-seeking endeavors.

Limitations for making judgments and decisions about components of a therapeutic self-care demand or about the regulation of the exercise or development of self-care agency are associated with individuals' views of themselves, their habits of investigation and reflections before making decisions about what action to take, their desires to take action that is appropriate and beneficial, and their having requisite knowledge and skills. Eight factors or conditions that set limitations on individuals' judgment and decision making with respect to self-care matters are expressed.

Set one

• Lack of familiarity with a situation and lack of knowledge about appropriate questions for investigation
• Insufficient knowledge or lack of necessary skills for seeking and acquiring appropriate technical knowledge from individuals or reference materials
• Lack of sufficient and valid antecedent and empirical knowledge to reflect and reason within a self-care frame of reference

Set two

• Interferences with the direction and maintenance of voluntary attention necessary to investigate situations from the perspective of self-care, for example, limitations of consciousness, intense emotional states, sudden or strong likes and dislikes, overriding interests and concerns
• Inability or limited ability to imagine alternate courses of action that could be taken and the consequence of each

Set three

• Reluctance or refusal of individuals to investigate situations of self-care as a basis for determining what can and should be done
• Reluctance to stop reflection and make a decision once a desirable and suitable course of action is identified and understood
• Refusal to make a decision about a possible course of self-care action or about the exercise or development of self-care agency

Limitations expressed in sets one and two interfere with individuals having or getting an adequate base of information for judgment and decision making. Limitations in set three indicate avoidance of decision making. Such limitations may reflect patterns of behavior typical of individuals, or they may reflect individuals' attachment of meaning to a situation and movement away from involvement in it.

Limitations for engagement in result-achieving courses of action within the investigative and production phases of self-care, including limitations for self-management, are associated with human functional states and with environmental conditions and circumstances. The following examples of limiting factors and conditions are expressed in four sets.

Set one

- Lack of knowledge or developed skills needed to operationalize decisions about self-care
- Lack of resources for self-care

Set two

- Lack of sufficient energy for sustained action in the investigative and production phases of self-care
- Inability or limited ability to control body movements in the performance of required actions in either or both phases of self-care
- Inability or limited ability of individuals to attend to themselves as self-care agents and to exercise vigilance with respect to existent and changing internal and external conditions

Set three

- Lack of interest in meeting self-care requisites
- Lack of desire to meet perceived needs for self-care
- Goal orientations and value placed on self-care inadequate to sustain engagement in the investigative and production actions essential for knowing and meeting therapeutic self-care demands

Set four

- Family members' or others' deliberate interferences with the performance of the courses of action necessary for individuals to know and meet their therapeutic self-care demands
- Patterns of personal or family living that restrict engagement in self-care operations
- Lack of support systems needed to sustain individuals when self-care is complex, time-consuming, and stressful
- Crisis situations in the family or household that interfere with self-care
- Disaster situations that interfere with engagement in self-care and with the usual ways for meeting self-care requisites

The first three of the four sets of interferences with engagement in courses of actions required in the phases of self-care express absence of conditions necessary for self-care. The fourth set of interferences is associated with individuals' conditions of living.

The approach to the formulation and expression of types of self-care limitations was taken because it fits the conditions found in concrete situations of practice. The presence of evidence of the named types of limitations singly or in various combinations in persons under nursing care provides one basis for nurses to determine the amount and kind of nursing required. It provides a basis for nurses' judgments about valid methods of helping and judgments about interpersonal processes to foster or maintain readiness on the part of patients to receive help through nursing.

SELF-CARE DEFICITS

The term self-care deficit refers to the relationship between self-care agency and therapeutic self-care demands of individuals in which capabilities for self-care, because of existent limitations, are not equal to meeting some or all of the components of their therapeutic self-care demands. Self-care deficits are associated with the kinds of components that make up the therapeutic self-care demand and with the number and variety of self-care limitations.

Self-care deficits are identified as complete or partial. A complete self-care deficit means no capability to meet a therapeutic self-care demand.

Partial deficits for self-care may be extensive or may be limited to an incapacity for meeting one or several self-care requisites within a therapeutic self-care demand. Nurses' knowledge of the distinctive features of self-care deficits in individuals in concrete situations of nursing practice is a result of nursing diagnostic activities to determine individuals' self-care abilities and limitations and of identification and particularization of their self-care requisites. However, experienced nurses in their initial contacts with patients habitually make observations to answer one of the initial questions of nursing practice: Is there gross evidence of a self-care deficit that is health-derived or health-related? This question could be phrased differently: Is it reasonable to assume, in light of known conditions, that there is an existent or emerging self-care (or dependent-care) deficit?

Presence of one or some combination of the following named conditions would constitute gross evidence of a self-care deficit:
- Absence of ongoing engagement in self-care or gross inadequacy of what is done to meet self-care requisites
- Limited awareness or loss of awareness of self and environment, excluding that due to natural sleep
- Inability to recall past experience in the control of conduct
- Limitations for judgment and decision making about self-care associated with lack of knowledge and unfamiliarity with internal and external conditions

***Exercise* to aid in understanding self-care limitations**

1. Read and think about the three kinds of self-care limitations described in the section entitled, "Self-Care Limitations."
2. For nurses to make judgments about the absence or presence of these limitations, nurses must obtain particular kinds and amounts of data, facts about reality conditions, and events on which to base their judgments.
3. Think about the question: How would I know if such limitations were or were not present in a particular patient?
4. Then consider the kinds of data and the sources of data that would be necessary to make judgments about the absence or presence of:
   a. Limitations of knowing
   b. Limitations for making judgments and decisions
   c. Limitations for engagement in result-achieving courses of action
5. Select one of the kinds of self-care limitations, *a* or *b* or *c* above, and develop a tool for use in obtaining data about one or more limitations named in a set, for example, limitations of knowing, set one, limitations 3 and 4. In developing the tool, seek answers to these questions for each limitation:
   a. To what do I attend?
   b. What information do I need?
   c. How can I obtain the information?
   d. What will be the form of my data?
   e. How much data will I need?
6. As part of the process of finding answers to these questions, talk informally to *individuals* about their having experienced such limitations and to *nurses* about their identifying such limitations in their patients.
7. Refine the tool. Have it reviewed to get answers to this question about each limitation: If I obtain the kinds of data indicated in the tool, will I have an adequate basis for making a judgment about the presence or absence of the limitation?

- Events indicative of disordered or impaired functioning giving rise to new health-deviation self-care requisites and for adjustments in one or more or all of the universal self-care requisites
- Needs of individuals to incorporate newly prescribed, complex self-care measures into their self-care systems, the performance of which requires specialized knowledge and skills to be acquired through training and experience

In seeking understanding of self-care agency, self-care limitations, and self-care deficits, it is important to recognize two dimensions of self-care. One dimension relates to the deliberate action operations of self-care involving self-awareness, rational thought, conscious purpose, plan of procedure, and willingness and resolution in proceeding according to an initial or revised plan. This is the personal, purposive dimension of self-care in the full human and psychological sense. The second dimension of self-care relates to the events that occur within individuals and their environments as a result of the joint presence of particular inputs and the existent human or environmental conditions. When particular inputs, for example, some amount and quality of ingested food, correlate directly with human or environmental conditions to bring about sought-after and desired focal conditions, the self-care measures performed have validity (pp. 143-147).[6]

In individuals' development of self-care agency, both dimensions of self-care must be learned. This includes knowing the kind and amount of data needed to make judgments about internal and external conditions, knowing how to obtain the data, and making judgments on the basis of particular kinds and amounts of data. It also includes knowing what should and should not be done under certain conditions. Thus the development of self-care agency goes beyond learning culturally prescribed self-care practices. Self-care deficits are associated not only with individuals' limitations for performing care measures, but also with the lack of validity or effectiveness of the self-care in which they engage.

DEPENDENT-CARE AGENCY

The terms **dependent-care, dependent-care agency,** and **dependent-care agent** were introduced within the frame of self-care deficit nursing theory when the need for them became evident during the 1970s. The terms were introduced in the course of curriculum revision deliberations by nursing faculty of Incarnate Word College, San Antonio, Texas. Since then, the terms have come into wider use. There are increased needs for dependent-care agents with the growth in the aging population; in numbers of persons with chronic illness, debilitating illnesses, and disabling conditions; and in the number and complexity of health-deviation-type self-care requisites to be met by or for individuals after hospital discharge.

The concept **dependent-care agency** is in the process of formalization. Like self-care agency, its broad conceptual structure is formed by capabilities to perform estimative, transitional, and productive operations in knowing and meeting the therapeutic self-care demand of another (or components thereof). There are enabling power components specific to the operations as operations relate to knowing and meeting components of the other's therapeutic self-care demand. Both of these depend on foundational capabilities and dispositions with adjustments to focus on meeting needs of another and working with the bodily parts of another person.

Dependent-care agency described

Dependent-care agency is the complex, acquired ability of mature or maturing persons to know and meet some or all of the self-care requisites of adolescent or adult persons who have health-derived or health-associated limitations of self-care agency, which places them in socially dependent relationships for care. With respect to infants and children, **dependent-care agency** is the complex acquired ability to incorporate knowing and meeting health-deviation self-care requirements of infants and children and needed adjustments in universal and developmental-type self-care requisites into ongoing systems of infant care, child care, and parenting activities.

Dependent-care agents may work in close association with the physician of the persons they help or take care of. They may be contributors to an ongoing nursing system or work with nursing supervision and consultation.

The development of dependent-care agency by individuals is usually a response to needs of family members or friends for help with their continuing self-care. Dependent-care agency is developed to meet known existent and, at times, emerging needs of the persons to be helped or taken care of. More likely than not the primary focus for development is mastery of production operations of self-care, for example, maintaining cleanliness of wounds, including dressing changes as well as meeting requisites for maintenance of sufficient intake of water and food. When production operations must be adjusted to specific human and environmental conditions, as in the administration of some prescribed medications, there is need for development of capabilities for performing estimative and transitional operations of self-care. There is always need for development of capabilities to recognize emergency situations and to act promptly and effectively.

Dependent-care agents

Nurses are increasingly placed in positions where they must work with families or individuals to identify and select persons psychologically and physically able and willing to function as dependent-care agents for family members or friends. This is a demand on both nurses in hospitals and in home care nursing programs. Nurses recognize the importance of protecting the health and well-being of dependent-care agents. They understand the energy-depleting effects of maintaining systems of dependent-care in the home and the stress associated with it. Therapeutic self-care demands of dependent-care agents must be calculated and means for meeting them established.

The amount of instruction needed for persons to develop dependent-care agency requisite for situations where they will function varies with their life experiences, their knowledge, and their developed skills that can be adjusted to the care situation. The relationship of the dependent-care agent to the person to be helped, the willingness of this person to accept help, and the sense of duty on the part of each will affect what can be accomplished. Studies of situations where dependent-care agents function are ongoing, as well as studies of ways and means to assess the potential of individuals for this function or their developed dependent-care capabilities.

REFERENCES

1. From Nursing Development Conference Group, Orem DE, editor: Concept formalization in nursing: process and product, ed 2, Little, Brown, & Co., 1979, Boston, pp. 135-141, 183, 192-193, 195-196, 205.
2. Backscheider JE: Self-care requirements, self-care capabilities and nursing systems in the diabetic nurse management clinic, Am J Public Health 64:1138-1146, 1974.

3. Parsons T: The structure of social action, New York, 1937, McGraw-Hill, pp. 44-45.
4. Pridham KF: Instruction of a school-age child with chronic illness for increased self-care, using diabetes mellitus as an example, Int Nurs Stud 8:237-246, 1971.
5. From Arnold MB: Emotion and personality, vol II, Neurological and physiological aspects, New York, 1960, Columbia University Press, pp. 54-55.
6. See Sommerhoff G: Analytical biology, London, 1950, Oxford University Press, pp. 143-147.

SELECTED READINGS

Evers GCM: Appraisal of self-care agency, A.S.A.-Scale, Assen/Maastricht, The Netherlands, 1989, Van Gorcum & Co.

Gast HL, et al: Self-care agency: conceptualizations and operationalizations, Adv Nurs Sci 12:26-38, 1989.

Meade CD, Byrd JC, and Lee M: Improving patient comprehension of literature on smoking, Am J Public Health 79:1411-1412, 1989.

Moore JB, and Gaffney KF: Development of an instrument to measure mothers' performance of self-care activities for children, Adv Nurs Sci 12:76-83, 1989.

Nursing Development Conference Group: Self-care agency: a conceptual analysis and self-care agency: diagnostic considerations. In Orem DE, editor: Concept formalization in nursing: process and product, Boston, 1979, Little, Brown & Co., pp. 181-231.

Pletcher MS: Nutrition self-care: an adaptation and component of the therapeutic regimen. In Riehl-Sisca J, editor: The science and art of self-care, Norwalk, 1985, Appleton-Century-Crofts, pp. 132-141.

Taylor SG, and Robinson-Purdy AV: Assessing self-management and dependent-care capabilities of hospitalized adults and care givers in preparation for discharge. In Clinical and cultural dimensions around the world, Papers and abstracts presented at the First International Self-Care Deficit Nursing Theory Conference, Kansas City, Missouri, October 15-18, 1989, Columbia, Missouri, 1989, School of Nursing, University of Missouri-Columbia, The Curators of the University of Missouri, pp. 4-16.

CHAPTER 8

A consideration of health, health care, and nursing

Nursing is recognized as one health service within a family of health services. The term *health* is used in a variety of ways, and it is necessary to sort out the meanings attached to it before addressing the question: What is it about nursing that affords it recognition as a health service?

THE TERM *HEALTH*

Health and **healthy** are terms used to describe living things—plants, animals, human beings—when they are structurally and functionally whole or sound. Individual human beings are said to be healthy or unhealthy. The same words are used to describe parts of the body, physiologic mechanisms, control of emotional reactions, and mental functioning as well as attitudes and motives. Individuals evaluate their own states of integrity or wholeness, appraising each day, or sometimes more frequently, whether they feel well or sick. They also make judgments about the health of others with whom they have direct or even indirect contact. These evaluative judgments imply that individuals have ideas of what health means, at least to them, as well as ideas of the evidence needed to judge that a person is healthy or unhealthy.

In light of the complexity of human functioning and its relationships to environmental elements and conditions, the term *health* has considerable general utility in describing the state of wholeness or integrity of human beings. However, temporary indispositions, such as not feeling well today, having a brief illness, or being injured, do not necessarily place the individual in the unhealthy category. Some structural and functional changes do not seriously interfere with human integrated functioning or else interfere with it in a circumscribed fashion. For example, a healthy child or adult with a fracture of an extremity may feel well though not structurally or functionally whole because of the break in the bone and the limitations of movement. Individuals in this state would be referred to as "injured and disabled" rather than as "sick" or "in poor health." However, any deviation from normal structure or functioning is properly referred to as an absence of health in the sense of wholeness or integrity.

Human beings are distinguished from other living things by their capacity (1) to reflect upon themselves and their environment, (2) to symbolize what they experience, and (3) to use symbolic creations (ideas, words) in thinking, in communicating, and in guiding efforts to do and to make things that are beneficial for themselves or others. Health, then, must include that which makes a person human (form of mental life), operating in conjunction with physiologic and psychophysiologic mechanisms and a material structure (biologic life) and in relation to coexistence with other human beings (interpersonal and social life). The meaning of the term *health* changes as views about people's human and biologic characteristics change.

Members of the health professions realize that they should be concerned with health in relation to integrated human functioning, including the contribution of their roles to its attainment. The health professions are in a position where members must have knowledge from a number of different fields if they are to use and develop the health sciences and health technologies that are valid in bringing about the kinds of changes in human beings that move them toward, rather than away from, a state of wholeness, a state of human integrity. With the extension of the term *health* to include psychological, interpersonal, and social aspects of living, as well as the commonly emphasized physical aspect, the health professions are beginning to recognize that, ideally, health is the responsibility of a society and its individual members and not of any one segment of that society.

The physical, psychological, interpersonal, and social aspects of health are inseparable in the individual. For example, consider a mother of several small children who has learned that she has tuberculosis. Her husband is employed full time in a local factory, and the family lives in a crowded flat in a large city. Her income from a part-time job has been important in providing some of the essential family needs. Her medical treatment, in addition to drug therapy, requires a prescribed amount of rest, a nutritious diet, and fresh air. The family's socioeconomic situation will affect the mother's ability to obtain the care she needs to arrest the tuberculosis. Her concern for her family and herself, in turn, will affect her mental state and thus her ability to rest and to participate in her own therapy. The maturity of the husband and wife, their creative abilities, the availability of resources, and the support received from family members, friends, neighbors, and persons in the helping professions will affect the well-being of the family. The abilities of the husband and wife to cooperate and to coordinate their efforts toward designing and producing a system of effective self-care for the wife that is integrated with dependent-care systems for the children and the husband's self-care system will be a determining force in providing restorative health care for the mother and primary preventive health care for the children and father.

Adversity in the form of ill health, scarcity of resources, or widespread disaster brings human suffering. But adversity may also bring people increased understanding of themselves and others. The human qualities of courage, patience or self-possession, and willingness to give of oneself to others are often revealed by people who suffer adversity.

The hypothetical example illustrates in a general way that various aspects of human functioning are interrelated. Accepting that an individual is an integrated whole is often difficult, perhaps because the sciences split humanity up; that is, they focus on different aspects of human structure or functioning to develop bodies of knowledge about human beings. Lay persons and some health workers tend to think of the individual human being as having one part called a *body* and another part called a *mind,* with the two parts interacting. A more acceptable image is that a human being is a unity that can be viewed as functioning biologically, symbolically, and socially.

Deliberate action by adults to maintain a state of health for themselves and their dependents involves the components of self-care discussed in Chapter 6. Self-care as action requires a base of education in the home, at school, and from practical experiences in self-care. Self-care is only one aspect of healthful living, but without continuous self-care that has therapeutic quality, integrated human functioning will be disrupted. Good health habits are essential in maintaining health, but the ability to change old habits to meet new requirements may be as essential. Education in self-care, not just training in self-care practices, is necessary for the development of knowledge, skills, and positive attitudes related to self-care and health. Children, adolescents, and young adults have interests in health and health care. All too frequently, adults with whom young people have contact are unable, unwilling, or uninterested in providing adequate help. In modern society parents and other educators should be concerned with what can be done to enable children to learn to direct themselves toward a state of integrated functioning and well-being that would promote human dignity and beauty even in illness and disability.

HEALTH AS A STATE

Dictionaries as well as the World Health Organization, an agency of the United Nations, use the term **state** in defining health. Human health or well-being is defined as "the state of being whole or sound." Although the word **health** is especially used to refer to the state of being free from "physical disease or pain," it is also used to refer to "soundness of mind and soul." The World Health Organization emphasizes that health is a state of physical, mental, and social well-being and not merely the absence of disease or infirmity. To conceptualize health, it is necessary to explore the term *state* in relationship to being sound or whole.

The term *state* applied to people is defined as the way a person reveals his or her existence. State is used in a very general fashion when applying it to well-defined conditions of persons that are considered as a whole without specification or analysis of components, for example, the states of being calm or anxious, asleep or awake, acutely ill, debilitated, depressed. State is also defined as a compound state. The term is used in this sense, for example, when a person's health state is expressed as a set of determined values of specified human characteristics that simultaneously reveal some aspects of the person's existence. The specified characteristics are worked with as a compound entity (a vector) having a definite number of components, which, when taken together as a set, describe the state of the person at a particular time.

Examples of the use of the term *state* in the health field in the sense of compound state include the taking of the vital signs of temperature, pulse, respiration, and blood pressure and considering these together as an index of the state of selected vital processes. The component parts of and the findings of a complete or partial physical examination can be considered a compound entity useful in specifying an individual's health state to some desired completeness (pp. 30-31).[1] Since the usefulness of the vital signs or physical examination findings may differ from time to time, it is necessary to monitor events or seek evidence of characteristics during a particular time period to have knowledge of (1) the actual frequencies of the occurrence of events and (2) their determinate probabilities (pp. 63-64).[2]

The term *sound* means possession of full vigor and strength and the absence of signs of disease and morbidity. The term *whole* means that nothing has been omitted, ignored, or lessened. These terms, when used together in regard to health, signify human functional and structural integrity, absence of genetic defects, and progressive integrated development of a human being as an individual unity moving toward higher and higher levels of integration (pp. 469-479).[2] Each human being as a complex unity is often described as having physical, psychic, and intellectual characteristics that become more highly integrated with progressive development. It is obvious that health, defined as a state of being sound or whole, is a state of human perfection that includes continuing human development. It is also obvious that bodies of accumulated knowledge about humankind are necessary for making determinations of the health states of individuals. Furthermore, time-oriented norms are required if judgments are to be made about structural, functional, and genetic integrity and about human development.

A person's general appearance is often the basis used for making judgments about the person's health state, for example, making the judgment that this or that person appears to be in good or poor health or that his or her health has improved or worsened. A scientific appraisal of an individual's health state requires that the term *state* be used in the compound sense. This approach necessitates that persons with the requisite knowledge search out the sets of human characteristics that will be useful in specifying health state to some desired completeness. Within the health field, biologists and physicians have contributed substantial bodies of knowledge about the physical aspects of human health. Norms have been established and approaches to determining anatomic, physiologic, genetic, and psychophysiologic components of the health state have been developed and refined (including specifying the kinds of information needed, data-gathering techniques, and rules for inference).

Psychic and intellectual components of an individual's health state viewed in the compound sense include (1) inner experiences, (2) behaviors and conduct (deliberate action) that can be observed in interpersonal and group situations, and (3) solitary endeavors. Concepts of mental health are not as firmly structured as those of physical health. Physical examinations, psychological tests, and the eliciting of subjective information from individuals about their behavior in interpersonal and group situations are used as means for obtaining information as a basis for making judgments about health states along these mental health dimensions. The development and use of these means is apportioned among a number of disciplines.

Health workers, including nurses, obtain and use information that describes and explains selected aspects of human structure and functioning. For example, nurses will use information obtained and expressed in terms of the disciplines of physiology and pathology in making judgments about self-care requisites and self-care agency of patients. Nurses are responsible for defining the components that describe health states of individuals and the quality and quantity of information about these components that are sufficient for nursing purposes. In order to deal with the many kinds of information obtainable about human developments and structural and functional states, some nurses and other health workers use the concept of "field," as Kurt Lewin defined it with respect to the life space of an individual or group (pp. xi and 45).[3] Field theory is essentially a method useful in analyzing relationships and organizing information. Those who use this approach must identify and describe the component parts of the field (the vector) that they are examining.

When health is described as a state of being whole and sound, it is necessary to link human growth and development to human structure and functioning. A person's state of growth and development changes over time. At a specific time, a person will exhibit a degree of structural and functional integrity according to his or her stage of development. Genetic factors can affect the development as well as the structural and functional integrity of individuals.

For nursing purposes, it is more practical (1) to recognize that at any one time an individual has reached a particular stage of development, which means that certain developments have occurred or are occurring and that specific developments are or are not in accord with established norms and (2) then to attend to the person's functional and structural integrity. For this reason and for purposes of this text, health state and developmental state are considered as separate entities. Nurses often *assume* that the developments of a person of a particular age are in accord with norms, for example, accepting the mature appearance of an individual as a basis for the judgment that he or she is mature. If a nurse *observes*, for example, that an individual cannot read or write, the nurse begins to examine various developments (e.g., cognitive developments) in order to know how to help the person understand and deal with meeting the therapeutic self-care demand.

For practical reasons, members of the various health professions must be able to take an approach to the health of individuals that will enable them to fulfill their purposes as health professionals in the social group. Ideally, members of the health professions view persons for whom they provide care as complex unities but view components of the health states of individuals from the perspectives of their own disciplines. This means that they know the meaning components have for their own specialized work.

Throughout life, individuals tend to learn that some combination of components usually will serve them well as an index of their health state. Persons with certain diseases and those under certain forms of medical diagnosis or therapy must learn to collect data as a basis for judging their own human functioning. Learning to determine and determining what combination of components will serve as an index of health state may be a part of the patient role in health care situations. Nurses should seek information about how patients perceive their own health states and the meanings they attach to these states or to various components.

POSITIONS ABOUT HEALTH AND WELL-BEING

In development of the self-care deficit theory of nursing the terms **health** and **well-being** are used to refer to two different but related human states. *Health* is used in the sense of a *state* of a person that is characterized by soundness or wholeness of developed human structures and of bodily and mental functioning. **Well-being** is used in the sense of individuals' perceived condition of existence. Well-being is a state characterized by experiences of contentment, pleasure, and kinds of happiness; by spiritual experiences; by movement toward fulfillment of one's self-ideal; and by continuing personalization. Well-being is associated with health, with success in personal endeavors, and with sufficiency of resources. However, individuals experience well-being and their human existence may be characterized by features of well-being even under conditions of adversity, including disorders of human structure and functioning.

Conceptualizations of health and well-being are related to points of view about human beings. These points of view should be made explicit for purposes of understanding human health and well-being.

Nurses in their writings express a variety of ways of viewing human beings. Emphasis is placed on the unity of human beings, on human beings as psychosomatic unities, on human beings as being greater than the sum of their parts, on human beings as open systems, on human beings as having various modalities of functioning, and on human beings as persons. Some nurses, as well as others in the health field, tend to search for an all encompassing way of viewing human beings and their health states. For nursing purposes it may be more effective to consider human beings from more than one point of view. The Nursing Development Conference Group held the position that in nursing there are practical advantages to viewing human beings as *persons,* as *symbolizers* and *agents,* as *organisms* and as *objects* subject to physical forces (pp. 122-123).[4]

The view of human beings as *persons* subsumes the views of human beings as agents and symbolizers and organisms. However, for practical purposes one or more of these views can be taken at different times without considering all that characterizes human beings as persons.

Before taking this or that view of human beings, it is a safeguard to posit that each human being like other living things is a *substantial or real unity* whose parts are formed and attain perfection through the differentiation of the whole during processes of development. The unity of living things stands in distinction to the unity of artifacts.

Since human beings have discernible parts (for example, arms, legs, stomach, lungs, functional systems such as urinary systems or neural circuits or neuroendocrine systems), it is essential to recognize them. Each developmentally differentiated structure or functional system is an existent entity with its own operations, with relations to other differentiated parts and to their operations, and to the unitary functioning of individuals who coexist in a world with other human beings. If there is acceptance of the real unity of individual human beings, there should be no difficulty in recognizing structural and functional differentiations within the unity.

Two points of view about human beings that afford considerable meaning to states of human health and well-being are that of human beings as *persons* and that of the *structural and functional differentiations of human beings.* Both are considered briefly.

The point of view of human beings as persons is a moving rather than a static one. It is the view of personalization of the individual, that is, movement toward maturation and achievement of the individual's human potential. This process of coming to be a person involves individuals in communications with their worlds; in action; in the exercise of the human desire to know, to seek the truth; and in the giving of themselves in the doing of good for themselves and others. Personalization is not a condition of individuals but a task in process while they live in coexistence with others.

Personalization proceeds as individuals live under conditions favorable or unfavorable to human developmental processes. Individuals learn to set their goals and choose among many goals as they move toward maturity. The process has two intertwining aspects. There is striving by individuals to achieve the potential of their natural endowments for physical and rational functioning while living a life of faith with respect to things hoped for and to perfect themselves as responsible human beings who raise questions, seek answers, reflect, and come to awareness of the relationship between what they know and what they do. *Self-realization* and *personality development* are terms used at times to refer to the process of personalization.

Individuals coming to view themselves as self-care or dependent-care agents, their exercise of responsibility for and engagement in self-care or dependent care, and their deliberate engagement in action to develop or redevelop the capabilities for self-care and dependent care are facets of the process of personalization. These facets of personalization relate to fulfillment of the potential of individuals for regulating their functioning toward soundness or wholeness (health of body and mind) within an existent potential and to their experiencing of well-being.

Some psychologists speak of persons who have progressed along the path of personalization to a high degree of maturity as *mentally healthy* and view *psychological maturity* and *intellectual maturity* as components of maturity proper. The signs of a mature or maturing person are accepted by these psychologists as signs of *mental health.* The humanities and the sciences of psychology and theology are helpful in the development of insight about human beings as persons.

The second view of human beings that focuses on structural and functional differentiations within the unity that is a human being is the view that has been developed by various human and life sciences. These include the sciences of biochemistry, biophysics, human anatomy, and human physiology with its various branches, psychology, psychophysiology, and social psychology. These sciences organize validated knowledge about human structures and functions at different levels of integration, including their ranges of variation by age and other factors. The medical sciences of pathology and its various branches structure knowledge about disorders of human structures and human functions.

The detailed approaches of the human and life sciences are coalesced and organized by the identification and naming of modalities of functioning. This process is accomplished in a number of ways. For example, bodily functions are distinguished from mental functions; organic, psychic, and intellectual functioning are specified sometimes with more specific differentiations or with additional differentiations such as psychosocial functioning. An individual's state of health, when *state* is used in the *compound sense,* can be investigated along one or more of these dimensions. For example, a routine complete physical examination is an investigation of organic functioning, and various types of psychological tests are used to investigate psychic functioning. The particularized self-care requisites of individuals and their prescribed therapeutic self-care demands are regulatory of one or a number of modalities of human functioning toward soundness or wholeness of functioning of individuals.

Nurses' use of knowledge in practice situations about specific structural or functional aspects of the human existence of their patients, since it is knowledge of parts and not the whole, demands the asking and answering of a number of questions: Are other functions affected? Will they be affected? Can the effects of particular structural disorders or levels of functioning on the life and well-being of the individual be projected? How will efforts to regulate this aspect of functioning affect other aspects of functioning and the state of well-being of the patient? Nurses should understand that the two represented views of human beings are related and that nurses should develop facility in the use of both views in practice situations.

The represented positions about human health and well-being and the described views of human beings are not attempts to answer questions about the nature of health or the nature of humankind. They are expressions of approaches that when prudently used by nurses have practical value in the attainment of nursing goals in practice situations.

NURSING AS HEALTH CARE

Nursing practice as related to individuals has become fixed or institutionalized around the process of one person (the nurse) giving direct help to another person (the patient) when that person is wholly or partly unable to help himself or herself in the accomplishment of daily health-related care because of the existing health situation. This help includes medically prescribed therapy in the treatment of disease and injury that is part of the patient's daily self-care. Nursing, then, is a helping or assisting service to persons who are wholly or partly dependent — infants, children, and adults — when they, their parents, guardians, or other adults responsible for their care are no longer able to give or supervise their care because of the nature of their therapeutic self-care needs.

Every nurse must be qualified to provide nursing to individuals, adults, or children who have demands for nursing assistance. As a helping art, nursing is the complex ability to accomplish or to contribute to the accomplishment of a person's usual and therapeutic self-care by compensating for or aiding in overcoming the conditions or disabilities that cause the person (1) to be unable to act, (2) to refrain from acting, or (3) to act ineffectively in self-care. From the viewpoint of the patient, nursing care is always something received; it is personal assistance or help from a person who is qualified and able to help. From the viewpoint of the nurse, however, nursing care is help effectively given. It is help that facilitates regulation of the patient's functioning through meeting the therapeutic self-care demand as well as movement toward responsibility for self-care. The points where nursing converges on the health state of an individual can be described in terms of self-care, self-care requisites, therapeutic self-care demand, the constituent elements of self-care agency, and the performance of self-care operations. Self-care has been described as deliberate action that enables the individual to survive in a variety of states of well-being or health or to move from one state to another. The person who has self-care agency and activates it in the performance of particular self-care operations can be said to be a *regulator* (pp. 195-218).[1] Such a person is a good regulator if his or her self-care actions bring about internal and external conditions necessary to maintain life processes and environmental conditions supportive of life processes, integrity of human structure and functioning, and human developmental processes.

Self-care actions are deliberately performed; they can be reproduced from one time to another, and they are selected and performed with the goal of keeping internal and external conditions constant according to some standard. The universal, developmental, and health-deviation self-care requisites are expressions of the types of regulatory actions that should be performed by self-care or dependent-care agents.

Identification and description of types of self-care requisites supply nurses, other health workers, and the public with what is important and what is wanted with respect to regulation. The calculation of an individual's therapeutic self-care demand provides information about regulatory actions, which would ideally be performed because of the known values of selected health state components and the probability of constancy or change in these values.

Information about the values of health state indicators and the probabilities attached to their values allows nurses to make judgments about the current and projected effects of these indicators on the individual's performance of self-care operations. Furthermore, such information provides nurses with knowledge about conditions that require use of particular helping methods to meet self-care requisites and to regulate the exercise or development of self-care agency. Nurses should also seek information about the stages of cognitive and moral development of individuals whenever they are significant for the development of the constituent parts of self-care agency and for their exercise in performing self-care operations. One broad index of health (including development) is an individual's view of self as a self-care or dependent-care agent and the freedom with which the individual accepts and acts with responsibility in matters of self-care or dependent care.

The impending birth of a child, a construction worker's hospitalization after a fall from a building, a young man's paralysis sustained in an automobile accident, or a mother's prolonged illness are a few examples of some of the health-related situations in life that require the assistance of the nurse in helping an individual or family compensate for or overcome the limitations in self-care activities imposed by an existing health situation. The goal in nursing, like the goal in all other health services, is to achieve movement toward integrity of functioning for individuals or groups, sick or well, when they need help. Commonly heard expressions describe quite clearly, if not in scientific terms, what is meant by health goals: "to stay well," "to get well," "to be cured," "to get stronger," "to get back to work," "to get over my nervousness," "to regain the use of my hand," "to have a healthy baby," "to have [Eddie] able to run and play again," and "to be able to live like other people again." These and similar expressions, heard many times a day by health care workers, describe the health goals sought by and for patients. They are associated with a movement of the patient away from abnormalities and the restriction of normal human activity due to disease, injury, or unsound relationships toward a goal of normalcy or wholeness. Health results sought for patients also may mean stabilizing the condition of a patient who is chronically ill or easing the suffering of the patient who is dying.

The provision of health services has become increasingly complex with the broadening concept of health, with advances in the sciences and in technology, and with the increasing numbers of health care workers and supportive and administrative personnel. Achieving health results for individuals, families, and communities within health services as presently organized is costly and often inefficient for the providers as well as the seekers and receivers of service. Financing health services, availability of services needed, quality of health care provided, communications among health workers, and coordination of services are some of the problem areas. Both the public and organized health services must become more involved in finding solutions to problems in the delivery of health services in order to avoid serious breakdowns in service, to provide service when and where it is not presently available, and to improve the quality of service when needed. Nurses must continue, and in some instances begin, to assume their part in this effort. To do this, nurses must be able to differentiate their focus in health care situations from that of physicians and other health care professionals.

The nursing focus versus the medical focus

Healthy adults perform many of the universal components of self-care without direct help. They feed, wash, dress, and perform many health-related actions for themselves, including seeking medical care when they recognize the need for it. These and other activities usually become a fixed part of daily living and are scarcely noticed. The sick or injured adult, however, may find that he or she is unable to accomplish usual self-care tasks. The universal components of self-care may have to be modified because of an individual's health situation. The person may have little or no knowledge about the new care components that are required because of illness or injury. The person requires nursing assistance, and the nurse contributes to his or her well-being by providing that assistance. The following example demonstrates the focus of nursing and the part the nurse shares with others in achieving health results for patients.

> A man has sustained serious burns of the face, neck, chest, and arms. He is suffering considerable pain, and certain movements intensify his pain. He is very ill. Some of his body tissues have been destroyed; he is extremely anxious about his condition; he fears disfigurement, disability, and even death. He does not question his hospitalization, his need for medical care, or his wife's continuous presence. He accepts without question the ministrations of the attending doctors and nurses, including the pain they may unavoidably cause him as they care for him. The doctors and nurses know their roles in assisting him. They have learned what they must do for him and how to do it most effectively through initial and continuing specialized education and training. This knowledge includes medical knowledge of burns and treatment techniques; a background knowledge of anatomy and physiology, chemistry, microbiology, pharmacology, nutrition, psychology, and sociology; and experience in observing and working under the supervision of experienced doctors and nurses caring for burn patients.

The focus of the nurse's activities in this example is the man with burns who requires assistance to prevent further deterioration of his health and to recover and return to his normal or a near normal way of life. But the doctor has the same focus for his or her activities. What then is specific to the nursing objectives for the patient?

First, one must look closely at the interests shared by doctor and nurse. Both see the patient as a human being—as a person who is unique, who has rights and responsibilities for self and others, who has motives and values, and who has a way of life that has been disrupted by the accident and present states of illness and dependency. Both see the patient as they see other human beings—as a rational living being, vulnerable to disease and injury, but with great capacity to combat disease and injury, to recover, or to adjust and find ways for compensating for lost abilities and to be courageous.

The doctor's special interests in this situation are the patient's life processes as they have been disrupted as a result of the burns. They may be further disrupted by improper or careless treatment, by invading microorganisms resulting in infection, and by failure to support the patient psychologically and help sustain the will to live during the initial and critical phase of his illness and in the recovery phase when disfigurement must be faced. The doctor is specially prepared to evaluate the physical and psychophysical aspects of the patient's condition and progress and to prescribe appropriate therapeutic measures to prevent or alleviate complications that may develop.

The nurse's special interest is the continuing therapeutic care the patient requires. The nurse is concerned with the universal components of self-care, now modified by the burns and their effects upon the man's integrated functioning, and with all the health-deviation components of care that may arise as a result of the burns. The nurse assists the patient on a continuous basis with his personal care, which he can no longer manage for himself, and sustains him during the periods of great suffering and mental stress resulting from his pain and fear.

The nursing focus takes into account both the medical point of view and the patient's point of view. The doctor's prescribed measures for the treatment and control of the patient's condition will have been instituted promptly as a part of the patient's continuing care, as well as other measures designed to aid the doctor in diagnosing and instituting early treatment to prevent complications. The doctor requires information about the physiologic and behavioral state of the patient during the time he or she is not present to observe them. Continuing observation and recordings of the patient's condition throughout each day are important components of therapeutic care made necessary by the patient's specific health situation. The nurse must be alert to the patient's condition to adjust care to immediate needs, including the possibility of a need for immediate or emergency medical care because of a worsening of the patient's condition.

Recognizing an emergency situation and securing immediate medical assistance is an important component of self-care that the patient in the example can no longer manage. It necessarily becomes a part of the nursing focus. The patient may not be aware of the need for observation and may not even be able to recognize the need for emergency medical assistance. The nursing focus, from the patient's point of view, requires recognition and acceptance by the nurse that it is the patient who is living with burned tissues, that it is the patient who must cope with the effects of physiologic changes and of fear and pain on integrity as an individual. The patient perceives the situation and thinks about the future. He imagines what it may be and is afraid. A nursing focus is unrealistic if it does not take into account how the patient views and is personally affected by his illness. The nurse's recognition and acceptance of the patient's point of view is essential if the patient is to be assisted through nursing to live with his illness and disability, to cooperate with those who assist him, and above all to be motivated to direct his energies toward recovering a normal or near normal state of health.

Parts of the nursing focus

There are six components of a nursing focus. These components include the physician's perspective of the health situation, the patient's perspective of the health situation, and four central patient components: (1) state of health, (2) health results sought, (3) the therapeutic self-care demand, and (4) present abilities and disabilities to engage in self-care. The parts of a nursing focus and their interrelationship are shown in Fig. 8-1.

Each of the six components is in itself complex. Both the physician's medical perspective of the patient's health state and health care needs and the patient's perspective of his or her health situation should be seen as encompassing all or parts of each of the four central patient components. The four patient components are complex and interrelated. Both physician and nurse contribute to the identification and delineation of these components, which requires securing and validating information about the patient's health state and health-derived care requirements. The patient's health state not only gives rise to requirements for health care, but also affects the patient's ability to engage in self-care activities.

One foundation for the basic design of a system of nursing for a patient is determined by identifying and describing the nursing focus for the patient. The parts of the nursing focus and their interrelationships are the elements from which the nursing design is formed. The design changes as the components change; for example, as a patient's health state improves, the health-deviation self-care requisites may decrease and self-care ability increase, thus increasing the patient's self-care activities and decreasing the number of care activities that nurses perform for the patient. Identification and description of the six components of the nursing focus and their interrelationships for individual patients make explicit the *health dimension of nursing* for each patient. This information serves to guide the nurse in maintaining a nursing perspective on the patient that is defined in health terms.

In developing a nursing perspective, the components of the nursing focus become the guides for nursing action to the degree that the nurse understands each component, acquires information relating to it in specific nursing situations, and is

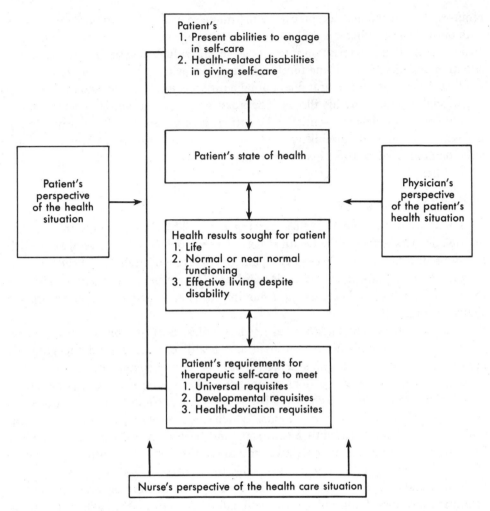

Fig. 8-1 Parts of a nursing focus.

able to interpret this information and attach nursing meaning to it. Consider a healthy adult woman who has sustained a fracture of a lower extremity and is immobilized in a cast. The patient is unable to do many things for herself because of her lack of mobility. The nursing focus in this situation should consider the patient's lack of mobility in its relationship to her general state of health and the health results sought. It will be clear to the nurse, in the light of nursing knowledge, that nonuse of the fractured extremity is both a component of the patient's therapeutic self-care and the underlying cause of the patient's inability to perform other usual self-care measures. It will also be clear that, objectively, the health results sought are (1) the healing of the fracture, (2) a return of the normal functioning of the extremity, and (3) the patient's recovery of mobility. The health results sought, however, are in turn directly related to and depend on the patient's age, general state of health, nutritional state, and physiologic capacity for forming the new bone growth necessary to the healing of the fracture. (The physiologic capacity for forming new bone tissue is frequently reduced in aged or undernourished patients.) The physician may view the patient's health situation primarily from an orthopedic point of view, with a primary concern for the effectiveness of the method of immobilization used and other aspects of the therapeutic regimen to promote healing. The patient may be primarily concerned with the effects of the fracture — pain, discomfort, disability, disruption of activities — and with the probable duration of the treatment.

When nurses enter nursing relationships with patients, they must distill from the mass of patient characteristics those that are relevant to the nursing focus. Nurses do not ignore the nonrelevant factors but view them in light of the influence they may exert on the factors that determine the specifications for nursing action. Further, nurses must keep in mind that the nursing focus for a patient may be either relatively stable or undergoing continuous change. In the earlier example of the patient with severe burns, the nursing focus probably would require adjustment from hour to hour or even more frequently during the critical periods of the patient's illness. The frequency of change in both the physician's perspective and the patient's perspective during these critical periods would necessarily affect the nursing perspective as well. Changes in the nursing perspective probably would occur less frequently after stabilization of the patient's condition, but the nurse would need to know and understand how change in one component of the nursing focus would affect the other components. For example, if there is a sudden and dramatic improvement in the condition of the patient who is burned or if he suffers a sudden relapse and becomes comatose, his requirements for therapeutic care and his ability to engage in self-care would change dramatically. The sudden change in one component of the nursing focus (the patient's state of health) may set off a chain reaction in all the other components that would make it essential for the nurse to completely revise the nursing focus for the patient.

The nursing focus is also the index or key in estimating the complexity of a nursing situation and thus in determining the kinds of nurses (e.g., level of education and training) that will be needed to meet the patient's requirements for nursing care. The complexity of a nursing situation is determined by (1) the rapidity of change in the components of the nursing focus, (2) the elements of the components, and (3) the number and kinds of relationships between the components. The complexity of a nursing situation is increased whenever the nursing focus is not clear-cut or obvious, for example, a situation in which the patient is critically ill; but the reasons for the illness are unknown. A clear-cut or obvious nursing focus is one that can be validly established by means of readily available information about the components and their relationships.

The ability to develop and maintain a valid nursing focus in nursing practice is directly related to the nurse's educational preparation and experience. The mark of the expert in nursing is the ability to see a health care situation from a nursing perspective and to recognize personal capabilities and limitations in establishing and maintaining a valid nursing focus. Because of their educational preparation, some nurses are not prepared to design, establish, and maintain a valid system of nursing for a patient without the supervision of a nurse with advanced preparation and experience. These same nurses, however, may be qualified by their educational background and well prepared to work in cooperation with another nurse, or they may be prepared to care for a patient in keeping with a design preestablished and maintained by another qualified nurse (see Chapter 12).

REQUIREMENTS FOR HEALTH CARE

Health care is based on systems of knowledge about human development and functioning and on practices with some demonstrated value in promoting health or in preventing, curing, or regulating disease. Concepts descriptive of systems of *preventive health care* are useful in unifying the meaning of health, disease, and health care for individuals. For this reason, prevention is the concept used as the means for presenting and interpreting variations of health care requirements and their meaning in nursing situations. Prevention as described in Leavell, et al. (pp. 14-38)[5] is based on (1) knowledge of the natural history of human disorders, (2) knowledge of the combination of causes of specific disorders of human structure and functioning, and (3) an identified rational basis for methods of intercepting or counteracting causative factors before the onset of a disease or at some period after its onset. Preventive health care thus requires knowledge of specific interferences with normal human structure and functioning at various stages of the life cycle in particular environments.

Systems of preventive health care recognize three levels of prevention: primary, secondary, and tertiary. Primary prevention is appropriate before the onset of disease and is directed to the *maintenance and promotion of integrity of structure and functioning* and the *prevention of specific diseases.* Secondary prevention is appropriate after the onset of disease and is directed to the *prevention of complications* (disease that occurs concurrently with other disease) and of *sequelae* (disorders of structure or function that follow or are caused by an attack of a disease) and *prevention of prolonged disability.* Tertiary prevention is appropriate when there is disability with a demand to function in society with limited human capacities. It is directed toward bringing about *effective and satisfying human functioning in accord with existing powers for human functioning.* The reader should refer to works in preventive medicine for detailed explanations of these levels of prevention.

Requirements of individuals for the three levels of preventive health care vary with age, states of development and health, and external environmental conditions. Care

> ***Exercise* to clarify the meaning of primary care and nursing's part in it**
>
> 1. Read statements, articles, or papers about primary care as described by the World Health Organization, by the Institute of Medicine of the National Academy of Sciences, or in articles in nursing, public health, or medical journals.
> 2. Record the various descriptions of primary care by sources from which they were taken.
> 3. Think about the meanings that are attached to the term primary care and consider these questions:
>   a. Does nursing have a contribution to make to primary care? Should nursing be recognized as a primary care service?
>   b. Should nurse practitioners in primary care settings be viewed as "physician extenders"?

at the primary level of prevention is a requirement of each individual throughout life. With the onset of disease or when a person is disabled, there will be requirements for care at the secondary and tertiary levels of prevention. Each person in a health care situation can be viewed, therefore, as having one of the following kinds of preventive health care requirements:

- Care at the primary level of prevention
- Care at the primary and secondary levels of prevention
- Care at the primary and tertiary levels of prevention
- Care at the primary, secondary, and tertiary levels of prevention

These four kinds of health care requirements have meaning for nursing because of their implications for life, health, and effective living on the part of the patient and the health care role responsibilities that each level of care specifies for patients, health workers, and others who provide care and services. They further impose demands for specific attitudes, knowledge, and skills on the part of patients, health workers, or others who provide care and services. Each level of prevention is considered so that some implications for nursing are made explicit.

Health care requirements at the primary level of prevention

Requirements for health maintenance and promotion and disease prevention are specified in relation to what is known about (1) human structure and functioning and (2) specific diseases or interferences with the normal human condition. The effective meeting of the universal self-care requisites adjusted to age, environmental conditions, and the individual's health and developmental state is health care at the primary level of prevention.

The adult has a major instrumental role in health care at the primary level of prevention because it is a continuous requirement. When the person is young, aged, ill, unknowing, or unskilled, the role of agent for meeting that person's universal self-care requisites should be taken by a responsible and qualified adult. The nurse may be this adult or may help another adult fill the role competently. The physician's or dentist's role is that of diagnostician in periodic health examinations, prescribed of preventive therapy (for example, diet adjusted to age), or instrumental agent in giving preventive therapy (e.g., specific preventive therapy after exposure to but before the onset of a specific communicable disease). The community role in health care at the primary level of prevention is a large one and relates to control of environmental conditions and adequacy of essential resources. It provides health services in the form of education to prepare individuals and families to fulfill their personal care roles. It also provides private or public health services to protect individuals from specific disease or to help them with problems of health maintenance and promotion.

General rules to guide nurses in identifying some of the nursing dimensions of health care requirements at the primary level of prevention include the following:

- Every individual under nursing care has health care requirements at the primary level of prevention
- Universal self-care and developmental self-care (Chapter 6), when therapeutic in quality, constitute health care at the primary level of prevention. They include practices to maintain and promote health and development and to prevent specific diseases. Practices to promote health are based on rationales of resources and conditions essential for survival and development and for normalcy of structure and functioning. Practices to prevent specific diseases are based on rationales of how to prevent or interrupt relations between causative agents of disease and factors in patients or the environment that together establish the conditions necessary for the disease to develop.
- In assisting individual patients, nurses are able to select and use or guide patients to select and use methods for meeting self-care requisites that promote and maintain health and development and prevent specific disease. Methods are properly adjusted to the factors of age, health, individual modes of functioning, and environment.
- Nurses apply factual information about the patient, the environment, and the patient's life-style and routine of daily living in their selection or use of universal and development self-care practices at the primary level of prevention. Health care at this level should be incorporated into each patient's system of daily living and be a permanent part of it.
- Nurses assist patients in health care directed to the goals of health maintenance and promotion and disease prevention with an awareness of the essential role of the patient or a responsible adult in the continuous provision of this level of preventive health care.

Health care requirements at the secondary and tertiary levels of prevention

Requirements for (1) prevention of complicating diseases and adverse effects of specific diseases and prolonged disability through early diagnosis and treatment (secondary prevention) and (2) rehabilitation in the event of disfigurement and disability (tertiary level of prevention) are specified in relation to what is known about the nature and effects of specific diseases, valid methods of regulating disease, and the human potential for living with and overcoming the disabling effects of disease. Health-deviation self-care of a therapeutic quality includes practices at either or both of these levels of prevention.

Health care at the secondary level of prevention is accomplished through accurate diagnosis and effective treatment at the onset or in some later stage of a disease. Periodic health examinations; accurate observations of signs and symptoms of health disorders by patient, family, or nurse; and the selection of further health care as indicated by observed signs and symptoms facilitate early diagnosis and treatment when adequate health services are available. Case finding in public health practice also facilitates early diagnosis and treatment.

During the course of a disease, health care requirements and the instrumental role of the patient as self-care agent vary with the effects of the disease and with the methods of diagnosis and treatment used. Health care is effective at the secondary level of prevention if (1) the disease is cured, the pathologic process arrested, or the effects of the disease kept under control; (2) complicating diseases are prevented; and (3) the dissemination of the causative agents of the disease is prevented.

Rehabilitation, as previously indicated, requires deliberate action on the part of the patient and health workers to adapt or adjust functioning to compensate for or overcome disorders that restrict human functioning in specific ways. Rehabilitative health care varies with the nature and the effects of the disorder, including the stage of the life cycle when the condition occurred. It also varies with the methods used for determining the extent of the disorder, patient's remaining functional capacity, and the techniques used to enable the patient to function effectively with some degree of satisfaction. This level of health care requires a belief in the human potential to overcome functional disorders and disability, effective techniques for determining functional loss and remaining functional capacities, and effective restorative or compensatory techniques. It also requires willingness on the part of the patient, the family, health workers, and communities to work toward the goal of rehabilitation. Many types of specialists and provision for special education, recreation, travel, and work must be available on a community basis. This level of preventive health care is effective whenever an individual is able to live or is making progress in living as an active member of a social group.

General rules to guide nurses in identifying the nursing dimensions of situations where patients have requirements for the secondary or tertiary levels of preventive health care include the following:
- Persons who suffer from disease or disorders of health or their effects have health care requirements at the secondary or tertiary levels of prevention that are specific to an active disease and its continuous dynamic effects or to a state of disfigurement or dysfunction.

- Health-deviation self-care (Chapter 6), when therapeutic in quality, is health care at the secondary or tertiary level of prevention in the form of self-care measures to regulate and prevent adverse effects of the disease, prevent complicating diseases, prevent prolonged disability, or adapt or adjust functioning to overcome or compensate for the adverse effects of permanent or prolonged disfigurement or dysfunction.
- In assisting individual patients, nurses must be able to use and to guide patients in the use of medically prescribed or endorsed measures of diagnosis, treatment, and rehabilitation to be incorporated into self-care, including adjustments of universal and developmental self-care requisites to the health and disease state of the patient.
- Nurses gather and apply factual information about the patient, including results of medical evaluations that specify level of functioning measured against norms for healthy individuals in the patient's age group, medical orders, environment, life-style, and routines of daily living.
- Health care at these levels becomes a temporary or a permanent part of a patient's daily life.
- Nurses assist patients in health care directed to the goals of secondary and tertiary prevention with the awareness that the role of the patient as responsible instrumental agent in health care varies not only with age but also with the nature of the disease and its effects. It also varies with the measures and techniques of diagnosis, treatment, and rehabilitation used in health care, their effects on the patient, the resources and services available to the patient, and his or her state of readiness to give or manage self-care with or without guidance and supervision.

CLASSIFICATION OF NURSING SITUATIONS BY HEALTH FOCUS

Since the same totality of things, persons, or situations may be classified in more than one way, it is necessary to consider the methods of establishing classifications. For example, if one has a box of red and yellow beads and if some of these beads are round and the others square, the beads may be grouped according to color or shape. The groupings are red beads and yellow beads when classified by color and round beads and square beads when classified by shape. If some red beads and some yellow beads are round and others square, then it is possible to group them according to both schemes of classification by placing red ones into separate groups of round and square beads and yellow ones into similar groups.

Classification is useful not only in organizing information or facts but also in serving practical purposes. In practical endeavors, considering each of the varying factors (e.g., color and shape of the beads) is necessary whenever the variations have an effect on the desired result. For a very simple example, consider that the red and yellow beads in the box are to be used in making two necklaces of the following design — beads of the same color, alternating round and square beads. Both color and shape must be considered in the planning. The number of round and square beads of each color for making two necklaces of specific lengths must be determined. Size of the beads and the number of beads available are other relevant considerations. Arrangement of the beads into color groups and of each color group into two shape groups would facilitate making judgments about the number of beads available as well as stringing the beads. This simple example of the beads illustrates how classifications are developed in terms of characteristics and how useful classification is in identifying and naming things and in accomplishing a task or a series of tasks. To function effectively, nurses require knowledge of both the health and helping aspects of nursing situations. A classification system that would assist nurses in understanding the health aspects of nursing situations is presented.

A person in need of nursing care can be described from a health perspective with reference to (1) the presence or absence of disease, injury, disability, or disfigurement; (2) the quality of general health state described in the general sense as excellent, good, fair, poor, or in terms of the values of sets of selected characteristics that together define the person's health state; and (3) the life-cycle-oriented events and circumstances that indicate current changes and existing needs for health care. These dimensions of health, when accurately described for a patient, indicate appropriate health care goals, specify the kinds of health care required, and may also indicate the kinds of obstacles to self-care that are present or could be present. A classification system based on these dimensions of health is suggested, and seven groupings of nursing situations according to the health focus of the situation are proposed. The suggested variations in each group identify subgroups. The classification is generally useful, that is, not just useful to nurses. It is essentially a classification of health care situations from which inferences about the nursing aspects of health care can be made.

- **Group 1**   The health focus is oriented to events and circumstances in relation to the *life cycle* that give rise to anatomic, physiologic, or psychologic changes associated with periods of growth and development, maturity, parenthood, aging, and old age. General health is within the range of excellent to good.
- **Group 2**   The health focus is oriented to the process of *recovery* from a specific disease (e.g., measles) or injury (e.g., a fracture of the pelvis resulting from a fall) or to overcoming or compensating for the effects of the disease or injury. Permanent *dysfunction, disfigurement,* or *disability* may or may not be present or expected. General health is within the range of excellent to good.
- **Group 3**   The health focus is oriented to *illness or disorder of undetermined origin,* with concern for the degree of illness, specific effects of the disorder, and effects of specific diagnostic or therapeutic measures used. General health is within the range of good to fair.

- **Group 4**   The health focus is oriented to *defects of a genetic or developmental nature,* or the *biologic state of the premature infant,* or the *low birth weight* infant. The state of general health may be affected by the direct or indirect effects of the defect or the biologic state.
- **Group 5**   The health focus is oriented to *regulation through active treatment of a disease or disorder or injury of determined origin,* with concern for the degree of illness; the specific effects of the disease, disorder, or injury; and the specific effects of the therapeutic measures used. Temporary or permanent disfigurement or disability may or may not be present or expected. The state of general health is or may be affected by direct or indirect effects of the disease, disorder, or injury.
- **Group 6**   The health focus is oriented to the *restoration, stabilization, or regulation of integrated functioning.* A vital process may have stopped or be seriously disrupted, or, in a newborn infant, breathing may not have started.
- **Group 7**   The health care focus is oriented to the regulation of the effects of processes that have disrupted human integrated functioning to the degree that quality of life is gravely affected or that life cannot long continue. Rational processes may be disturbed or relatively unaffected.

VARIATIONS IN HEALTH CARE AND NURSING

Because of differences in health focus, each of the seven groupings of nursing situations, indicates requirements for different kinds of combinations of health care directed to one or more of the goals of preventive health care. For example, in nursing situations with a life cycle focus, the requirement for health care is at the primary level of prevention with the goals of maintaining and promoting health and preventing specific diseases and injuries. Awareness of these goals guides nurses as well as other health workers in the selection of measures of care and assistance for individuals or groups within specific environments.

In the descriptions that follow, health care goals and health care needs are specified and variations indicated for each health focus. It should be understood that although the life cycle orientation to health care represents a type of nursing situation, in nursing practice the guides suggested for care with this focus are used along with guides for each of the other six situations, since every person is in one of the phases of the life cycle. The life cycle focus validates and provides the base for both universal and developmental self-care requisites. Health-deviation self-care requisites are associated with groups 2 to 6. The helping focus of nursing must be linked to the health care focus (Fig. 8-2). The linking of the helping and health focuses in nursing practice is mediated by patient variables, therapeutic self-care demand and self-care agency, and the relationship between them.

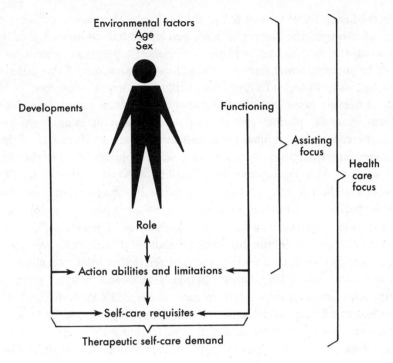

Fig. 8-2 Two focuses of nurses in health care situations.

Life cycle

In a nursing situation where the health focus is oriented to the life cycle, the care is designed for promoting and maintaining health and for protecting against specific diseases and injuries. Environmental conditions and internal changes connected with intrauterine growth and development, infancy, childhood, adolescence, and maturity and related events and conditions such as pregnancy, menopause, and aging determine the specific kinds of health care that will be needed.

A nursing case of this type is one in which the patient's behavior indicates well-being rather than illness and in which there is evidence that the patient is in good to excellent health. The general health care needs would include:

- Periodic health evaluation to determine the normalcy of the patient's growth, functioning, and development and the quality of general health
- Health maintenance and promotion adjusted to the specific phase of and events in the patient's life cycle and to general health
- Protection against environmental factors, with specific concern for growth and development
- Assistance to the patient and the family in assuming appropriate roles in continuing health care through self-care

When the health focus is oriented to the life cycle, therapeutic self-care consists primarily of meeting the universal and developmental components of self-care adjusted to age; to sex; to the conditions of puberty, pregnancy, menopause, and aging; and to environmental factors. The self-care limitations of the patient would arise from age or from lack of knowledge, skills, or essential resources.

Types of nursing cases with the life cycle focus include cases where the specific health focus is on (1) normal growth and development of infants, children, and youth; (2) the continuing psychological and intellectual development of the adult; (3) pregnancy in girls, young women, and older women; and (4) the anatomic, physiologic, and psychological changes of middle age and advanced age. The four general kinds of health care appropriate for the life cycle orientation would be adjusted to specific demands represented by the four types of nursing cases. The four types of cases require that a nurse have knowledge of growth and development as related to the phases in the life cycle; validated health care practices in the area of primary prevention; cultural practices related to infant or child care and to adolescent and adult life, family living, sexual and marital relations, and prepartum, intrapartum, and postpartum care; social and economic forces affecting the individual and family; and the influence of physical, biologic, and social agents in the environment on individual, family, and community health. The life cycle focus, including its specific types of cases, is inherent in the health focus of the other five groups of cases. In a sense, it may be considered the core of any type of nursing situation.

Recovery

Recovery from disease, injury, or a functional disorder is the focus of health care. Medical treatment for the disease or injury has been instituted and has been effective in cure or regulation. Vital functions are stabilized. The characteristics of the medical therapy and its effects on the individual and the residual effects of the pathologic process prescribe the needs for health care.

Specific cases within group 2 would be instances in which complete recovery is expected with no residual defect or disability, cases in which there will be a permanent structural or functional defect through loss of or defect in an organ or a part of the body, and cases in which a functional disorder is regulated by continuous therapy. Cases may also vary as to the degree of illness; there may be normal functioning, except for the affected structures or functions or degree of illness experienced. Health care needs would include:

- Continued control of the recovery process through medical evaluation to determine the presence of sequelae and complications, the progress in recovery, and the effectiveness of disease regulation
- Continued medical therapy and self-care specific for the cure or regulation of the disease, injury, or functional disorder and its effects

- Specific protection when needed and possible in order to prevent sequelae and complications, defect, or disability resulting from the disease, injury, or functional disorder or from care measures
- Early detection and medical diagnosis of complications with prompt treatment
- Rehabilitation of the patient including the patient's self-image in the event of disfigurement, including loss of bodily parts or temporarily or permanently impaired functions
- Health maintenance and promotion and specific protection from the actual or possible effects of the disease, injury, or functional disorder on general health and growth and development
- Assistance to the patient and the family in assuming appropriate roles in health care, including self-care as related to the overall health care needs

In nursing cases of the group 2 type, therapeutic self-care would include care measures related to and derived from the disease process or functional disorder and measures derived from and related to medical diagnosis and therapy. Universal and developmental self-care requisites would require adjustments, not only to age and sex and environmental factors, but also to the effects of the disease or injury and to the prescribed medical therapy. Self-care limitations may be caused by the effects of the disease process, the therapy used, the lack of necessary knowledge and skills, or a lack of resources.

Illness of undetermined origin

In group 3, health care is organized around signs and symptoms, degree of illness, and the need for medical diagnosis of the disease or disorder causing the signs and symptoms. A nursing case of this type is one in which the patient is suffering from a disorder with evident signs and symptoms and is either seriously ill and incapacitated, moderately or mildly ill, or functioning normally except for the presenting signs and symptoms of the disorder. The unknown causes of the signs and symptoms indicate that medical diagnosis and health evaluation is a principal health care need. The health care needs would include:

- Prompt medical diagnosis of the nature, causes, and effects of the disease or disorder
- Alleviation of symptoms through medical therapy and self-care measures with precautions for not masking symptoms
- Prompt treatment and other protective care to prevent further structural or functional impairment or permanent defect and disability
- Health maintenance and promotion required as a result of the nature of the signs and symptoms, the degree of illness, and actual or possible effects on the patient's general health
- Assistance to the patient and the family in assuming appropriate roles in continuing health care, including self-care

The nursing aspects of group 3 situations would be similar to those of group 2 situations. Participation in health evaluations and medical diagnostic measures could be a major component of self-care in group 3 situations, since the undetermined nature of the disorder would be a major concern of some patients that would affect both self-care and nursing.

Genetic and developmental defects and biologic immaturity

The health focus is oriented to the care and treatment of patients with structural and functional defects or a state of immaturity present at birth. The defects may be hereditary or congenital. Immaturity may be a consequence of a premature birth or associated with low birth weight or other factors. Health care is oriented to making adjustments and adaptations necessitated by the defect or undeveloped state and to supplying the environmental conditions necessary to support life, facilitate integrated functioning, and contribute to present and future normalcy in daily living.

The characteristics of each structural or functional defect or behavioral disorder would determine how human functioning and daily living are impaired. For example, an infant with a cleft palate presents a different requirement for health care than does an infant with an inborn error in metabolism (in which certain biochemical reactions necessary for health and integrated functioning do not occur). Both the nature and extent of the effects of specific defects — for example, a cleft lip as compared with a cleft palate — on life, health, and effective living must be considered. Health care requirements in group 4 would include:

- Continuous health care (including provision of a therapeutic environment) to achieve the adjustments and adaptations the patient needs for support of life processes and integrated functioning
- Continuous health evaluation to determine the effects of the defect, behavioral disorder, or biologic state on general health, growth, and development and functioning
- Continuous diagnosis to determine the extent and the effects of the defect or disorder and the effects of therapy
- Specific protection against complications or extension of present impairments into more disabling limitations
- Rehabilitation of patient or parents of patient as indicated
- Health maintenance and promotion and specific protection from actual or possible effects of the defect or disorder on general health, growth, and development and functioning
- Assistance to the patient and family in assuming appropriate roles in continuing health care, including self-care

Nursing care is focused on contributing to the necessary adaptations and adjustments required as a result of the defect or biologic state and for maintaining essential environmental conditions. Rehabilitation may be of great importance in cases of this type. In some instances, major adjustments in family life are required. When defects are extensive and affect self-direction and behavioral control or mobility, provisions for continuing care within or outside the family setting are necessary.

Cure or regulation

Health care in the form of active treatment for the cure or regulation of the effects of an injury, or disease, or functional disorder, including behavioral disorders not existent at birth, may be required during any period of a patient's life cycle. Major variations within this pattern relate to (1) the nature and extent of the injury and its effect; (2) the manner in which the disease or disorder manifests itself, including presenting signs and symptoms; (3) whether vital functions are stabilized or not stabilized; and (4) the degree of illness.

The following factors should be considered: Are the effects of the condition localized or generalized? Is the disease acute or chronic? If it is chronic, is it in an acute phase or in a phase of remission? Can the disease be cured? If not, can it be regulated with continuous therapy? Is some degree of regulation possible when the disease process is progressive and cannot be cured or entirely controlled? Is palliative and symptomatic therapy required? Health care requirements would include:
- Continuous care and medical therapy to cure or regulate the disease process or the functional disorder, to heal injured tissues, to alleviate symptoms, and to prevent disability
- Therapy to stabilize or to protect vital functions and integrated functioning
- Continuous control through evaluation of the progress of the disease process, the disorder, or the progress of recovery from the injury
- Specific protection to prevent complications or the extension of present effects of the disease, disorder, or injury that might result in disability
- Early diagnosis and prompt treatment of complications
- Health maintenance and promotion of general health, growth, and development
- Care to assist the patient in coping with suffering and disability when present
- Rehabilitation
- Assistance to the patient and family to assume appropriate roles in continuing health care, including self-care

The nursing aspects of the cure or regulation type of situation range from relatively simple to extremely complex. The specific symptoms, the degree of illness, the prognosis, the effects of the disease process on vital functions and integrated functioning, the amount and type of stress, as well as the form(s) of medical diagnosis and therapy and the effects of these measures, determine the kind and amount of self-care required by the patient. Self-care and nursing care are adjusted according to the changes in the patient's health state and to changes in medical diagnosis and therapy.

Stabilization of integrated functioning

In this type of case, health care is oriented to stabilization and control of the vital processes that have been disrupted by disease processes or by injury or by impaired respiratory and cardiac functioning at birth. Variations in the individual case should be identified. What is the extent to which integrated functioning has been affected? Has an injury or its effects directly involved vital organs or affected integrated functioning? Is there immediate danger of death? Can any degree of control be established? If there is suffering, what is its nature and degree? Is the patient aware of the probable effects of the condition on life and health? Is there an anticipation of death or an uncontrolled fear of death? Whether the patient is an infant, child, adolescent, or adult is of great importance in nursing patients in this category. General health care requirements would include:

- Immediate institution of therapy to initiate, restore, or stabilize and support vital functions and facilitate integrated functioning
- Continuous control through nursing and medical evaluation to determine the degree of functional deviation in the life processes and to adjust or institute therapy as required
- Nursing care and medical therapy to alleviate distressing symptoms and relieve suffering
- Nursing care and medical therapy to prevent complications, to diagnose them early, and to institute prompt treatment
- Assistance to the ill or injured patient and family to sustain themselves in their suffering and to assume appropriate roles in the health situation
- Care to enable a dying person and the family to face the reality of death

Quality of life is gravely and irreversibly affected (group 7)

Nursing is the essential health service for persons whose quality of life is gravely and irreversibly affected because of serious disruption of integrated functioning. Medical supervision, rather than active medical care, is required except in emergency situations. Care is directed to overcome obstacles arising from the effects of pathology to meet the universal self-care requisites. In many situations, the major focus is on meeting universal self-care requisites particularized for the conditions and circumstances under which persons live. Developmental self-care requisites would be concerned with learning how to live with some degree of effectiveness and satisfaction under the disrupted and abnormal conditions of human functioning. Health care requirements would include:

- Effective nursing management of patients and their environments
- Continuing medical supervision and active medical care as required
- Continuous effective meeting of the universal self-care requisites
- Finding ways and means and their use in supporting patients' development, for example, finding new ways of communicating, management of fear, and feelings of despair or rejection

- Continuous symptom management
- Appropriate assistance to family members (and to patients when appropriate) to help them understand patients' functional states, including the stability or instability of their states, their roles in care, and realistic planning for care in the present and the future
- Continuing support to patient and family to enable them to sustain themselves and to have a measure of security

In situations where the quality of life is gravely and irreversibly affected because of the effects of disease and injury, nurses work with patients and their families, are in communication with physicians, and collaborate with other health workers about goals being sought. The provision and maintenance of a safe and developmental-type environment is an essential aspect of health care.

Terminal illness (group 7)

Health care is frequently oriented to the comfort and security of those who are in the terminal stages of illness. Care is directed to the control of persistent pain (if present) and to the regulation or control of other distressing symptoms (e.g., anorexia, dyspnea, frequency of urination, depression). Patients suffer increasing weakness and total distress (p. 14).[6] Variations result from the natural history of the disorder, the types of symptoms being experienced, and the methods used for the regulation of symptoms. The aims of health care are to enable individuals with a terminal illness to live as themselves, to understand their illness and how to participate in care, to approach death in their own particular way, and to be with family, friends, and health care workers in an environment of security and trust. General health care requirements would include:

- Effective medical management of the terminal illness
- Active medical treatment as advisable
- Continuous regulation of presenting sets of symptoms
- Continuous effective meeting of the universal self-care requisites
- Assistance directed to control of feelings of despair or rejection
- Assistance to the patient and family to understand the patient's illness and its projected outcome and their roles in care and in preparation for the future
- Continuing support to patient and family to enable them to sustain themselves and to have a measure of security
- Development of care measures to support the patient at the time of death and ensure that family members know what help to secure and how to secure it

In situations of terminal illness, nurses ideally function with patients and family; physicians; paramedical personnel; and priests, ministers, or rabbis to institute and maintain a developmental environment for patients and all persons involved in their care.

HEALTH CARE SYSTEMS

Health care systems, including nursing systems, are constituted from actions deliberately selected and performed by individuals. Health care systems include self-care and dependent-care systems created within the context of daily living. They also include care and service provided by ever-increasing numbers and types of health care personnel. People make health care systems; they are not naturally existent entities. The failure of nurses and others to recognize that health care systems must be made often results in inadequate communication with patients, families, and other health workers toward attaining the goal of coordination of human efforts.

Health care systems generated in part by physicians, nurses, and other health workers should be viewed as being constituted from the contributed actions of persons who have different social statuses and roles in social groups. Positions and roles in the field of health service indicate the kinds of actions that the persons filling them should be able to contribute to the formation of effective health care systems. What persons do contribute varies with their education, training, willingness, and other factors. The organizational charting of positions for a community health service, a hospital, or a nursing home is not necessarily a measure of the kind of health service being provided to consumers.

Nursing may be one of a number of health services needed by and provided to persons with health care requirements. The mix of health services being provided, the essential relationships among the services, and the individual and the combined contributions of the services to the health of an individual or a group constitute the health care system. From a service perspective, persons who seek and are provided with health care from institutionalized services have the *role* of consumer and purchaser of an available service. From the perspective of their relationship to the actual providers of care, they are in the *patient role*. In the role of consumer and purchaser, people pay for what they receive through taxes, third-party payments, or direct payment. In the role of patient, individuals should be helped to actively participate in their health care to the degree that their health and developmental states permit.

To provide nursing that is relevant to a patient's health care requirements, a nurse must be able to define his or her nursing role, including role relationships to the patient and to other health workers. Role definition requires awareness of the general dimensions of a patient's health care situation. It is a task that nurses perform at the time they enter health care situations and periodically thereafter. The seven groups of nursing situations organized according to differences in health care focuses and the general formulations of health care needs for each group can be used as an aid to the nurse's role definition.

Nurses require information to describe (1) the roles of the patient in each of the health services received (each service may be approached as a separate system or as a subsystem of the total health care system), (2) the contribution that each health service is capable of making to the patient's existing or projected health state, (3) the favorable or unfavorable effects of particular care measures on the patient, and (4) the way the various services must articulate when specific health care technologies are used or when specific results are sought. Further, since a patient may be affected favorably or unfavorably by an aspect of the health care situation or by the impact of the total system of health care, nurses as well as physicians must be alert not only to the effects of specific care measures on the patient but to the patient's level of tolerance for the health care systems as a whole.

When the demands of using particular forms of health care on a patient become sufficiently burdensome, the patient may withdraw. Withdrawal may take a number of forms, for example, psychological withdrawal, as in depression, or making the decision and taking action to remove oneself from the health care situation. Patients sign releases or simply walk away without informing health workers of their plans. Withdrawal may be evidence of the ineffectiveness or inefficiency of the system of health care.

Nurses seek information to describe why an individual has sought and received health care. Two questions are suggested as guides in securing information: (1) Why and from whom did the patient seek (is the patient seeking) health care? (2) Why and by whom was the patient accepted (is the patient being accepted) as a recipient of health care? The *subjective measures* of a person's need for health service include (1) state of satisfaction or dissatisfaction with his or her own structure and modes of functioning; (2) judgments about what is normal or abnormal, tolerable or intolerable; and (3) judgments about existing abilities to cope with the effects of perceived disorders of structure or functioning. Adults and older children have data on how they now appear, function, and feel to compare with their state at some previous time. In making these judgments, individuals use two sets of norms—what is usual or "normal" for them and cultural norms about what is "normal for the group," which may or may not be based on scientific knowledge.

Persons who seek health services may want help to find out what is "wrong" with them, to feel better, or to be cured. They may be seeking a health evaluation, assistance with a specific health problem, or the performance of some diagnostic or preventive health care measure such as vaccination. Health workers accept and take into account an individual's request and his or her evaluation of the need for health care as they engage in assessment of the health situation. The modes of delivery of health services to the people of a community will determine from whom health care is sought initially and who accepts individuals or groups for health care, thus affording them the positions of patient in the health care system.

The *objective measure* of a person's need for health services of various types is either the overt presence of or some indication of disordered structure or functioning or evidence of a need for assistance in coping with a usual or unusual health care requirement. Assessment of health state or health care needs is a health service that traditionally has been provided by physicians. Today, some technologies for securing evidence to describe normality or abnormality of human structure and functioning are highly developed. These procedures are performed by a variety of health workers who have specialized preparation in the use of one or more of these technologies.

Specific medical diagnostic procedures initiated by a physician may be preceded by a general health assessment. There is a developing trend for persons seeking health care in hospital outpatient departments or community health centers to have their needs for health care evaluated first by a physician's assistant or by a nurse. Nurses and physician's assistants sometimes perform routine physical examinations. This initial objective assessment of health is not a substitute for the medical diagnostic process conducted by the physician or the detailed evaluation conducted by other specialists including nurses. When a nurse is the first health worker to see a person seeking or requiring health care, the nurse should attend to the patient's view of the need for care, to gross evidence of normality or abnormality of structure and functioning, and to what the individual indicates is the usual mode of functioning. The nurse may act at this time to meet the person's obvious needs for nursing assistance, as well as to refer the person to a physician for care if appropriate.

The initial seeking of subjective and objective information to measure a person's need for health care provides data to aid in formulating the purpose of the individualized health care system to be instituted for the patient. There may be a need at this time or later for cooperative action to resolve differences between the patient's subjective view of his or her needs and the objective views of the physicians, nurses, or other health workers. When the rights and responsibilities of individuals for their own health care are respected, each patient is permitted and encouraged to participate in the formulation of the purpose of the health care system to be produced and in the identification and clarification of roles. The purpose to which health care is directed serves to unify the efforts of physicians, nurses, and others who contribute to the patient's health care. If physicians and nurses and others do not communicate with the patient and among themselves, individuals in the health care situation may be working toward results that are not compatible with results being sought by other persons who are contributing to health care.

Seeking and analyzing data to aid in selecting constituent care elements for a system of health care that would be valid for the patient should be started when a person first seeks health care. It should be continued as long as the individual is under health care. This endeavor is necessary to provide persons seeking care with the care they need now as well as to foresee what they will need at some future time. Each health care facility (hospital, nursing home, clinic) that accepts a person or group as a recipient of service is responsible for the quality and amount of care provided. There should be established means for an initial and continued examination of the dimensions of each patient's health care situation in relation to the patient's view and the health worker's view of reasons why health care is needed.

REFERENCES

1. Ashby WR: An introduction to cybernetics, London, Chapman & Hall Ltd., 1956, pp. 30-31.
2. Lonergan BJF: Insight, a study of human understanding, New York, 1958, Philosophical Library, 1958, pp. 65-66, 195-218, 469-479.
3. Lewin K: Field theory in social science, selected theoretical papers, Cartwright D, editor, Harper Torchbooks, New York, 1951, pp. xi and 45.
4. Nursing Development Conference Group, Orem, DE, editor: Concept formalization in nursing: process and product, ed. 2, Boston, 1979, Little, Brown, & Co., 1979, pp. 122-123.
5. Leavell HR, et al: Preventive medicine for the doctor in his community, ed 3, New York, 1965, McGraw-Hill, pp. 14-38.
6. From Saunders C: Hospital Medicine Publications, The management of terminal illness, London, 1967, p. 14.

SELECTED READINGS

Bateson MC: Health as artifact, J Prof Nurs 5:322-325, 1989.
Benenson AS, editor: Control of communicable diseases in man, ed 14, Washington, DC, 1985, American Public Health Association.
Bowlby J: Maternal care and mental health, and Ainsworth MD, et al: Deprivation of maternal care, ed 2, New York, 1966, Schocken Books (originally publications of the World Health Organization).
Callahan D: Adequate health care in an aging society: are they morally compatible, Daedalus, The Aging Society, 115:247-267, 1986.
Cassell EJ: Ideas in conflict; the rise and fall (and rise and fall) of new views of disease, Daedalus, America's doctors, medical science, medical care, 115:19-41, 1986.
Christakis NA: Responding to a pandemic: international interests in AIDS control, Daedalus, Living with AIDS, 118:113-134, 1989.
Cutler JC, and Arnold RC: Venereal disease control by health departments in the past: lessons for the present, Am J Public Health 74:372-376, 1988.
Evans RG: "We'll take care of it for you," health care in the Canadian community, Daedalus, In Search of Canada, 117:155-189, 1988.
Friedland GH: Clinical care in the AIDS epidemic, Daedalus, Living with AIDS, 118:59-83, 1989.
Kapp MB: Medical empowerment of the elderly, Hastings Center Report, 19:5-7, 1989.
Nelson LJ, et al: Taking the train to a world of strangers: health care marketing and ethics, Hastings Center Report, 19:36-43, 1989.
Rivlin AM et al: Caring for the disabled elderly: who will pay? Washington, DC, 1988, The Brookings Institution.
Saunders C: The management of terminal illness, London, 1967, Hospital Medicine Publications. (extensive bibliography).
Selye H: The stress of life, New York, 1956, McGraw-Hill Book Co.
The Swedish Ministry of Health and Social Affairs: Health in Sweden, facts from basic studies under the HS 90 programme, Stockholm, Sweden, 1982. (HS 90 – The Swedish health services in the 1990s).
Walsh M: The patient with behavioural problems. In Accident and emergency nursing, a new approach, London, 1985, William Heinemann Medical Books Ltd., pp. 225-280.

CHAPTER 9

Nursing practice, nursing cases, and nursing agency

To practice nursing means to be regularly engaged in and responsible for the nursing of one or more persons (singly or in groups) in their time-place locations. Nurses' engagement in the practice of nursing may be continuous; however, often there are changes in persons for whom nursing is provided. To practice nursing means to enter into the life situations of others (usually strangers) to function as nurse with social and nursing legitimacy.

Persons provided with nursing during the same time duration measured in days, weeks, or months constitute the **case load** of a nurse. The amount of time necessary to provide the kind and amount of nursing required continuously or periodically by nurses' patients affects the number of persons or numbers of groups of persons constituting nurses' case loads. The extensity and intensity of nursing requirements of individuals affect the time requirements for providing nursing and, therefore, the number of patients that nurses can nurse effectively.

Nursing persons in health care situations classed in groups 5 and 6 (Chapter 8) at times may require the continuous presence of not one but more than one nurse at the same time and over the twenty-four hours of each day. At the other extreme, nurses who practice in nurse managed clinics who work primarily with ambulatory patients with therapeutic self-care demand components associated with pathologies or with the results and effects of medical treatments that must be met continuously (a subgroup of group 5, Chapter 8) may have very large case loads. Patient clinic visits are scheduled periodically according to need or on request and visits do not consume the major portion of a nurse's day.

NURSING CASES

Nursing cases are concrete instances of persons requiring and receiving nursing because of health-derived or health-related self-care deficits. Each nursing case has a history of events that precipitate requirements for nursing, events that occur during the period of being nursed, events that precipitate change from one system of providing nursing to another, and events that terminate the provision of nursing. Each concrete nursing case presents two challenges to the practicing nurse. The first challenge is to resolve the question: How can this person(s) be helped through nursing? The second challenge is for nurses to provide within time and place frames the kind and amount of nursing judged to be essential, including recognition and management of contractual problems, interpersonal problems, role problems, and the technologic problems arising during the course of providing nursing.

Nurses who enter into the life situations of others who are in need of nursing are professionally obligated to accept these persons and become informed about them and their conditions and circumstances of living. Empirical knowledge is sought not only from the views of "taking care of" and "helping" but from the view of nursing science, theoretically and practically practical nursing sciences, including views provided by the articulating life sciences.

What nurses seek to know about persons under their care is limited to information relevant to their nursing. Observations of nurses are guided in each instance of nursing by their antecedent theoretical and empirical knowledge of nursing as it is generally or specifically relevant to the patient. There is a nursing basis for nurses obtaining particular kinds of information and not other kinds of information in each instance of nursing practice.

Nurses must be able to attribute nursing meaning to information obtained and to use it as the basis for making nursing judgments and decisions. All information, both relevant and nonrelevant, about patients is held in confidence. According to its nature, information may be referred back to the patient, the patient's significant others, or to the physician or other health worker whenever the information is specific to their domains. In the latter situations nurses may help patients convey the information, record it in the official patient record, or communicate it verbally in emergency situations.

Nursing-specific and nursing-relevant information is set forth by the theory of self-care, the theory of self-care deficit, and the theory of nursing system. Information is specified within each of the theories as it pertains to persons in space-time matrices; properties of persons and properties of their relationships; motion or change that occurs in persons, their properties, or their operations; and to products made through deliberately performed actions (see Chapter 3, Table 3-1).

Information about these entities is sought and obtained at specific times over some time period. Nurses' location of the information in one or more of the six nursing design units (Chapter 5) indicates the *nursing meaning* of the information. The foci of the six nursing design units described in Chapter 5 are repeated here for purposes of understanding their place in the affording of nursing meaning to information about entities specified by the self-care deficit theory of nursing. Nurses reflect on time-specific patient information and make judgments about its relevance to:
- The contract for nursing and nursing's jurisdiction in the case
- The formation and operation of a legitimate functional unity of persons for the provision of nursing and the provision of self-care or dependent care

- The current or prior system of self-care or dependent-care
- The therapeutic self-care demand
- Valid self-care roles based on self-care capabilities
- The design of a system(s) of nursing

Chapter 5 indicates the kinds of information that is appropriate for the six nursing design units. Nurses' allocation to design units of information about patients and their conditions and circumstances of living mentally or in some recorded form by time periods shows the stability or instability of significant features of nursing cases. Initial data and changes in the data over time provides a descriptive picture of design features of a nursing case.

SUMMARY DESCRIPTION – DESIGN OF A NURSING CASE

Information about patients under nursing care because of cerebrovascular accidents was organized as a typical case. The six design units were used in assigning nursing meaning to relevant available information. There is no suggestion that the exposition of the design features of the presented "case" is complete or even adequate. The presentation illustrated the attachment of nursing meaning to information and the relevance of information to nursing system design and production. The case is presented by design units A-F. The case material presented is for a time period when health state was relatively stable. The case description by design units should be read with understanding of the grave potential for unfavorable changes in health state that can occur at any time. There is no focus on all possible conditions that appear in cases of this type.

A – Contract for and jurisdiction of nursing

Information, judgments, and decisions specific to this design unit are presented under ten headings.

Person to be nursed

Mary Doe, a 70-year-old wife of Harry and mother of adult married children, resides in the family home as part of an extended family.

Reason for seeking nursing

Mrs. Doe has a complete self-care deficit following a second cerebrovascular accident.

Prior care givers

Previous care givers, in regressive order, are nurses in Hospital X; husband in home; nurses at rehabilitation center; nurses at Hospital X; self before first stroke.

Request for and projected requirements for nursing

Hospital referral to Home Care Association after Mr. Doe and family (in collaboration with Mrs. Doe's physician) had made the decision to take care of Mrs. Doe in her home. Proposal: A dependent-care system in the home that would be articulated with a periodic system of nursing produced by association nurses who would be responsible for instruction of family members. Nursing will be provided by association nurses until home care is no longer appropriate for Mrs. Doe. Nurses and assistants will provide direct nursing of Mrs. Doe. Nurses will provide instruction, guidance, and direction that is needed by family members contributing to the dependent-care system. This would include monitoring Mrs. Doe's condition, monitoring results of care, and evaluation of adequacy of the combined systems. Nurses will make referrals about needs for special services or equipment to the association or to other agencies.

Position in health care system

Mrs. Doe is under the care of a physician who is a specialist in internal medicine because of diabetes mellitus and two cerebrovascular accidents, the second of which affected the brainstem.

Nurses' knowledge of impact on family

The hospital social worker advised the family to have Mrs. Doe provided with care in a nursing home. Despite stress associated with Mrs. Doe's previous illness, the family said the only acceptable course was to have Mrs. Doe in her own home.

Number and qualifications of nurses and assistants to nurses

A primary nurse is required with provision for a replacement nurse. The primary nurse has educational qualifications for entry to professional level practice with 10 years of nursing practice experience. A home health aide, with provision for replacement, is also required. The aide is trained vocationally with 8 years of experience in the association. The primary nurse will provide nursing daily or adjust schedule in accord with Mrs. Doe's nursing requirements. The home health aide will provide care for Mrs. Doe daily.

Contracting parties

Mr. Doe (in collaboration with Mrs. Doe's physician) and the Home Health Care Association are the contracting parties.

Resources required and obtained

Resources include a hospital bed, lift, suction equipment, and other standard equipment.

Method of financing

Third-party payment is available.

B — Legitimate functional unity of care providers

Mrs. Doe has no active participatory role and limited awareness, but does react to some events. Legitimate care providers are the Association nurses and home health aides, the three family members, and association personnel, such as a physical therapist and speech therapist, who provide for Mrs. Doe's special requirements.

C — Current or prior self-care or dependent-care system

Not relevant at this time period.

D — Therapeutic self-care demand

Mrs. Doe's therapeutic self-care demand is conditioned primarily by her health state and by her condition of living, that is, confinement to bed. Her state of health is characterized by impaired neuromuscular functioning resultant from cerebrovascular accidents including inability to speak, to swallow, or to manage the position of her body and its parts. Her cardiac and respiratory functioning are stabilized but there have been periods when breathing was in the Cheyne-Stokes pattern. Cough reflex is diminished with inability to handle her own secretions. There is no bladder or bowel control. Mrs. Doe has a gastrostomy tube that is sutured in place. Mrs. Doe has diabetes mellitus with a care regimen of prescribed morning dose of insulin and prescribed diet, which family understands and manages. Level of awareness fluctuates during the day and over time periods from alertness to grogginess.

The components of Mrs. Doe's therapeutic self-care demand are universal-type self-care requisites and health-deviation requisites. Developmental-type self-care requisites are not considered apart from the universal requisites of prevention of hazards and promotion of normalcy.

The factors that condition each universal and health-deviation self-care requisite are presented along with summary listings of technologies and actions. Technologies and actions are not presented in the precise fashion described in Chapter 6, but as action statements without detailed development of action sequences.

Maintaining a sufficient intake of air

Normal pattern of inspiration and expiration is obstructed at times by the following conditioning factors, each of which may affect sufficiency of air intake: Cheyne-Stokes pattern of breathing; diminished cough reflex with inability to manage secretions; confinement to bed and inability to manage self, to turn, to sit up.

Technologies and actions include the following:

- Position in bed to facilitate breathing; transfer to upright position in chair; change position in bed.

- Observe for open airway.
- Suction to remove secretions.
- Regulate air flow and humidity in room.
- Observe for respiratory distress.

Maintaining a sufficient intake of water

Securing and consuming water is affected by inability to speak, move, and swallow. Technologies and actions include the following:
- Know and maintain standard for fluid intake for Mrs. Doe.
- Adjust fluid intake to fluid loss.
- Give water through gastrostomy tube at intervals throughout the day other than after prescribed feedings.
- Give water after each gastrostomy feeding.
- Observe for signs of dehydration or overhydration.

Maintaining a sufficient intake of food

The securing and consumption of food by Mrs. Doe is interfered with or conditioned by her inability to speak, move, or swallow.

Technologies and actions include the following:
- Have available the medically prescribed, prepared formula for feeding Mrs. Doe the caloric and protein adequacy of which has been evaluated by the dietitian associated with the Home Health Care Association.
- Prepare the formula and feed Mrs. Doe through her gastrostomy tube four times daily; administer water after feeding.
- Administer prescribed insulin dose each morning.
- Observe for signs of hypoglycemia and hyperglycemia.
- Observe for signs of hunger.
- Observe for signs of inadequate nutrition.

Providing care associated with eliminative processes and excrements

The meeting of this universal self-care requisite is affected by absence of bladder and bowel control, inability to move, composition and consistency of tube feedings, and amount and sufficiency of water intake.

Technologies and actions related to urinary output include:
- Urine elimination through Foley catheter involving periodic change of catheter and a routine of catheter care to ensure safety, effectiveness, and prevention of infection.
- Ensure that the standard for intake of water is met.
- Observe urine for color, clearness, and odor; measure urine output and record amount as well as observed features.
- Dispose of urine in a sanitary manner.

- Care for urine drainage bag.

Technologies and actions related to bowel evacuation include the following:

- Develop and maintain a regimen for bowel evacuation. This may require medication to counteract the effects of the composition and consistency of gastrostomy tube feedings on bowel evacuation.
- Stimulate activity spaced throughout the day such as turning and repositioning.
- Hygienic care of body parts and surfaces after bowel evacuation; maintain clean clothing and bed linen.
- Use sanitary procedure to dispose of feces and to handle soiled linen.
- Observe and record consistency of the stool, its color, and amount of fluid in the evacuation.
- Record time of evacuations.
- Taking appropriate action when diarrhea or constipation occurs.

Technologies and actions related to the excretory activities of the skin include the following:

- Perform regular personal care related to insensible perspiration, including bathing of all body surfaces, keeping clothing and linen clean.
- Know patient's body temperature and the environmental temperature.
- Regulate room temperature; adjust weight and amount of clothing and air flow to maintain a physical environment that supports normal body temperature.
- Observe for sweating and its associated signs and symptoms. Act to ensure that patient is warm and dry. Act to determine the underlying reasons and institute appropriate regulatory action.

Maintaining a balance between activity and rest and between solitude and social interaction

Maintaining these balances for Mrs. Doe are affected by her inability to move and speak and by alternating periods of alertness and extremely limited awareness during the course of a day or over a period of days. Mrs. Doe can hear and see and reacts or responds to events by gaze.

Technologies and actions related to maintenance of a balance between activity and rest include the following:

- Support Mrs. Doe's diurnal wake-sleep pattern.
- Provide for periods of stimulation and rest during the day.
- Prepare for sleep at night.
- Select stimulation to which Mrs. Doe responds favorably such as television or persons who Mrs. Doe wants to be with her and who relate to her with speech.
- Provide for physical movement: passive exercises of the extremities; move from bed to chair at least once a day.

- Recognize and respond appropriately to signs of fatigue brought about by care activities.

Technologies and actions related to maintenance of a balance between solitude and social interaction include the following:

- Recognize and respond to Mrs. Doe's signals for solitude (wanting to be left alone) with knowledge of what she preferred when well.
- Interact with Mrs. Doe during each care-giving contact. Limit verbalization during care in the interest of preventing fatigue.
- Show interest in and concern for Mrs. Doe at the same time affording her rightful independence as a person.
- Demonstrate a "caring about" attitude as "taking care of" activities are performed.
- Allow Mrs. Doe to select visitors through the use of the picture communication board to which she responds with a specific gaze.
- Provide for television viewing.

Preventing hazards

The meeting of this universal self-care requisite is viewed as related to the meeting of the previously described requisites. It is affected by Mrs. Doe's lack of self-management capabilities, limited awareness, inability to swallow, absence of bladder and bowel control, use of a Foley catheter, gastrostomy tube, and insulin-dependent diabetes mellitus.

Technologies and actions for meeting this requisite include the following:

- Recognize signs of clinical emergency situations and respond appropriately.
- Take action to prevent untoward events associated with Mrs. Doe's confinement to bed for the major portion of every day and in moving from bed to chair to bed.
- Maintain conditions to prevent respiratory distress and respiratory infections.
- Maintain actions to prevent hazards associated with the use and care of the Foley catheter, including infection.
- Maintain actions to prevent hazards associated with use and care of Mrs. Doe's gastrostomy tube and administration of feedings. These include infection, tube displacement, and feeding associated diarrhea.
- Maintain action to minimize stress and physical exhaustion resultant from performance of care measures by others without ability to participate.
- Know fluid intake and fluid loss (sweat, urine, bowel evacuations) and take action appropriate to maintain fluid balance.
- Maintain observations relative to Mrs. Doe's safety and to the occurrence of emergencies with immediate reporting to physician, the Home Health Care Association, emergency medical services as appropriate.

Being normal

All the conditioning factors identified in prevention of hazards are relevant to Mrs. Doe's normality. The lack of self-management capabilities and the limitation of awareness are most significant.

The following technologies and actions are important:
- Recognize when Mrs. Doe is aware; approach her and respond to her as a person.
- Maintain features of family living familiar to Mrs. Doe, including Mrs. Doe in accord with her family roles.
- Maintain Mrs. Doe's contacts with friends, church members, and other social contacts that she prefers.
- Contribute to development and to Mrs. Doe's use of a pictorial system of communication.
- Recognize evidence of discomfort and pain and act to relieve these experiences by elimination of causes, soothing care measures, and use of prescribed medication if needed.
- Know Mrs. Doe's religious orientations and practices and assist appropriately in their maintenance.
- Foster Mrs. Doe's maintenance of her sense of self.
- Provide care to maintain Mrs. Doe's integrity to the degree possible with respect to, for example, grooming, body alignment, body temperature, fluid balance.

All of the described universal self-care requisite components of Mrs. Doe's therapeutic self-care demand are adjusted to factors derived from the results and effects of two cerebrovascular accidents, to her condition of insulin-dependent diabetes mellitus, and to health care system factors such as the fixed gastrostomy tube and use of insulin. Other health-deviation self-care requisites to be met continuously are identified.

Health-deviation self-care requisites

Mrs. Doe's other health-deviation self-care requisites that would constitute components of her therapeutic self-care demand at a minimum include the following:
- Securing appropriate assistance from Mrs. Doe's physician by telephone or visit in the event of occurrence of signs and symptoms of another cardiovascular accident; substantial neurologic change; elevated blood pressure; signs and symptoms of hyperglycemia, hypoglycemia, urinary tract infection, or infection in the area of the gastrostomy tube; respiratory distress; fever; unexplained pain; a fall.
- Effective conduct of the medically prescribed diabetes mellitus management regimen including morning insulin in the prescribed dose, observation of blood glucose levels, calculation of insulin dose within the prescribed range if afternoon insulin is required, administration of prescribed feed-

ings by gastrostomy tube, and observation for signs of hypoglycemia or hyperglycemia.

• Observe for the status of and changes in Mrs. Doe related to specific aspects of her functioning and her known pathologies, including attention to features of and changes in cardiac functioning, kidney functioning, circulation, neurologic functioning, the integrity and condition of skin and mucous membranes, and bowel functioning.

E — Self-care capabilities and roles, dependent-care capabilities and roles

Mrs. Doe has no known operational capabilities to engage in self-care. There is no known potential for restoration of prior capabilities or for development of new capabilities. Mrs. Doe has some ability to convey her reactions through her gaze.

Adult members of Mrs. Doe's family have learned and continue to learn to meet components of Mrs. Doe's therapeutic self-care demand by performing some care measures that must be performed at specific times, as well as ones that may need to be performed any time of the day. They provide care consistently, safely, and effectively. Dependent-care capabilities of family members are not adequate for meeting all components of Mrs. Doe's therapeutic self-care demand or for knowing when and how to make adjustments or major changes.

Some family members experience psychological and physiological dependent-care limitations. Other family members recognize when this occurs and are flexible compensating for what one family member cannot do at a particular time.

All family members are subject to fatigue and what they can endure relative to the dependent-care situation.

F — Design features of the nursing system

The nursing system for Mrs. Doe is a periodic system that is in operation each day but not continuously. The nursing system articulates with a dependent-care system for Mrs. Doe that is in continuous production. There is provision for communication of dependent-care agents with the primary nurse or the Home Care Association at times when nurses are not present in Mrs. Doe's home.

The nursing system and the dependent-care system were initiated upon Mrs. Doe's return home from the hospital. Both systems have achieved a degree of operational stability but continue to develop as nursing problems are recognized, resolved, and solutions found. The nursing system is produced and managed by the primary nurse with assistance of the home health aide(s). The dependent-care system is produced and managed primarily by three members of Mrs. Doe's family working collaboratively.

Broad role responsibilities of the primary nurse

The primary nurse has two broad responsibilities: (1) to govern, produce, and manage the nursing system in accord with its constituent action elements, articulating primary nurse contributions with those of the home health aide and the person and action elements of the dependent-care system; and (2) to determine the elements and the relations among elements of the dependent-care system, to identify signs of its adequacy and effectiveness, and to confer with family members to guide them in their endeavors and in effecting needed adjustments and changes.

Specific role responsibilities of the primary nurse

The following is a development of these responsibilities:

- Instruct and guide family with respect to meeting components of Mrs. Doe's therapeutic self-care demand.
- Guide and direct the home health aide as changes occur in Mrs. Doe's condition; be accessible to the home health aide for supervision and consultation.
- Assess Mrs. Doe's vital signs. Conduct a physical assessment for Mrs. Doe once a week or more frequently as indicated. Do blood glucose checks to determine effectiveness of care measures for management of diabetes mellitus.
- Obtain information about and judge the nursing or medical relevance of the Cheyne-Stokes pattern of breathing when it occurs.
- Obtain information from home health aide and dependent-care agents about the presence or absence of respiratory distress or airway problems and their management when present.
- Observe for and make judgments about matters that should be referred to Mrs. Doe's physician. Advise family about nurse-perceived needs for contacting physician.
- Make judgments about situations where the nurse should communicate directly with the physician.
- Instruct family about signs of emergency situations and emergency care, including notification of Mrs. Doe's physician or emergency medical services when emergencies arise.
- Manage care related to use of the Foley catheter and its periodic replacement. Observe for sign of urinary tract infection.
- Observe for the integrity of patient's tissues with concern for the condition of mouth and the skin, with attention to tissues surrounding the permanent gastrostomy tube.
- Know nutritional and fluid intake and make judgments about its adequacy.
- Know urinary and bowel output and assess and judge quality and quantity.
- Observe for hazardous conditions in Mrs. Doe's environment and in care performance and work with home health aide and dependent-care agents to remove them or to institute safety measures.
- Work with home health aide and dependent-care agents to identify new and emerging self-care requisites and to design means for meeting them.
- Work cooperatively with speech therapist in the development and use of picture charts to aid Mrs. Doe to communicate.

- Work cooperatively with the physical therapist with respect to rules of body alignment, passive exercise, protective measures, transfer from bed to chair and return, and use of needed equipment.
- Consult with dietitian associated with Home Health Care Association for reevaluations of Mrs. Doe's diet.
- Document immediately observations and measures of care performed and problems encountered with recommendation for follow-up.
- Work with family members to guide and support them with respect to knowing and meeting components of their therapeutic self-care demands associated with or affected by their dependent-care activities.
- Consult with dependent-care agents about their assessments of the quality and effectiveness of Mrs. Doe's care and problems they are encountering.
- Endeavor to know what Mrs. Doe's family is experiencing and support them in ways that are helpful but not intrusive.
- Assist the family to become an operational unit with the nurses and home health aide in designing and providing care for Mrs. Doe with understanding of areas of independence and interdependence.
- Be judicious in the use of nursing supplies and equipment and in protecting household furnishings that are used in Mrs. Doe's care.
- Periodically assess personal capabilities and actions in governing, producing, and managing the periodic system of nursing for Mrs. Doe and in cooperative functioning with Mrs. Doe's family. Identify needs for knowledge, new skills, or improvement of skills.
- Seek nursing consultation and supervision from the assigned nurse in the Home Health Care Association.

Role responsibilities of the home health aide

The following is a development of these responsibilities:
- Communicate with patient as care is provided.
- Bathe patient; provide mouth care; care for hair; exercise concern for Mrs. Doe's privacy.
- Perform range of motion exercises.
- Position Mrs. Doe to facilitate comfort and support unobstructed breathing; protect extremities.
- Inspect skin and report problems of skin integrity to nurse.
- Use clothing and coverings for Mrs. Doe that are appropriate for maintaining normal body temperature under prevailing environmental conditions.
- Provide Foley catheter care according to the specified regimen.
- Empty and care for urinary drainage bag; record urinary output.
- Provide care within the regimen for bowel evacuation and note features of bowel movements, including fluid content of evacuations.

- Provide care in a manner that prevents psychological stress and prevents or minimizes the occurrence of physical exhaustion for Mrs. Doe.
- Cooperate with family members who provide care.
- Be judicious in the use of resources and protect the household furnishings in Mrs. Doe's room.
- Document immediately care provided and report information to the primary nurse and nursing supervisor.
- Seek supervision as needed.
- Assess personal capabilities and contributions to Mrs. Doe's care. Identify need for additionl skills and supporting knowledge.

Broad role responsibilities of dependent-care agents

These responsibilities include taking care of Mrs. Doe twenty-four hours of each day safely and effectively and being with her and performing care measures at specified times or when the need for them occurs. Dependent-care agents must be flexible in accepting changing responsibilities for performance of care measures to ensure continuity of care and operational unity in the provision of care. There is the broad responsibility to accept Home Health Care Association nurses into the household and to work with them, not as strangers or intruders, but as professionals to be collaborated with in the care of Mrs. Doe.

Specific role responsibilities of dependent-care agents

These responsibilities are developed as follows:
- Give fixed prescribed dose of morning insulin; give afternoon dose if needed according to the prescribed sliding scale.
- Prepare and give prescribed feedings by gastrostomy tube four times a day; give water after and between feedings.
- Empty urinary drainage bag; measure and record amount of urine; observe characteristics of urine, noting changes in color or clarity.
- Change Mrs. Doe's position in bed; position to facilitate inspiration and expiration.
- Keep Mrs. Doe clean and dry after bowel evacuation; note color and consistency of stool and the amount of fluid in the evacuation; record.
- Maintain weight of Mrs. Doe's clothing and covering in accord with environmental conditions to prevent chilling and sweating.
- Manage environmental conditions and Mrs. Doe's position in bed or chair to provide some balance between activity and rest.
- Manage social conditions to provide for a balance between solitude and social interaction.
- Act to prevent development of hazardous conditions and to ensure Mrs. Doe's safety if they occur.

- Maintain environmental conditions to assure Mrs. Doe that she is in the home with her family.
- Work with nurses and home health aide to ensure that Mrs. Doe's self-care requisites are known and met.
- Seek guidance and direction from primary nurse when courses of care action are unclear or instruction is needed.
- Notify the primary nurse or the Home Health Care Association when nursing help is needed.
- Communicate with Mrs. Doe's physician as requested by the physician; convey information to the physician that the primary nurses identify as important for the family to report.
- Know the indications of emergency situations; observe for such evidence; report and seek help from Mrs. Doe's physician or from emergency medical services.
- Perform family related role responsibilities including (1) supporting one another in providing care to minimize stress and prevent fatigue, (2) ensuring that each family member's therapeutic self-care demand is calculated and met, (3) observing family members for signs of stress and fatigue and act to provide relief, (4) observing effects of providing home care for Mrs. Doe on individual family members and the family as a structural and functional unity, and (5) taking action to prevent family dysfunction or to restore family stability.
- Maintain a care record.

NURSING PRACTICE FEATURES

The foregoing example of design unit information for a type of nursing case reveals the social, interpersonal, and technologic features of the case. It also highlights the active conditioners of self-management abilities, self-care agency, and therapeutic self-care demand components of patients in those cases. The contractual and interpersonal features of the case represented through design units information were conditioned by the patient's complete self-care deficit and by loss of self-management capabilities associated with the results and effects of two cerebrovascular accidents (health state factors). The contract for nursing was not with the patient but with the patient's husband who would be legally responsible for her. Interactions of nurses with the patient were one-sided, with patient reactions as the only contributions to the process. Nurses interacted with family members in the initiation, development, and maintenance of interlocking nursing and dependent-care systems.

The factor actively conditioning the patient properties of self-care agency and therapeutic self-care demand was health state with age and development state, both stable and affecting therapeutic self-care demand to a minimal degree. Age in this case was not actively related to developmental state as it would be with infants and children because maturation had been achieved. If or how psychological or personal development could proceed in cases of this type is unclear. Health state factors expressed as the results and effects of two cerebrovascular accidents imposed on the patient a style of living that did not permit movement from one place to another unless moved or transported physically by other persons. It also required the patient to remain in a health care system for the duration of life.

Family system factors, sociocultural factors, socioeconomic factors, and available resources were family relevant. They would be conditioners of the willingness and the developing ability of the family and its members and the availability of time, labor, and resources to provide a continuous system of dependent care in the home and to articulate it with a periodic system of nursing. This case can be summarized as well as typed according to its health care focus, the causes and the extent of the self-care deficit, the components of the therapeutic self-care demand, the complexity and stability of the therapeutic self-care demand, and by the type of nursing system that would be the product of the work of nurses expressed in terms of the compensatory or educational features of the action system and its continuous or periodic production.

Nursing practice features of nursing cases fall roughly into two groups. Operational features are broadly grouped as societal, interpersonal, and technologic features. These features identify, in analogous terms, the players in the drama of nursing and their places in families and the larger society, what the play is about, the roles of each player, relation of players to one another, the time-place localization of players, and the playing out of roles by each player. Second, are characterizing features of the players themselves and their environments. In the real world of nurses, nurses' patients, and nursing operations distinguishing features of individuals and their environments are associated with a number of factors named *basic conditioning factors*. In the case example, health state and the imposed pattern of living were major conditioning factors. Basic conditioning factors also affect nurses and their property of nursing agency.

Practicing nurses must have the capabilities to identify and organize information about patients in each nursing case in terms of its societal, interpersonal, and technologic meanings for nursing. They must have detailed, authoritative, antecedent knowledge about *basic conditioning factors* and their relevance to individuals and properties of individuals and to the behavior of individuals singly or in groups. Nurses' knowledge of basic conditioning factors ideally is both theoretical and experiential. For example, nurses know from the fields of human development and human behavior specific developments that are associated with different periods of the human life cycle. They know from the fields of sociology, cultural anthropology, and economics that there are life-style differences and differences in the availability of resources in social groups within societies. But nurses also know from their practice of nursing the features that some patients probably would have in common with other patients, for example, the well-developed manipulative skills of male veterans of a particular war, who live in rural areas and are farmers or mechanics.[1] Nurses, for example, also know from experience the effects of high-stress, high-demand households on patients, and what is and is not possible for nurses to do to help them maintain an adequate system of self-care. Nurses learn what nursing adjustments must be made to help educationally deprived persons with arrested cognitive development before such adjustments and technologies can be validated and become a part of practically practical nursing science.

Attention is now given to these two kinds of features of nursing cases considering them from a practice perspective. There is some overlap and repetition but this is necessary in order to emphasize the practice perspective rather than a nursing content or nursing science perspective.

Operational features of nursing practice

The central idea of the theory of nursing system (Chapter 3) stated that "nursing systems are formed by nurses through their deliberate exercise of specialized nursing capabilities (nursing agency) within the context of their interpersonal and contractual relationships with persons with health derived or health associated" self-care deficits. This central idea specifies that nurses engage in the technologic operations of nursing practice within the framework of a social contract or agreement that initially relates persons who need nursing with nurses and within a continuing interpersonal relationship. Both relationships are necessary because they are enabling for nurses to design and produce nursing systems.

The social relationship of nurses to patients or their next of kin is contractual. The interpersonal relationship is professional, helping, and nursing. These relationships must be brought about and maintained deliberately throughout the time period when nursing is provided. Because social, interpersonal, and technologic operations are necessary, nursing practice has three dimensions, and nursing systems can be thought of as tridimensional.

Components or elements that affect the societal and interpersonal operations of nursing practice and in turn the technologic operations are described.

Social and interpersonal components

The *social components* of nursing practice bring nurses into contact with persons who are their patients, locating these persons in larger social structures. The society provides the mechanisms for relating persons who need nursing to persons who are qualified, able, and willing to provide it. The social component includes the agreement under which nursing will be provided, including the parties to the agreement and the duration of the agreement.

The legitimacy of occupancy of positions of nurse and nurse's patient derives from societal standards, laws regulating the practice of nursing, and from qualifying conditions possessed by persons with the statuses of nurse and patient. Nurses and nurses' patients who are related under some type of agreement for the provision of nursing seek a relationship of instrumental effectiveness between the nursing capabilities of nurses and the nursing requirements of patients as defined by the nature of and the reasons for the existence of patients' self-care deficits. It is nurses' initial and continuing judgments about the presence of and reasons for patients' self-care deficits that establish and maintain the linkages between the social and technologic components of nursing practice.

The *interpersonal components* of nursing practice are enabling for both the social-contractual components and the technologic components of practice. Contact, association, and communication are essential interpersonal components required for bringing particular nurses into a nursing relationship with particular patients and for effecting arrangements for the provision of nursing. One result sought from interpersonal relations of nurses and patients and their families is a level of coordination that is enabling for the performance of the technologic work of nursing practice (Table 9-1).

The level of cooperation attained among nurses, their associates, their patients, and persons with significant relations to patients is a function of the quality of the interpersonal relations among them and the effective designing of nursing systems. Mutual cooperation and effectively managed division of labor within nursing practice situations is *high-level* coordination. A high level of coordination allows considerable independence of cooperating individuals. Such a level of coordination requires role differentiation; acceptance of role responsibilities; knowledge of role articulations; and developed social, interpersonal, and communication skills of involved individuals. The world of the nurse is not the world of the patient. Nurses and their patients ideally search for some common ground from which they can move to relate and communicate so that what patients need is revealed and how nurses can help is communicated.

Nursing students are sometimes instructed that the *role of nurse* is to care for the "whole person" or the "whole patient." This advice may confuse or mislead students who are not helped to understand that the persons who are nurses' patients have requirements for nursing and at the same time have requirements for other kinds of care and help, for example, support from family and friends, spiritual care and instruction, and medical care. Nurses associate and communicate with the *persons* who are their patients and provide the specialized kind of care that is named nursing. They also cooperate with patients and their families to ensure that other kinds of care needed or desired are provided. Nurses sometimes elect to help persons who are their patients, as people commonly help one another as needs arise. When this occurs, both nurse and patient should know that what is done is outside the nurse role. Nurses must exercise prudence in not taking on professional role responsibilities from other fields of human service.

Contact and interpersonal exchanges between nurses and patients in practice situations vary in frequency, duration, and initiator of contact. Nurses need to manage

Table 9-1   Three dimensions of nursing practice

	Element		
Features	Person in Role	Person in Role	Type of relationship
Social	In position of *nurse* who can legitimately enter into negotiations for providing nursing	In the position of becoming a nurse's patient	Contractual for nursing
Interpersonal	*Active role* as person who is qualified and functioning as nurse	*Active role* to *no instrumental role* as person who is, was, or can be his or her own self-care agent	Professional, helping, nursing
Technological	*Nurse role set* defined by (1) the work operations of professionals and (2) the presence of a self-care deficit in the patient, including extent and causes	*Patient role set* as defined by (1) the process of diagnosis to determine needs for nursing assistance and (2) the presence and characteristics of an identified and described self-care deficit	Nursing as specified by role sets of patient and nurse

the interpersonal components of practice toward the production of required nursing and at the same time to protect and foster the well-being of patients. Interpersonal contact and communication require effort and energy expenditure by both patient and nurse. This is illustrated by a seriously ill patient who said to his nurse, "Don't tell me one more thing; just take care of me." Patients vary in their tolerance for contact and associations in accord with their temperament, their degree of illness, and their available energy.

Ideally, the interpersonal relationship between a nurse and a patient contributes to the alleviation of the patient's stress and that of the family, enabling the patient and the family to act responsibly in matters of health and health care. A relationship that permits a patient to develop and maintain confidence in the nurse and in himself or herself is the foundation for a deliberate process of nursing that contributes positively to the patient's achievement of present and future health goals.*

---

* Ida Jean Orlando, The dynamic nurse-patient relationship, Putnam, New York, 1961, and Ernestine Wiedenbach, Clinical nursing, a helping art, Springer, New York, 1964, focus on behavior of nurse and patient during the nursing process. Dorothy Johnson, The nature of a science of nursing, Nurs Outlook 59:291-294, 1959, and Dorothy Johnson, A philosophy of nursing, Nurs Outlook 59:198-200, 1959, indicate the nurse's role in alleviation of the patient's stress.

The three dimensions of nursing practice in concrete situations of practice yield systems of relationships among individuals and systems of actions performed by nurses and persons under their care. The systems of relationships establish the structure of nursing practice situations, and the systems of actions (the nursing systems) determine the movement toward goals sought by nurses and their patients.

Background information

Background information about patients is relevant to the three dimensions of nursing practice: social, interpersonal, and professional-technologic. Such information facilitates nursing along all dimensions. Background information is about (1) the larger social frame of reference in which nursing is provided, (2) factors that can affect or are affecting the development and maintenance of an effective interpersonal system(s) and (3) factors that can influence the extent and intensity of the interaction of nurses with persons under nursing care and others, and (4) factors that are likely to affect the quality and degree of patient participation in nursing situations and thus influence the *amount* of nursing required. Factors of the latter type affect both the technologic and the interpersonal dimensions of practice.

Background information may be accumulated by nurses in first or early contacts with patients and their families or with multiperson units under the care of nurses. Other information may be obtained over the duration of the nursing situation, and some information may need to be brought up to date.

Social

Information that permits nurses to place the person(s) under nursing care within a larger social frame of reference includes the following:
- The unit of service of the nurse, an individual patient, or a multiperson unit, for example, a family or a residence group (Chapter 10)
- The place(s) where the person(s) under nursing care resides and the place(s) where nursing is provided
- Events that preceded and the reasons for seeking or being under nursing care
- The next of kin or legal guardian or person responsible for managing the affairs of persons under nursing care
- The parties to the initial or continuing agreement about providing and receiving nursing and the level at which the agreement is instituted; for example, and as previously indicated, the agreement may be between the person who is a nurse's patient and the agency where the nurse is employed
- Overt evidence that persons under nursing care have health-related or health-derived self-care deficits and that nurse capabilities are in conformity with nursing requirements of patients

Such background information is essential if nurses are to know and develop some insights about the social dimensions of each practice situation.

Interpersonal

Information about factors that are likely to facilitate or hinder the development and maintenance of effective relationships in nursing situations and the extensity and intensity of interactions may be obtained during early contacts of nurses with patients and persons significant to them as well as throughout the duration of nursing situations. Some of these factors remain relatively stable throughout the duration of nursing situations; others are subject to change. Those that do not vary should be accepted by nurses as *conditions of action* that must be taken into account when nurses select ways and means to achieve adaptive exchanges with patients or others significant to the patient or when nurses calculate the amount and kinds of contact that will be required with patients and others within nursing situations.

Factors identified as likely to influence the possibilities for and the quality of adaptive exchanges between nurses and patients and nurses and others within interpersonal situations include the following:
- Arousal level and ability to attend
- Age and gender
- Levels of emotional and intellectual maturity
- Present emotional state and degree of emotional control
- Communication modalities — reading, writing, spoken word
- Primary language
- Sensory deficits that limit sensory consciousness
- Cultural prescriptions about roles
- Knowledge of present and past events relevant to action

These nine factors presented here as essential background information about persons under nursing care are significant for nurses' understanding of patient behaviors and for adjusting their own approaches in interpersonal situations with patients and others.

Factors that are determinants of the *extent and intensity of interactions* of nurses and patients and nurses and others related to patients include the following:
- Ages of patients
- Physical, emotional, and intellectual development
- Arousal level and ability to attend, as when:
  Awake and aware, generally alert, drowsy, asleep
  Anesthetized
  Confused, stuporous, comatose, delirious
  In intense emotional states of fear or anger with attention narrowly focused
- Behavioral state when awake, for example, calm, restive, preoccupied, excited, uncomfortable, fearful, anxious
- Degree of illness and nature of illness (acute, chronic)
- Degree of debility

- Degree of uncompensated disability, physical or psychological
- Stability of various dimensions of patient functioning and degree to which life and health are endangered
- Complexity and frequency of change in patients' therapeutic self-care demands
- Patients' existent or emerging needs for and the giving of social and emotional support by persons significant to patients

Nurses who have insights about the effects of the named factors on the frequency and quality of nurse-patient interactions and nurses' interactions with others have *one basis* for judging the time requirements for nursing; the importance of nursing for the life, health, and well-being of persons under care; and the meaning that nursing has for patients and those related to them.

Factors affecting the quality of patient participation

Patients' participation and cooperation with nurses in the receiving and giving of nursing care is influenced by age, developmental state, degree of maturity or personalization, and arousal levels and abilities to attend to themselves and their environments. Given values of these factors are enabling for participation, however, other factors also affect patient participation. These factors include the following:

1. Self-image as responsible person and as self-care or dependent-care agent identified from:
    a. Self-reference expressions, for example, "I have been doing my best to manage my care," or "I have been taking care of myself for eighty years"
    b. More specific expressions about role in current health care situation; role expectations of others; role relationships to others
    c. Expressions of patients about how they are affected by what they are or have been experiencing
    d. Explicit statements about what has been done in self-care or dependent care, what can no longer be done, and the effectiveness or ineffectiveness of care
    e. Explicit statements about present requirements for care
2. What patients attend to voluntarily; what they are preoccupied with
3. Interests and concerns as revealed by recurring conversational themes or as deliberately communicated by patients or persons related to them:
    a. Expressions of interest in and concern for their health state or specific features of it
    b. Expressions of interest in and knowledge of health and health care
    c. Expressions of interest and concerns about personal matters other than their health care that precludes their attending to self-care matters, for example, family affairs
4. Evidence of developed and operable human powers that indicate how patients do conduct themselves in situations where they must act deliberately to attain

sought-after results. Such evidence need not be related to self-care or dependent care. Evidence would relate to what patients do and do not do with
respect to:

a. Initiating action sequences and carrying them through to completion of
   the task, including:
   (1) Eliciting aid as needed to complete a task
   (2) Directing and maintaining attention on self, on actions in process,
       and on relevant environmental conditions
b. Modes of thinking about reality situations, for example, at the level of
   the concrete or abstract*
c. Being reflective about actions performed and expressing judgments about
   them
d. Making decisions
e. Conserving available energy
f. Controlling positioning, ambulating, and engaging in manipulative
   movements

Information about these factors that affect the quality of patient participation are
important to nurses in all situations where patients are adult and capable of managing
themselves in their environments. Information about named factors reveals action
abilities and action limitations of a general nature that are indexes of how patients can
participate and the adjustments that nurses need to make in using various methods
of helping. For example, when patients think concretely, directions and instructions
should be phrased in terms of specific things to be done and the sequences in which
they are to be done.

The suggestions about kinds of background information focus on *patients as persons*
and are phrased in terms of factors that reveal or affect self-direction and
self-management by persons under nursing care. Background information of the
kinds indicated when obtained and used by nurses is relevant to the effectiveness of
nurses functioning within the social and interpersonal areas of practice and
contributes to the attainment of nursing results through the technologic operations
of nursing practice.

Technologic components

Professional-technologic components of nursing practice are designed for the
attainment of nursing results for patients. Their attainment occurs within the frame
of a social-contractual relationship and an interpersonal relationship or in some
instances intergroup relationships. The technologic components include the profes-

---

* See Nursing Development Conference Group, *Concept Formalization in Nursing: Process and Product*, ed.
2, Orem DE, editor, Little, Brown & Co., Boston, 1979, pp. 215-229, esp. pp. 219-229, for an account of Joan
Backscheider's work in classifying intellectual operations of an adult ambulatory nursing population with
indications of meaning for nursing.

sional operations and the management operations of nursing practice. The professional operations are collectively referred to as the nursing process. The management operations of planning and controlling (including evaluation) are interspersed with the technologic operations of nursing diagnosis, nursing prescription, and nursing regulation or treatment. These operations are described in Chapter 10.

BASIC CONDITIONING FACTORS AND NURSING PRACTICE

The self-care deficit theory of nursing suggests that features of persons nursed including some specific properties are affected by human and environmental factors pertaining to them as individuals and as members of families and social groups. Nurses must understand the nature of the ten basic conditioning factors named and briefly described in Chapter 6 if they are to be used by them in the practice of nursing. The use of the factors within the design operations of nursing practice is evident in the case material presented in this chapter, especially in Design Units A, B, D, and E and in the section Background Information.

To further clarify the use of the factors in nursing practice, an example of use by clinical nursing specialists in one hospital is presented. This is followed by a description of the 10 basic conditioning factors as they pertain to the operational elements of nursing practice and the conceptual elements of the self-care deficit theory of nursing.

Nurses' use of basic conditioning factors, an example

Basic conditioning factors can be used and grouped in a number of ways. One organization of factors was revealed by an analysis of material descriptive of nursing cases reported by clinical nursing specialists in a hospital serving a population, the members of which had many characterizing features in common.[1]

In analysis of described cases it was found that information about basic conditioning factors was used and organized in four sets in the process of describing nursing cases. The first set of factors described the person who was nursed. The factors in the set included the following:

- The age and gender of the patient and age by dates of admission for health care in the specific hospital
- The residence of the patient and its environmental features (an environmental factor)
- Family system factors including patient's position in the family and information about other family members with relevant details about residence and relationship with the patient
- Sociocultural factors including education, occupation, occupational experiences, or life experiences
- Socioeconomic factors including resources currently available or potentially available

These factors describe the person who is in the position of nurses' patient and provide one empirical knowledge base that nurses use in nursing patients.

The second set has only one factor, that is, the pattern of living of the patient. Information sought included usual and repetitively performed daily activities, including self-care measures performed daily; activities performed at other intervals of time including recreational activities and self-care measures; amount of time spent alone and with others; adjustments in pattern of living imposed by health state or health care system factors; and responsibilities for other persons, for a household, for pets, or a garden, or responsibilities for a business or farm.

The third set of factors included the factors of health state and health care system factors. Health state was conceptualized as having anatomic, physiologic, and psychological features. Attention was given to the following:

- Documented conditions of health before and during current care period and on discharge: (1) physician's medical diagnosis and named documented conditions and (2) nurse-determined, -named, and -documented conditions
- Health state features identified and described by (1) patient or (2) patient's family members
- Health care system features described by discipline (nursing, medicine, others by name) and by form of care (active, supervisory, consultative) before admission for care or during current care period

The fourth set included the factors of developmental state (adult oriented) in its relation to the existence and the meeting of developmental type self-care requisites under known environmental conditions. The focus of the set was on:

- Nurse-observed and patient-described current and future self-management capabilities in relation to current and projected conditions of living within specified physical and social environments and under conditions imposed by health state features
- Patient- and nurse-identified factors necessary for self-management or factors that adversely affect self-management
- Personal developmental potential evidenced by
  (1) patients' views of the future and goals held and
  (2) objective appraisals

Practical value of basic conditioning factors

Basic conditioning factors as understood and worked with by members of the Nursing Development Conference Group "increased the ability of members to deal with the complexity of concrete complementary elements in concrete situations of practice" (p. 170).[2] For example, a person under nursing care is a concrete element in a nursing practice situation but to know the person as a concrete element the nurse must know the person's health state because of its conditioning effects, that is, the way the person is affected. As "insights about the functions of basic conditioning factors increased so did Group members' understanding of how to sort out and relate patient data in nursing practice situations as well as their understanding of points of articulation of the subject matter of nursing with the subject matter descriptive and explanatory of the . . . factors" (pp. 170-171).[2]

The selection and use of named basic conditioning factors is based on the premise that persons who seek and receive nursing are individuals who at the same time are members of families — families that are units of larger sociocultural groups living in some place or places during the period of each individual's existence in the world.

The basic conditioning factors group themselves into three categories: (1) factors descriptive of individuals who are nurses' patients singly or in groups, (2) factors that relate these individuals to their families of origin or families of marriage, and (3) factors that locate these individuals in their worlds and relate them to conditions and circumstances of living.

Factors descriptive of individuals include age, gender, and developmental state. Factors that locate persons within family constellations and socioculture groups are broadly expressed as sociocultural orientations and family system factors. The factors that describe individuals in their worlds of existence include health state, health care system factors, patterns of living, environmental factors, and resource availability and adequacy.

Information that describes basic conditioning factors in each nursing case must be obtained by nurses initially and on a continuing basis as necessary throughout the duration of the provision of nursing. Some factors will remain stable; others will fluctuate or change. Relationships among factors must be understood. With infants and children age is actively related to developmental state and health state to both age and developmental state. With mature adults both age and developmental state have achieved their own stability and health state may be the most active conditioning factor. With persons in advanced age, the condition of aging and health state factors will be seen as related factors.

In nursing practice situations nurses obtain information about basic conditioning factors in a variety of ways. Information is obtained from patient records, including medical history and the medical diagnosis and medical prescriptions, by direct questioning of patients or members of their families, by observing what patients and family members say and do, and more formally by taking a nursing history. Nurses obtain such information in order to have it available for use in making nursing judgments and decisions and in guiding the practical endeavors of nurses.

The use by nurses of information about basic conditioning factors relative to the societal, interpersonal, and interactional aspects of nursing has been described in some detail. The use of such information as it affects the patient properties of self-care agency and therapeutic self-care demand has been developed. To further understand this, the relationships of basic conditioning factors to the substantive structure of self-care agency and therapeutic self-care demand should be made explicit.

Information about each of the 10 basic conditioning factors may be necessary for use in calculating patients' therapeutic self-care demand. The information is necessary for (1) particularizing universal self-care requisites and (2) identifying obstacles to be overcome if universal self-care requisites are to be met as well as factors that condition the selection and use of particular technologies or methods for meeting requisites. See the Appendix for listing of factors that affect the meeting of universal self-care requisites. Information about health state, health care system factors, pattern of living, and environmental factors is relevant to the identification and description of the health deviation components of patients' therapeutic self-care demands. Information about age and gender, developmental state, and sociocultural factors may be relevant in some cases. The identification and description of developmental self-care requisites require information about the age and gender of individuals, family system factors, patterns of living, health state and health care system factors, and relevant environmental factors. Sociocultural factors may be of special relevance.

Information about basic conditioning factors to identify self-care capabilities and limitations of patients should be related to the substantive components of self-care agency, with a primary focus on use of information about health state and health care system factors. This process of relating basic conditioning factors to the substantive components of the patient property self-care agency can begin with the self-care operations (estimative, transitional, productive) or the power components of self-care agency or with the various sets of capabilities and dispositions foundational for engagement in self-care (see Chapter 7). For example, if there is health state information that a person is comatose, that person can engage in no self-care operations since the person cannot exert and maintain voluntary attention, and is not perceptive of his or her life situation. Or, persons who have not developed and incorporated a concept of self as self-care agent into their self-concepts may not be motivated and maintain willingness to consistently perform measures to meet components of their therapeutic self-care demand.

The conditioning factors of age and health state and health care system factors are now considered in some detail with respect to nursing situations and nursing cases.

AGE AS A FACTOR IN NURSING

A patient's age is an index of both the health care focus and the helping focus of nursing. Personal maturation and organic, psychic, and intellectual functioning vary with the periods of the human life cycle. Basic self-care in meeting universal and developmental self-care requisites varies with periods of the human life cycle; however, the types of universal and developmental self-care requisites to be met remain the same. The variations are in the values at which the requisites should be met (e.g., the kind and amount of rest distributed by these time periods), in how they can be met, and in who will meet them.

Age is one index of the amount and kind of help needed from nurses or others. This results from the association of chronological age and developmental state. Capabilities for management of self in one's environment; psychic habits and dispositions; the attachment of meaning to what is perceived; as well as powers of understanding, reflection, and judgment vary by stages of development.

Both a basic health care focus and valid modes of helping can be inferred from information about a patient's age. Individual differences including developmental differences are recognized and taken into account by nurses. When individuals are in good to excellent states of health, age-relevant care and helping methods suffice other than in periods when special self-care is required, for example, because of an injury or a change in environmental conditions. Care of newborn infants is an example of the need to adjust care to age, to health state of infants, and to the process of infants' adjustments to new environmental conditions. As indicated previously, the basic conditioning factors of age and gender, developmental state, health state, and conditions of living in combination influence both the therapeutic self-care demands and the abilities and limitations of individuals for self-care.

Individuals who can benefit from nursing may be of any age and any state of development and health. When multiperson units such as families become the subject of care and service from nurses, the constituent members of the unit may be of similar or dissimilar ages and states of development and health. Nurses' descriptions of persons who are seeking or under nursing care must consider age, developmental state, and health state. If these three factors are not investigated and characterizing data are not obtained, nurses will not have an adequate basis for understanding the helping and health aspects of nursing, since they influence both aspects of nursing. Age as a factor in the production of variety in nursing situations will be discussed. The influences of age and other factors on the production of variations in the therapeutic self-care demands and the self-care agency of patients will then be addressed.

Age of the patient is an important factor in every nursing situation. It normally is closely related to the characteristics of a person's behavior, and it has meaning in relationship to the self-care behavior of the patient and the nursing behavior of the nurse. Age also has a number of meanings in a given society, and these meanings will have a variety of influences on the lives of the members of that society. Nurses must be aware of these meanings and their influences, since such knowledge is related to the consideration of age in every nursing situation.

The meaning of age

Age is most frequently thought of in terms of chronological age, the period of time between birth and succeeding time periods. Chronological age is measured in seconds, minutes, hours, days, weeks, months, and years. Nurses may care for infants whose age can be measured in seconds as well as for persons whose age can be measured in decades. In prenatal life, chronologic age is measured in time intervals within the 9-month gestation period (the first, second, and third trimesters).

A person at any age may show failure to grow and develop along organic, psychic, or intellectual dimensions. Every individual should be provided with a type of environment that promotes development not only toward physical .maturation but also toward emotional and intellectual maturity. Evidence of particular kinds of retardation of development should be considered as perhaps limiting but not as completely restricting personal maturation. Restraining persons with particular kinds of retardation from involvement in the human scene, for example, keeping them confined without education for self-care and other aspects of personal and community living, is a societal-imposed hazard on their development, health, and well-being.

Developmental age refers to the combinations of qualities, powers, and capacities that develop naturally in each person in light of hereditary factors and environmental conditions. The developmental age of an individual is determined by identifying physical and behavioral developments and comparing them with chronological age group norms. Characteristic growth and developmental pictures of individuals by chronological age periods are valuable guides to nurses in understanding health care requirements (including care to promote normal growth and development) and limitations for deliberate action. Each nurse must be constantly alert to advances in the knowledge of human growth and development and in technologies that foster normal growth, development, and health by age group.

Growth in physical size is readily observable and measurable. Since individuals grow at different rates, children of the same chronologic age may vary in physical size. Persons who are small or large because of hereditary factors or whose natural growth has been retarded in some way, such as through malnutrition, may have problems in accepting themselves and in being accepted by others. Problems may also arise from a child's degree of development or maturity, which determines what a child can do at a particular age. If development is slow, help may be needed in allaying the child's fears that he or she will not be normal or be able to do what other children of the same age can do. If the rate of maturing is rapid, the child may need guidance in accepting himself or herself and relating to other children.

Some societies establish the chronological age at which individuals, according to law, are capable of making certain decisions, of entering into contracts, and of being held legally responsible for their acts. In the United States, this age is part of either the common law of the country or the civil law of the states. According to common law, for example, the *age of majority*, or adulthood is 21 years for both men and women. In some states, however, it is 18 years for women. Before a person reaches the legal age of adulthood, the law recognizes other ages, such as the age of discretion, the age of consent, and military age. The *age of discretion* means that a minor at the age of 14 years is recognized as possessing sufficient knowledge to be responsible for certain acts and to exercise certain powers. A minor under 7 years of age is conclusively presumed incapable of criminal intent, and a minor between the ages of 7 and 14 years is considered incapable of criminal intent unless there is proof to the contrary. The *age of consent*, which varies by state, is the age at which a person is recognized as legally competent to consent to marriage and to other acts.

Laws also protect persons who have not reached adult status. These laws hold natural and adoptive parents legally responsible for the support of a child. Support includes the provision of food, clothing, shelter, education, and health care. Legally, parents are responsible for the protection of the health and well-being of their child, including the development of character and personal and social values.

A person's chronological age and sex relate to status within a family, for example, the status and roles of husband and wife, mother and father, son and daughter, and brother and sister. Status and role define the duties and responsibilities of the individual toward other members of his or her family.

Age as it is discussed here is a relatively important factor in cultural practices related to infant and child care and supervision, instruction of children in self-care and sex attitudes, education toward independence, teaching skills and beliefs, formal education, care of the aged, marriage, and the family. The respect and care given to the young, to the elderly, and to women during pregnancy and the assistance given to individuals in the transitional period from youth to adulthood all reflect how a society views the importance of these age-related events. A patient's attitude or the attitude of family members and the attitude of the nurse in these areas are important influences in each nursing situation.

Influence of age on nursing

The chronological and developmental ages of a patient affect the health and helping dimensions of the nursing situation in a number of ways. They influence (1) the social relations of nurse and patient, (2) techniques for assisting, communicating, and socializing to roles, (3) appropriate nurse responses to a patient's behavior, (4) frequency and duration of the contacts between nurse and patient, (5) the scope of the nurse's responsibility for protecting the patient as a person, (6) the nurse's relationship to members of the patient's family, and (7) the health and self-care needs of the patient. Understanding these influences requires knowledge of human growth and development, social networks, cultural practices, and communication and social interaction theories and technologies. This knowledge must be applied in collecting descriptive information about patients, interpreting the information, and using it in designing and providing nursing assistance for adults and children.

Nurses and nursing students may be in the adolescent stage of the life cycle, which is preparatory for access to specialized work in the society. They may also be adults preparing for or engaging in specialized work. Their patients may be of any age.

Ideally, the nurse's behavior should convey acceptance and respect toward all patients. This is, of course, mature behavior and requires that the nurse recognize each patient as a person, as a member of a family, and as one who has a unique heredity and life history. Mature behavior in interpersonal situations also demands from the nurse an awareness of the need for adjusting his or her behavior to practices in the patient's culture that regulate social relations by age and position in the family or community.

Providing nursing to a child differs in several ways from providing nursing to an adult. The age status of a patient as an adult, a neonate, an infant, a child, or a youth has important implications for nursing, regardless of the patient's state of health and disease. The adult's right and responsibility to make decisions is recognized by society, as is the child's inability to do this. The developed and developing powers of the child must be identified and fostered within the nursing situation. Nurses should be acutely aware of the limits for realistic behavioral expectations for children according to age. Nurses should also provide for differences in environmental needs and be alert to signals of health problems by age groups. Evidence of failure to grow and develop as well as evidence of regressive changes and dysfunction by age group must be understood by nurses.

Nurses should understand the quality of trust, including its importance in effective interpersonal relations and in human growth and development. The trust a patient has in a nurse, the nurse's acceptance of it, and the nurse's respect for the patient are interacting forces that aid in the maintenance of the nurse-patient relationship. The nurse at times will be required to set limits for the behavior of children, youth, and sometimes adults as it relates to the patient's or the nurse's well-being. When trust, acceptance, and respect prevail, limit setting is more likely to be viewed as help given and not as restraint or coercion.

Age-specific factors in nursing children

In nursing situations involving infants, children, and youth, the patient continues in his or her role of *a dependent who must be cared for or guided by a responsible adult.* Nursing of young patients is a mix of care measures, which each patient needs because of his or her (1) chronological and developmental age, (2) genetic heritage, (3) unique personality, (4) physical and social environment, and (5) health state and related health care needs. Nursing in situations where the patient is young may involve direct care of the patient by the nurse and assistance to parents or guardians in learning to give the continuous care needed by the child or to cooperate with health workers. The nurse's dual relationship to child and to parents makes the nurse role complex and requires that techniques of assisting be adapted to the needs of the child and the needs of the parents, who may be adolescents or adults.

In the direct nursing care of a young patient, the nurse selects ways of assisting that are in accord with the patient's age and stage of growth and development. *Caring for, acting or doing for,* and *providing an environment that promotes development* are valid ways for nursing infants and young children. *Guiding* and *supporting* the child in self-care action are appropriate methods of nursing older children to the degree permitted by the health state. Older children and adolescents can learn and want to be responsible for their personal health-related care. They will also want to and need guidance and supervision from a responsible adult, though at times they will resist these efforts. Sustained interest of the nurse in the health care efforts of the young patient can make a great contribution toward the patient's becoming an effective self-care agent. Nurses should endeavor to help adolescents develop beneficial self-care practices. When nurses know that the adult family members have incorporated practices harmful to health into their daily living, guidance of youth toward physical and mental health should be an important nursing concern.

When children have some continuing therapeutic self-care needs that the parents are incapable of meeting, care responsibilities for the child may be distributed between the nurse and the parents. The distribution should be based on an objective consideration of the parents' limitations for giving the needed therapeutic care. When infants and sick children are placed in hospitals or other health care institutions, parents should be permitted to be with the child and fulfill some of the care responsibilities for the child whenever possible and prudent.

When parents cannot be with their child, the child should have a person to whom he or she can relate during various periods of the day. In an institutional situation, this role may be assigned to a person trained in child care rather than in nursing. This practice is appropriate when most of the care needs of the infant or child are not of the specialized type of care required as a result of disease, injury, or defect. Nurses should be able to give both aspects of care to children, but they also should be able to work cooperatively with both parents and with persons trained for child care. In long-term care institutions or when children are ill at home for prolonged periods, their formal education should be continued under the direction of qualified teachers.

The nature of the interpersonal relationship between a nurse and an infant, child, or adolescent patient is of paramount importance. It should communicate trust. The young patient should be able to feel that the nurse is a responsible adult who is interested in him or her and to whom he or she can turn for help. The nurse fosters the child's growth and development and at the same time contributes to the achievement of other specific health results. It is thus essential that the nurse know about the present developmental state of the child and how children develop cognitively and use knowledge at various ages.

The relationships between the nurse and the mother, father, or guardian of a child also may be affected by the age of the nurse or of the parents as well as by cultural factors. In cases where parents have differing opinions about the care needs of the child, the nurse may find it necessary to work with both parents for the child's well-being. This situation is complex. Some nurses may not be sufficiently competent to cope with it.

A nursing situation in which the patient is an infant, child, or youth continues as long as the patient requires specialized therapeutic care or until the parents or guardians have overcome their limitations for giving the needed care or assistance. Nurses should select methods that will benefit both the child and the parents. For example, if an infant or child has to be fed using a technique adapted for a cleft lip or palate, it may be appropriate for the nurse to involve the parents early in learning to feed the infant. Parents may need periodic guidance and supervision from a nurse when they are giving and managing the continuous therapeutic care required by a sick or disabled child or when they are giving therapeutic care to a well child.

When a child's integrated functioning is seriously disturbed or the health care technologies are complex and interrelated and in situations where the child's suffering is intense, nurses should not involve the parents in the technical aspects of the child's health care. In situations where parents must become technically able to participate in or completely provide the continuous health care for their child at home, nurses must carefully determine how the parents can be assisted without harm to them or to the child. In situations where children have birth defects or an illness that places parents in an adverse light with or without reason, or when children are unwanted and rejected, parents may need health care for their own sake as well as for that of the child.

In infant, child, or adolescent nursing situations, there should be an open line of communication between nurse(s) and parents and nurse(s) and physician(s). This is necessary because of the legal status of the patient as a minor and the patient's limitations in understanding and decision making. Because children are immature, they cannot be expected to be responsible agents in their own health care or in coordination of the various parts of care. The role of the adolescent in self-care, including its coordination with other aspects of health care, may be extended with guidance and supervision. The nurse must be aware of prescribed roles, rights, and responsibilities. Parents sometimes may not be in contact with adolescent sons or daughters or assume responsibility for their care or support. Guidance and support from interested and accepting adults are essential to meet developmental needs of young people who have taken on or are about to take on the duties of adult members of a society.

In caring for a minor, physicians must be in direct communication with the child's parents and nurses. The physician has an ethical and legal responsibility to keep parents informed of the child's health state. Some physicians also accept responsibility for guiding parents in fostering the growth and development of the child. A failure in communication between a child's parents and the physician may have adverse effects on the total health care situation, including the nursing component.

In some child nursing situations, it is essential that the child's nurse talk with nurses in another agency in coordinating the care of a child. A nurse giving care to a child at home, for example, may want to discuss nursing information with a nurse in an outpatient clinic or in a hospital before a clinic visit or hospitalization. Nurses, too, may find it necessary to contact the child's teachers or assist the child's parents in doing this whenever the child's daily health care needs must be given attention at school. When two or more health care agencies are involved in providing health services, coordination of their activities is important for the effective health care of both children and adults. Channels of communication should be provided and kept open to facilitate interagency coordination of health care for individual patients.

Age-specific factors in nursing adults

From the viewpoint of the patient's age, adult nursing situations differ from child nursing situations in that adults have the right to decide about the kinds of health care they will accept and the responsibility to act for themselves in matters of self-care and health. Adults may be emotionally or socially dependent on other people as a result of inadequate physical or personality development or because of the effects of disease, injury, or disability. However, they are not dependent in the way children are because of their age.

In child nursing situations, the child's age is a signal to the nurse of how to care for and communicate with the child, of growth and developmental needs, and of effects of illness or environmental factors on development. The adult patient's age is a signal to the nurse that the patient is responsible for himself or herself and his or her dependents (unless the patient is incompetent from developmental or health state factors). A patient's age tells the nurse that the patient is able to communicate as an adult but at a level that is influenced by habits of perceiving and thinking and that needs for help in self-care arise from health state or health care requirements. Adult age also may point to needs for assistance in accepting and living in a state of social dependency resulting from illness or treatment, in becoming self-directing about matters of self-care, and in learning to seek and use nursing services, including guidance and consultation in self-care.

In adult nursing situations, a nurse-family relationship may or may not exist. When an adult patient is not physically or mentally competent to manage his or her own affairs to make decisions about health care, nurses may have frequent contacts with a responsible member of the patient's family. When family members in a home provide the continuous care needed by a patient, nurses may instruct, supervise, and consult with family members.

Sometimes adult patients who are incompetent have legally appointed guardians. Adult patients who may be seriously ill or aged may give another responsible adult the power of attorney to transact business for them in accordance with regulations established by law. If adults are unable to decide or act for themselves, a family member, preferably the closest relative, should act for them. Adult children often care for their aged parents, or a wife may care for a seriously ill husband or a husband for a seriously ill wife. When an adult has a legally appointed guardian, the guardian occupies much the same position as the natural parents of a child.

Other age-related considerations are of great importance in nursing situations. Adult patients who are aware of their experiences and of the events that occur in the health care situation serve as information and communication centers in the health care situation. They interact with health workers, other persons who provide services, and family members and friends. The frequency and duration of contacts, the variety of social contacts, the content of communications, and a patient's interpretation of and reactions to his or her experiences are influencing factors on health care and nursing. Health workers place demands on patients to make observations, to reveal information, and, at times, to give messages to other health workers and to manage their own care. It is important that adult patients be helped to become responsible agents in their own health care. It is also important that nurses, physicians, and other health workers not burden a patient with their own coordinating duties.

The nursing situation may also be affected by an adult's social responsibilities. The adult patient's health and health care may interfere with family life, work, and other aspects of adult living. The adult may be unable to finance health care, care for dependent children, or provide for family needs. An adult patient's motivation to overcome or compensate for limitations resulting from injury or disability may be greatly influenced by family and work responsibilities or conditions of living.

HEALTH STATE AS A FACTOR IN NURSING

Well-being, general health state, injury, and illness are critical factors in nursing situations, for they are the determinants of the appropriate health care focus and the types of health results sought. Nurses must have information about the general health states of patients as well as information about conditions and events associated with the specific health disorders from which patients suffer.

Information about the patient's health state is obtained from a number of sources: the patient, persons who live with the patient, the patient's physician, the medical history, and the recorded results of physical and other examinations and laboratory tests. Understanding the meaning of such information requires that nurses have knowledge of normal integrated human functioning, pathologic conditions, basic procedures of health evaluation, and the purposes of medical diagnoses and therapy in relation to health and disease. Nurses, in making observations of patients or of records and reports on patients, initially and continuously determine evidence that will enable them to understand patients' health states.

Specifically, the information the nurse seeks will include descriptions of (1) the degree of illness, its causes, and whether it is acute or chronic; (2) obvious injuries or defects; (3) the patient's present behavior patterns (what he or she does or does not do); (4) the effects of disease or disordered function being experienced by the patient (including pain, alterations of body temperature, alterations of respiratory and circulatory functioning, gastrointestinal functioning, genitourinary functioning, nervous and musculoskeletal functioning, alterations of the skin and its appendages, and bleeding and anemia); and (5) possible or known effects of the patient's present health state on integrated functioning and effective living.

It is important that nurses know if the disease or disorder the patient has is one of the common causes of death. Vascular diseases of the central nervous system, acute coronary disease, other heart diseases, and malignancy are leading causes of death. The effect a disease may have on the life of a patient is a factor that affects the outlook and behavior of the patient and family as well as that of the nurse. The effects of a patient's illness on the family is very important in all nursing situations.

The physician's view of the patient's health situation is reflected in the medical diagnosis and prognosis, the recorded medical history, and the results of the physical examinations and laboratory tests. The kind of therapy the physician prescribes and the diagnostic and other measures the physician uses are also significant for nursing.

In nursing situations where patients are under active medical care there is need for discussion between the patient's nurse(s) and the physician so that the nurse can determine (1) how the physician views the patient's health situation; (2) the aspects of the patient's medical care regimen that should become parts of the patient's self-care system on a long-term or short-term basis, including monitoring of selected aspects of human functioning; (3) which physician, if there is more than one, has the position of responsibility for integrating and coordinating the patient's medical care; and (4) the projected duration of active medical care for the patient. Only through the conscious and deliberate efforts of physicians and nurses to communicate with each other about the daily care of the patient can nursing care and medical care be coordinated to produce an effective health care system for the patient.

During the initial period of nursing, a patient may be relatively healthy; slightly, moderately, or seriously ill; injured; or suffering from defect or disability. Life experiences, present environmental situation, and interests and concerns will influence the patient's view of the health state and the need for health care as well as the patient's readiness or ability to cooperate with health care workers (pp. 180-193).[3] A patient's view of his or her health situation may be related to the characteristics of the disease process itself. There is a process of becoming ill. There are also modes of adaptation to illness and to the recovery process. The disease, the kinds of symptoms, and the rapidity with which they develop help to describe the process of becoming ill. One physician who studied patients who had cerebral vascular accidents or strokes described the patients as having been plunged within a relatively short time into "a rather unfamiliar and complicated life situation" that "is rapidly changing," a situation where the "full import and meaning cannot be readily grasped in the initial states."

In describing their experiences and reactions in the initial phases of the disease process, the patients' responses demonstrated (1) personality resources—for example, "courage, self-control, patience, and acceptance," (2) minimization and rationalization of initial symptoms, (3) resignation to the outcome of the illness, and (4) "mounting apprehensiveness and heightened dependency." In strokes, as in other illnesses where there can be extensive brain damage, there may be unawareness of illness or of deficits such as that resulting from a paralysis. The stroke patient's view of his or her illness during its early phases and the tendency to maximize or minimize difficulties rather than to see them realistically were indicators of reactions in later phases of the illness and in the recovery process (pp. 74-76).[4]

In studying diseases and patterns of illness, it is important for nurses and nursing students to learn what has been presently identified about patterns of adaptation. In studies of two types of disabling illness, the following patterns were noted: (1) insightful acceptance, (2) a struggle with conflicts brought on by disability through projection and other psychological mechanisms, (3) exaggeration of dependency and the demanding of more help than might actually be required, and (4) a slowly developing depression with loss of motor ability, a sense of failure in coping with events with resultant sadness, and feelings of helplessness that may be unrecognized by the patient initially. Once they are recognized, however, they are not denied (pp. 78-80).[4]

Patients' views of their health situation influence their own roles and nurses' roles in the nursing situation. What responsibility can the patient bear now and fulfill effectively in the future? In light of the patients' perception of and responses to their health situation, what kind of assistance is required to identify the patient role? How can patients be helped to face and accept the demands that illness or injury place on them? Nurses, especially those who have not experienced personal or family problems of a serious nature or who have not been victims of a natural disaster, may not be perceptive about the impact of personal loss or of excessive physical and emotional demands on the individual.

Illness and injury generally impose hardships on people. The outcome of illness and injury may be uncertain; a person is faced with the unknown and may experience anxiety, fear of permanent disability, life-long suffering, or even death. In some instances, patients must make decisions about the kinds of measures they will permit the physician to use. Nurses should be able to envision the meaning that illness or disability and being a patient have for individuals.

If a nurse sees only movements toward health—toward more effective living— without seeing the demands and burdens that injury, illness, and health care place on a patient, the basis for nursing diagnosis and prescription is incomplete. The nursing perspective will be inaccurate, and the nurse will not have a sound basis for proceeding toward the nursing goal of assisting the patient in responsible action in matters of self-care. The patient may be willing to accept care given by the nurse, may demand care from the nurse, or may be disinterested in or even refuse care. Patients may need help in understanding not only their self-care demands but also the rationale for particular self-care requisites or for sets of requisites. A nurse's investigations may reveal that a first task is to help the individual learn how to cooperate in the determination of needs that can be met through nursing.

Health results

Nurses' investigations of and judgments about the self-care requisites of patients take into consideration the reasons why patients are under health care and the health results to be achieved. The types of health results mentioned previously include the maintenance and promotion of health, including the prevention of disease, defect, and disability; the cure or regulation of disease processes; the preservation or restoration of vital processes; rehabilitation toward effective living in the event of disability; and being able to live and function with some degree of ease and personal satisfaction during a terminal illness.

When patients with health disorders are under nursing care, nurses must have or seek authoritative information about the natural history of specific diseases. The medical literature or physician and nurse specialists with extensive experience in caring for patients with particular diseases are sources. Such knowledge enables nurses to envision the kinds of health results associated with the disease. For example, through fact-gathering activities, the nurse finds that a patient has been diagnosed as having a stone in the right ureter. From observations of the patient and from the physician's notes, the nurse is aware that the pain is severe and the patient is in great distress. The nurse draws on knowledge from anatomy, physiology, and pathology in forming a mental picture of what is presently in process in the patient. The nurse understands the physiologic problem resulting from the presence of the stone and the mechanics related to the possible passage of the stone, considering the size and shape of the stone in relation to the diameter of the ureter and to its tissue structure and physiology. Causes of stone formation and of preventive measures come to mind. The nurse draws on his or her knowledge of pain and physiology, psychology, and pathology in making observations and judgments.

From reading the physician's medical orders for the patient and from talking with the physician, the nurse also becomes aware that the physician does not plan at this time to use surgical techniques but will first see if the patient can pass the stone, using drug therapy as indicated. The nurse becomes aware that the patient will be enduring the painful process of passing the stone, with all its distressing effects, and concludes that the desired, immediate health-related results needed by the patient are four in number: (1) the elimination of the stone, (2) prevention or control of complications, (3) relief from pain, and (4) reduction of physical and psychologic stress. The nurse knows the distressing effects produced by the passing of stones and is aware of the results to be sought and the kinds of care measures that will be effective while the patient lives through the process of passing the stone. Nurses' knowledge of health, disease, and medical diagnostic and therapeutic modalities should include their points of articulation with nursing. The patient variables, therapeutic self-care demand and self-care agency, provide appropriate linkages.

Patients' points of view

Patients see their health care situations from their own unique perspectives. Their education, experience, feeling and attitudes about life and people, and knowledge of health care and attitudes toward it color their views. Patients' insights about their own health care needs, the meaning they attach to presenting signs and symptoms, and their awareness of their ability or inability to engage in effective required self-care and to work cooperatively with nurses and physicians is essential information for nurses to have and use in helping patients. Individual nurses should develop approaches that are helpful to them in grasping quickly the views of individual patients about their health care situations and in identifying the interests and concerns of patients.

A woman being interviewed by a nurse-midwife about her obstetrical experiences expressed the following views of herself in relation to her first pregnancy: (1) not having knowledge of what to do because of the pregnancy; (2) requiring time to formulate and express questions to ask the nurse and the obstetrician; (3) being able to cope with some but not all of the demands for self-care and self-management during the pregnancy; (4) being in need of learning to live as a woman who is pregnant and who is in labor, to relate to health care professionals, and to provide infant care; (5) being ready or not ready to learn at specific times.* The woman noted that she was well educated, intelligent, and occupationally effective. She was aware of her own limitations for effective action within the health care situations associated with her first pregnancy. Time was viewed as a relevant factor.

Cooperation and coordination in health care

The achievement of health results for individuals is based in large part on the capabilities and motivation of health service personnel and their willingness and ability to cooperate and to coordinate their efforts. To *cooperate* is to act jointly in achieving some common goal. A situation that requires cooperation or a joint action of a number of persons sets up a demand that the persons acting together to reach a common goal regulate and combine their efforts so that action will be harmonious and will contribute to the achievement of the goal. This regulation and combination of effort is *coordination*.

If several people attempt to work toward a common goal but do so without coordination, duplication of effort, inefficiency, and even failure to achieve the goal may occur. Effective coordination of effort requires that persons involved reach a common understanding of their goal, know their respective roles in its achievement, perform in an agreed manner so that the activities will be properly related to the goal,

---

* From the record of an interview conducted by Mary E. Fitzpatrick.

and communicate developments and changes resulting from their actions whenever such information is necessary for the performance of other roles.

Learning to nurse includes learning to work in cooperation with patients and their families, other nurses, physicians, and other health care specialists. Nursing students and young nurses should have planned experiences designed to aid them in initiating and responding to contacts with other health workers as well as patients and their families. The language of the health and medical sciences facilitates communication between nurses and other health workers. Terms that are specific to a particular health service may need definition and explanation when used in interdisciplinary communication. The language of nursing is developing.

Beliefs of nurses and other health workers about their roles and the roles of others affect their interests and their willingness to function in cooperative relationships in health care situations. Some health workers have little insight about the specific characteristics of nursing and its significance in achieving health results. On the other hand, because of their continuous relationship with a patient, nurses often have considerable knowledge of the roles and contributions of other health workers. Nurses should have skill in representing to physicians, social workers, and others the characteristics of nursing and the nature of the health care contribution it makes in various types of health care situations.

Members of different health services who give help to the same person are sometimes collectively referred to as a health team. A health team is an organized group of health workers who have roles related to meeting the health care needs of a patient or a group of patients. A team does not exist unless there are common goals, cooperative relationships, and coordinated activities. In many health care situations there are no health teams in the usual sense. Frequently, patients are cared for by a number of health workers who cooperate on a one-to-one basis with the patient and with other health workers. An organized health team enables its individual members to see their respective roles in relation to achievement of health results for a patient, to establish a group identity, and to afford authority to and to respect group members in relation to their roles and capabilities.

The formal establishment of a health team may be the only way or the preferred way for giving care or designing and managing care. Team functioning requires time and specialized effort on the part of each person involved. When health teams are not formally organized, cooperation and coordination of effort must be initiated by individual health workers.

Health teams are essential to performing some complex diagnostic and treatment measures. Often some members of these teams work with extremely complex machines or equipment that must be brought into a functional relationship with a patient (e.g., the heart-lung machine during open-heart surgery). Whenever team members work in face-to-face relationships or when linked by highly effective communication devices, coordination of effort is facilitated. Analysis of the roles, the relationships, and the specific activities of members of a health team (e.g., a surgical team preparing for and performing a surgical procedure for a patient in an operating room) is a helpful exercise toward understanding health team functioning.

HEALTH CARE SYSTEM FACTORS

Variations in nursing situations that are parts of larger health situations arise from the number and kinds of health workers contributing care or service to patients. In some situations there are only nurses and physicians, but in others there are many types of health workers. For example, when persons suffer from an illness of undetermined origin or when medical treatment is complex, a large number and a variety of health workers may be involved. Forms of health care vary from one part of the world to another and, in some instances, within the same country. In the United States, the predominant form of health care is derived from scientific medicine as it has developed in the Western world.

This form of health care has traditionally had as its focus *disease*, which is defined as an abnormal biologic process with characteristic symptoms. The modern concept of disease describes it as a process involving alterations in human structure or functioning including integrated human functioning. The modern concept of disease also includes the concept that a specific disease has more than a single cause (concept of multiple causation). Medical scientists identify, describe, and name unique diseases, that is, distinct pathologic processes. Descriptions include the sequential series of changes that have been observed in individuals suffering from particular diseases.

The increasing knowledge about disease has been complemented by substantial increases of physiologic and psychological knowledge of value to physicians and other health workers in the diagnosis, treatment, and prevention of disease and in the maintenance and promotion of normal development and functioning. Information about the prevention of disease and the maintenance and promotion of good health has become a part of the general culture. Thus health has come into focus in scientific medicine not just as something to be restored but as a desirable state to be maintained. As a result, the social and economic dimensions of health and health care have been given increased prominence.

At the present stage of its development, scientific medicine includes what has become known as *preventive medicine*, which is defined as "the science and art of preventing disease, prolonging life and promoting physical and mental health and efficiency . . . through intercepting disease processes by community and individual action" (p. 11).[5] Preventive medicine recognizes (1) disease as a process of multiple causation, (2) the relationship of the process to disease agents, living or nonliving, (3) human characteristics, and (4) human responses to internal and external disease-producing stimuli.

The physician is recognized as the practitioner of scientific medicine, whose functions in society include the diagnosis and treatment of disease and its effects. Medical diagnosis, the identification of natural causes and natural effects of disease, precedes treatment. Medical treatment is extended not only to the cure and control of disease processes and the restoration of health and alleviation of symptoms, but also to the prevention of disease and to overcoming defects and disability. Physicians in private or group practice of medicine perform these measures for individuals and families. Other physicians may be associated with various organizations, such as hospitals or business and industrial organizations, to supply care to the clients or the members of these organizations and sometimes to their families.

Medical care refers to the care given to individuals by physicians. The term is sometimes used in a broader sense for services to individuals by agencies and members of the various health professions and occupations — hospitals, physicians, dentists, nurses, and pharmacists. Nursing as a health care service is properly referred to as a part of medical care when the term *medical care* is used with this broader meaning. Nonmedical systems of health care exist in addition to the scientific medical care commonly practiced in the United States.

The practice of scientific medicine requires a number of paramedical and technical services. Paramedical services contribute to some one aspect of medical practice. The major paramedical services are physical therapy, occupational therapy, speech therapy, and some of the services of medical social workers. The various paramedical services use specialized diagnostic and treatment techniques requiring skilled personnel.

Nutritionists and dietitians may have important roles in care directed toward the prevention, cure, or control of disease, working with both the physician and the patient whenever dietary treatment is involved. Clinical psychologists also perform functions that contribute to the diagnosis and treatment of mental and emotional disorders through psychological testing, counseling, and other therapeutic techniques.

In addition to the preceding services, other highly specialized technical services are essential in the physician's use of diagnostic and therapeutic measures. Physicians diagnosing and determining the course of a disease or a disorder and the effects of therapy require not only the efforts of physicians who are specialists in pathology but also the services of chemists, physicists, and clinical laboratory technicians. The physician in his or her medical practice may also require the services of other physicians who specialize in roentgenology (radiologists) and technicians skilled in the use of x-rays and other types of radiation.

NURSING AGENCY AND NURSES

Nurses are person elements in nursing practice situations. Within the self-care deficit theory of nursing and specifically within the theory of nursing system (Fig. 3-3) nurses are characterized by the property nursing agency which is enabling for their design and production of nursing for persons with health derived or health associated self-care deficits and for assisting persons with dependent-care deficits. Nurses should view themselves realistically. When nurses are knowing about themselves and about others and when nurses accept and respect themselves and others, it is easier for nurses to establish and maintain cooperative relationships with patients and their families and with co-workers.

Nursing agency, Nursing Development Conference Group

Nursing agency is a theoretical concept that was formalized in 1971 after a lengthy process of exploration by members of the Nursing Development Conference Group. Members were guided in their discussions and analyses of nursing cases by this simple idea: *under these given conditions and circumstances nurses will require these capabilities to nurse effectively.* To be guided by this idea it was necessary for group members to take the stance of conceptual theorists and not the stance of nursing practitioners investigating this or that concrete situation of practice. The history of the process of formalization of the concept nursing agency is enlightening. It was the last theoretical concept within the definition of nursing system to be formalized (pp. 155-167).[2]

The Conference Group's exposition of nursing agency is reproduced (pp. 120-122).[2]

Nursing agency is a complex set of qualities of a person acquired through specialized study and experiences in real-world nursing situations. This set of qualities enables a person to assist others (1) in the immediate exercise of self-care agency, in its initial or continuing development, or in making transformations in it, but always in relation to the person's usual pattern of self-care or the objectively established therapeutic self-care demand; (2) by determining the constitutive parts of therapeutic self-care demand and the essential relations among the parts, and by keeping therapeutic self-care demand adjusted to changes in the person or the environment (this includes the availability of valid and reliable technologies); (3) by evaluating the characteristics of the individual's self-care system(s) with respect to adequacy as related to an objectively established therapeutic self-care demand; (4) by designing and assisting with the institution and management of self-care systems that relate various abilities within self-care agency to parts, or to the totality, of self-care demand; and (5) by designing and providing systems of assistance that substitute for the total or partial absence of self-care agency or compensate for specific inadequacies of the constitutive parts of self-care agency.

The general characteristics of nursing agency are described as nursing abilities and limitations as related to the aforementioned types of assistance adjusted to conditions prevailing in some types of nursing situations. The characteristics of nursing agency at a specific time are the result of certain enabling and limiting factors related to a nurse's age and maturity, degree of development and perfection of the nursing art, structured nursing knowledge, state of health, and the environmental conditions under which the nurse exercises nursing agency.

The nursing behaviors that a nurse activates in a particular nursing situation at a particular time are only a portion of the total behavioral repertoire of nursing agency.

Nursing agency is activated initially by stimuli and signals relevant to establishing the characteristics of, and making judgments about, constitutive parts of *therapeutic self-care demand and self-care agency*. Subsequent activation of nursing agency results from judgments about: (1) the presence, the causes, and the dimensions of a *self-care deficit;* (2) the possibility or feasibility of *effecting transformations in self-care agency* as related to therapeutic self-care demand; and (3) effective methods to meet specific action requirements within therapeutic self-care demand now, in the immediate future, and in the more distant future.

These three sets of judgments establish the conditionality of changes in self-care agency and therapeutic self-care demand on the exercise of nursing agency. When the conditionalities are established, further exercise of nursing agency will be directed toward the achievement of some combination of results expressed in relation to therapeutic self-care demand and self-care agency. Results that accrue over time include the following:

1. Self-care agency is or is becoming proportionate to estimating and meeting therapeutic self-care demand.
2. Self-care agency is exercised in relation to therapeutic self-care demand, and this exercise produces a self-care system that exhibits effectiveness in meeting constitutive parts, or the totality, of the demand.
3. Therapeutic self-care demand at any point in time (a) describes factors in the patient or the environment that (for the sake of the patient's life, health, or well-being) must be held steady within a range of values or brought within and held within such a range, and (b) has a known degree of instrumental effectiveness derived from the choice of technologies and specific techniques for use in changing, or in some way controlling, patient or environmental factors.
4. Therapeutic self-care demand is met over time.

Nursing agency has been described as the power of one individual to provide for other individuals with health-related self-care deficits material and energy inputs essential for the self-maintenance and the health and well-being of these others. Nursing agency is exercised in the form of a dynamic system of human actions. The end product of the exercise of nursing agency is this dynamic system of action (a nursing system), which must be brought into existence, maintained in existence, and managed to accomplish for legitimate patients some or all of the four results described previously.

Nursing agency, an expanded conceptual structure

The theoretical concept nursing agency as it is defined by the Nursing Development Conference Group focuses on the professional-technologic features of this nurse property. Nursing agency is analogous to self-care agency in that both symbolize sets of human characteristics and abilities that are for specialized types of deliberate action. They differ in that nursing agency is developed and exercised for the benefit and well-being of others and self-care agency is developed and exercised for the benefit of oneself. Since nursing agency has its orientation to others, it is important to add to its professional-technologic component the societal and the interpersonal interactive components (Fig. 9-1).

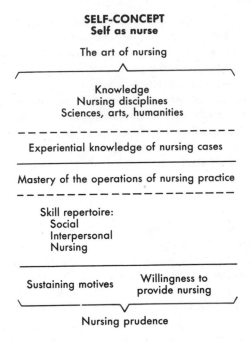

SELF-CONCEPT
Self as nurse

The art of nursing

Knowledge
Nursing disciplines
Sciences, arts, humanities

- -

Experiential knowledge of nursing cases

Mastery of the operations of nursing practice

- -

Skill repertoire:
Social
Interpersonal
Nursing

Sustaining motives   Willingness to
                         provide nursing

Nursing prudence

Fig. 9-1 Elements of the concept nursing agency.

When nurses activate nursing agency in relationship to persons they nurse, the result is series of discrete nursing actions or operations—societal, interpersonal, technologic. The static representation of nursing agency in Fig. 9-1 includes cognitive, affective, and volitional elements, as well as those that point to skilled performance of what is done. Nursing in the figure is identified as "the art of nursing" with foundations in theoretical and experiential knowledge and in developed skills.

Art and prudence

The art of nursing is the quality of individual nurses that allows them to make creative investigations and analyses and syntheses of the variables and conditioning factors within nursing situations in order to work toward the goal of the production of effective systems of nursing assistance for individuals or multiperson units. *Nursing prudence* is the quality of nurses that enables them (1) to seek and take counsel in new or difficult nursing situations, (2) to make correct judgments about what to do and what to avoid when particular conditions prevail or suddenly develop in nursing situations, (3) to decide to act in a particular way, and (4) to take action. Both nursing art and nursing prudence aid in and are essential for the production of effective systems of nursing assistance, but in different ways.

Through their art, nurses envision, design, and produce nursing assistance for others, assistance that is in accord with why and how persons can be helped through nursing. Art is concerned with creating systems of nursing assistance or care. Nursing prudence is concerned with doing this or that act at particular moments in light of one's knowledge of the situation. Both the art of nursing and nursing prudence develop with experience. The degree to which and the manner in which they develop in individual nurses are associated with nurses' talents, personality characteristics, developed and preferred modes of thinking, stages of personal moral development, abilities to conceptualize complex situations of action and to analyze and synthesize factual information, and the kinds of life experiences they have had, including nursing experiences. Nursing prudence also demands that nurses continue to advance themselves in the nursing sciences and in foundational disciplines. With the rapid advances in the sciences, it is unrealistic to think that prudence can be achieved by practical experience in nursing.

Characteristics of nurses

To be able to view themselves realistically as persons who render nursing care, nurses must have the time and preparation to give the patient care. Education and experience in nursing and the scope of responsibility for nursing patients should influence that view. Many factors affect the willingness of the nurse to render care. Some nurses frequently specify lack of time as a result of the many demands on them. Other nurses refer to patients as "difficult" or "easy," thereby implying the kind and degree of effort involved in rendering care. The patient's age, gender, race, culture, social status, or disease factors also have an effect on the nurse's willingness to render care. In fact, some nurses develop preferences about the types of patients for whom they are willing to render care. In the last analysis, the quality and availability of nursing care in specific nursing situations is based on the unconditional willingness of individual nurses to render care.

Socialization in nursing situations is required because nurses and patients are usually strangers and they must enter into helping relationships. A patient may need preparation in fulfilling the patient role in the nursing situation. Temperament, self-image, and pattern of living may affect the patient's ability to accept the role of patient. Further, the nurse's gender, age, culture, or socioeconomic status may facilitate or hinder the patient's performance in the patient role. Similarly, these same factors, as they relate to the patient, may have an effect on the nurse's performance of the nurse role.

The socializing process may continue throughout the period the patient requires nursing care. It is not merely an initial effort on the part of the nurse and the patient to adjust to their roles in the situation, but a continued effort to carry out their roles and to understand their relationships with other persons who are providing care in the situation. The nurse sometimes must ask: Is the patient able to participate in his or her own health care by giving essential information to the physician or to others? The following excerpts from recorded material about a nursing case present an example of a need for help in this direction. It is evident from these excerpts that the nurse and the patient had established an effective nurse-patient relationship and that the patient trusted the nurse. The progress made by the patient as a result of his own socializing efforts is also evident. The observations were made and recorded by Sister Gretta Monnig (pp. 89-90).[6]

> The patient was sitting in a chair when the surgeon made rounds. The doctor remarked that this was enema day. The patient said nothing about the enema but told the surgeon he felt fine. After the surgeon had left the room, the nurse remarked that she would get the enema. The patient replied, "I do not need an enema; I had a bowel movement this morning." The nurse asked why he had not told the surgeon.
>
> "I take a look at all those doctors and can't think of a thing to say. Do the other patients feel this way?" he asked.
>
> The nurse replied, "Most patients think of their questions after their doctor has been in to see them. It must be hard to ask questions in front of a large group of people."
>
> "All those people scared me. I was afraid that my questions would sound silly," replied the patient.
>
> The nurse asked, "Is it easier to talk to the doctor when he makes rounds to change your dressings?"
>
> "He always seems to be in a hurry," replied the patient.
>
> "How about the doctor who comes in the evening?" asked the nurse.
>
> "He is a fine doctor," said the patient. "I usually save my questions for him, but I still forget to ask him."
>
> "Would writing the questions on a slip of paper help you to remember what you want to ask the doctor?" asked the nurse.
>
> "I will try that," replied the patient.
>
> In the evening the patient said, "I wrote down my questions today. The doctor answered every one of them. He talked to me quite a while. I never realized how interesting doctors are." After that evening the patient appeared more at ease when the doctors made rounds (pp. 89-90).[6]

Ideally, then, the socializing efforts of nurses help them to know their patients and how to direct their efforts in encouraging patients to better cope with socializing activities in health situations. When children are involved, their developmental state and physical dependence on adults are of prime importance in the socializing aspects or the nursing situation. The nurse who gives care to children has a dual function in socialization activities. The nurse must continue, along with the parents, to aid the child in normal development. Under the conditions imposed by illness or special health needs, a child is confronted by physicians and other adults who place a variety of demands on both the child and the parents. Fostering the child's movement toward independence during illness through socializing activities is an important nursing task. Supervised contacts with other children may be of great importance in the socialization of children in institutional settings. Some 3-year-old children, for example, can effectively demonstrate to another child how to behave under conditions new to them—where and when to wash the face and hands, where to eat, and the proper use of utensils.

Closely related to socialization is the nurse's and the patient's awareness of overt and covert problems in health care situations. The case material on the socialization of the patient demonstrated that the patient was aware of his inability to communicate with the physicians attending him and recognized his need to change that behavior. It was up to the nurse to assist him in changing. The nurse cannot do this effectively unless he or she understands and accepts the nurse's and the patient's role in the nursing situation.

Personal factors that help to describe the nurse include (1) *age, gender, race, and physical and constitutional characteristics;* (2) *health state, socioeconomic status, culture, and roles in family and community;* and (3) *maturity as a person.* These personal factors are the ones most likely to influence nurses' relations to patients. The age and gender differences between the patient and the nurse are of considerable importance. A male patient, for example, may be either willing or reluctant to accept assistance from a female nurse. Health and the changes that normally occur with aging may limit what nurses can do regardless of what they are willing to do. For these reasons some norms related to personal factors are specified as pertinent considerations in certain types of nursing positions.

A nurse's socioeconomic and cultural background may influence the requirements for socializing efforts in a given situation. Nurses must be cognizant of the similarities and differences between the patient's pattern of living and their own that may have an influence on both the patient and themselves. Some nurses have a tendency to look at certain patterns of living as inferior merely because these practices are different from their own or from their ideal.

The nurse's maturity as a person determines how he or she will perceive himself or herself and the patient within a helping relationship. Mature nurses have a realistic view of themselves. Family and community demands may exert a desirable or an undesirable influence on a nurse. Lack of energy, lack of interest, and preoccupation with matters outside the nursing situation are some of the effects family and community demands may create. There are also positive effects; for example, the demands of family and community may stimulate the nurse's interest in people and in solving problems of living. Enlightened motivation and wisdom in helping and working with people in interpersonal situations are important positive effects that accrue to the mature nurse.

Included under nurse responsibilities are factors that, on the one hand, help to determine what the nurse is able to do and, on the other, what the nurse is permitted to do. Three groups of factors are suggested: (1) education and experience in nursing practice, (2) limitations set by the nurse's position and role as related to the patient, and (3) the status of the nurse as a responsible person.

Education and experience in nursing practice help to define what a nurse is able to do and what he or she can be expected to do. The system of nursing education that has evolved in the second half of the twentieth century provides education for a number of roles in nursing practice—professional, technical, and vocational. The experiences of a nurse and the pursuit of continuing education will determine in large part the degree of expertness attained. Expert nursing, of course, depends on the nurse's own development of the art of nursing, and this requires personal effort and guidance from expert nurse practitioners.

A nurse's abilities and limitations for designing, providing, and managing nursing care at any time arise from initial education, experience, continuing education, and developed nursing skills. No nurse can be expert in all types of nursing situations. Particular situations require specific knowledge and skills, and some situations require a depth of knowledge in a number of areas. Legal restrictions set by the nurse's license to practice also limit what the nurse can do. In nursing practice, what a nurse is able to do and permitted to do legally should be known by the nurse, by the health care institutions in which he or she works, and, in some nursing situations, by the nurse's patients. The nurse's case load of patients and the time allocation for their care should not be determined arbitrarily. Both should be determined in relation to the nursing requirements of the patients, the nurse's capabilities for nursing practice, and the nurse's expertness in particular types of nursing situations.

Nurses make judgments and decisions about themselves, their families, and their patients. The quality of the judgments and decisions they make gives expression to their personal commitments and their sense of responsibility in life situations. The state of personal moral development achieved by a nurse affects the characteristics of the decisions the nurse makes in nursing situations as well as in other situations. Nursing students should have learning experiences that will facilitate their moral development. Nurses in practice should examine the decisions they make in nursing situations in order to achieve understanding of themselves, the deliberate choices they made, their understanding of the options open at the times the choices were made, and the relationship between what they know and what they do. A nurse may know what should be done when particular conditions prevail in a nursing situation, but of vital concern to both nurse and patient is the actual decision the nurse makes.

Responsible nurses evaluate their own nursing performance in light of the patient's requirements for care. They seek and accept nursing supervision and strive to develop as nurses. They identify factors in nursing situations that interfere with patient progress and are able and unafraid to act to bring about change or represent these conditions to other responsible persons. Changes in nursing practice come about to the degree that nurses are both knowledgeable and responsible.

The relationships between nurses and patients vary in duration from hours to days to months to years. Nurses must be able to enter into short-term and long-term relationships with patients with a view toward rendering effective help for short periods of time or over a prolonged period of time with either periodic or continuous contact. Regardless of the duration of contact and the patient's specific nursing requirements, nurses must have the knowledge, the enduring attitudes, the willingness, and the skills necessary for helping their patients with self-care and with regulating patients' use or development of self-care agency. Desirable nurse characteristics in relation to the social, interpersonal, and technologic dimensions of nursing practice necessary for the design, production, and management of effective nursing systems are suggested below.

Suggested desirable nurse characteristics
Social

- Is well informed about and accepts the general social and legal dimensions of nursing situations; has specialized knowledge of the particular social and legal dimensions of some types of nursing situations
- Has knowledge of cultural differences between social groups and among members of social groups and understands the significance of people's cultural orientations in their contacts and communications with others
- Has a repertoire of social skills, including communication skills, sufficient for effecting and maintaining contacts with individuals and multiperson units from a range of social classes and culture groups
- Accepts and respects himself or herself and others as developing persons, recognizing that each person has characteristic ways of conducting himself or herself in interpersonal situations
- Is courteous and considerate of others
- Is responsible in the provision of nursing to individuals or multiperson units within defined types of nursing situations
- Understands the domain and boundaries of nursing as one of the health services provided for by society
- Understands the nature of contractual and professional relationships and is able to perform the operations of nursing practice within limits set by these relationships

Interpersonal*

- Is well informed about the psychosocial dimensions of human functioning
- Has knowledge of factors that facilitate or impede interpersonal functioning

---

* The identified characteristics pertain to interpersonal operations needed in all types of nursing situations. Some methods or technologic approaches to meeting certain self-care requisites or to regulating self-care agency are purely interpersonal in nature; such interpersonal methods are considered as being within the technologic operations of nursing practice. Mental health nursing specialists caution against the indiscriminate use of regulatory technologies that are valid for use in situations where patients have grave interpersonal problems.

- Has knowledge of conditions necessary for the development of helping relationships
- Is interested in identifying and resolving human problems that interfere with satisfying relationships with others and produce emotional pain or suffering
- Has a repertoire of interpersonal skills that can be adjusted to infants, children, and adults, including those who are ill, disabled, or debilitated, and that enable the nurse to:
  1. Be an active participant in relationships with patients and their significant others
  2. Be a participant observer in interpersonal relationships with patients and their significant others with the goal of identifying personality characteristics (e.g., being controlling or passive) significant in the relationship and the existence and degree of emotional suffering or emotional pain (anxiety) and physical discomfort and pain (if both are severe, they can interfere with the patient's observation of events, resulting in a lack of knowledge of the interpersonal situation and sometimes in misinterpretation of it)
  3. Reduce patients' emotional pain and physical discomfort and pain by effecting conditions that increase patients' comfort and satisfaction within the nurse-patient relationship
  4. Increase awareness of the interpersonal situation in terms of the desirable or undesirable factors that affect meeting patients' therapeutic self-care demands and regulating their self-care agency
- Is able to relate to patients and their significant others in a manner that conforms to the conventional form for human interactions (e.g., making eye contact when engaged in conversation, maintaining a conversational tone when seeking information)
- Has a repertoire of communication skills (adjusted to the age and developmental state of individuals, their cultural practices, and communication problems resulting from genetic defects and pathological processes) sufficient for effecting and maintaining relationships essential in the production of wholly compensatory, partly compensatory, and supportive-educative nursing systems for patients
- Accepts persons who are under nursing care and works with them in accordance with their roles in self-care and dependent care
- Identifies broader social and legal aspects of interpersonal situations (e.g., who is legally responsible for the patient) and is able to represent these in a prudent way to patients or their significant others

Technologic

- Has mastery of valid and reliable techniques for nursing diagnosis and prescription; for meeting the therapeutic self-care demands of individuals with

various mixes of universal, developmental, and health-deviation self-care requisites; and for regulating the quality and exercise of the self-care agency of individuals
- Is experienced or becoming experienced in using valid and reliable techniques in performing the technologic operations of nursing practice (see 1) in defined types and subtypes of nursing situations and in producing nursing systems within these situations
- Is able to integrate the social and interpersonal dimensions of nursing practice with the technologic dimensions (see 1) toward the production and management of effective nursing systems for individuals and multiperson units
- Is alert, at ease, and confident in nursing situations; is relaxed but able to mobilize for immediate and effective action to protect patients' well-being and to regulate the variables of nursing systems and the relationships among them
- Seeks nursing practice experience and supervision as well as specialized education and training to extend or deepen his or her area of nursing practice with respect to nursing populations
- Works toward the formulation and testing of methods and techniques for technologic operations of nursing practice within his or her nursing specialization
- Strives to increase ability to apprehend those factors in nursing situations that condition the values of the patient variables, self-care agency, and therapeutic self-care demand and thus set up requirements that nursing agency be of a particular value
- Identifies the results obtained in specific nursing situations from the use of specific methods in meeting patients' therapeutic self-care demands and in regulating their self-care agency; compiles results over time by types of nursing situations; isolates factors associated with types of results; and compares results in the different types of nursing situations.

The characteristics of nurses presented above represent a further development of the nursing agency. They can be used as a foundation for exploratory studies of nurses' qualifications for nursing practice, which in turn serve as bases for research to establish the associations between nurse characteristics and the design, production, and management of nursing systems.

REFERENCES
1. Nursing cases of clinical nursing specialists, The Harry S. Truman Memorial Veterans Hospital, Columbia, Missouri, presented at The School of Nursing, University of Missouri, Columbia, Summer Institute on Self-care Deficit Nursing Theory, June 12, 1986.
2. Nursing Development Conference Group, Orem DE, editor: Concept formalization in nursing: process and product, ed 2, Boston, 1979, Little, Brown & Co., p. 170.
3. Knutson AL: The individual, society, and health behavior, New York, 1969, Russell Sage Foundation, pp. 180-193.

4. Ullman M, "Health Deviations and Behavior. In Orem DE, and Parker KS, editors: Nursing content in preservice nursing curriculums, Washington, D.C., 1964, Catholic University of America Press, pp. 74-76.
5. Leavell HR, et al: Preventive medicine for the doctor in his community, McGraw-Hill Book Co., 1965, New York, p. 11.
6. Monnig Sr. NG: Identification and description of nursing opportunities for health teaching of patients with gastric surgery as a basis for curriculum development in nursing, Master's dissertation, School of Nursing, Catholic University of America, Washington, D.C., 1965, pp. 89-90.

SELECTED READINGS

Bassuk EL, and Rosenberg L: Why does family homelessness occur? A case control study. Am J Public Health 78:783-788, 1988.

Choi T, Josten L, and Christensen ML: Health-specific family coping index for noninstitutional care, Am J Public Health 73:1275-1277, 1983.

Das V: Voices of children, Daedalus, Another India, 118:263-294, 1989.

Gibson RC: Blacks in an aging society, Daedalus, The Aging Society 115:349-371, 1986.

Hagestad GO: The aging society as a context for family life, Daedalus, The Aging Society 115:119-139, 1986.

Kornblatt E, et al: Home-health care: who's where? Am J Public Health 77:733-734, 1987.

Loveland-Cherry C, et al: A nursing protocol based on Orem's self-care model: application with aftercare clients. In Riehl-Sisca J, editor: The science and art of self-care, Norwalk, 1985, Appleton-Century-Crofts, pp. 285-297.

Nursing Development Conference Group: Nursing knowledge and nursing practice. In Orem DE, editor: Concept formalization in nursing: process and product, ed 2, Boston, 1979, Little, Brown & Co., pp. 233-300.

Rodin J: Aging and health: effects of the sense of control, Science 233:1271-1276, 1986.

Swets JA: Measuring the accuracy of diagnostic systems, Science 240:1285-1293, 1988.

Taylor SG: The structure of nursing diagnosis from Orem's theory, accepted for publication by *Nursing Science Quarterly*.

Torres-Gil F: The latinization of a multigenerational population: Hispanics in an aging society, Daedalus, The Aging Society, 115:325-348, 1986.

Warner R: Deinstitutionalization: how did we get where we are? J Social Issues 45:17-30, 1989.

White M: The virtue of Japanese mothers: cultural definitions of women's lives, Daedalus, Futures, 116:149-163, 1987.

CHAPTER 10

Nurses and nursing practice

Nurses enter into agreements to provide nursing. They enter into interpersonal relationships with persons they nurse and with persons related to them. They interact and communicate with these persons. All of the activities, including information-gathering activities required for the societal and interpersonal aspects of nursing, are enabling for nurses to engage in the professional-technologic operations of nursing practice. These operations can be identified in a way that is common to the health professions that provide direct care and service to people.

OPERATIONS OF PROFESSIONAL PRACTICE

Professional practice within the health service professions varies in accord with the proper object of each health service, the state of development of each service's practical and applied sciences, and the kind of preprofessional and professional, including advanced professional education of its practitioners. Operations that are specifically professional-technologic are identifed as (1) diagnostic, (2) prescriptive, (3) treatment or regulatory, and (4) case management. These operations are directed to and performed for the sake of persons receiving the specific health services singly or in groups. Each of the named operations has a general meaning that becomes specific within the individual health service.

General description of operations

Diagnostic operations involve a process of careful examination and analysis of the facts that are descriptive of a particular person and the person's conditions and circumstances of living in an attempt to understand or explain the nature of existent or changing condition(s) for which health service is sought. What health service professionals diagnose and the diagnoses they make are specific to each service. Diagnostic operations precede prescriptive operations, which precede treatment or regulatory operations. Diagnostic operations result in answers to the questions: What is? What are the distinguishing characteristics of what is? What is its nature? Why is it as it is? Diagnostic operations follow or are concurrent with investigative operations to accumulate the facts that are relevant to the problems for which people seek care from specific health services.

Prescriptive operations are practical judgments followed by decision-making operations about courses of action to be followed in situations where particular diagnosed conditions exist. Prescriptive processes answer the questions: What can be done given the known present and the projected state of affairs and the means available? What should be done in light of the total situation of the person and the conditions and circumstances of living not just this or that single aspect of the situation?

Treatment or regulatory operations are the practical activities through which what is prescribed is executed and through which the diagnosed condition or problem is treated in order to remove it to control it or to keep it within boundaries compatible with human life, health, and well-being.

Case management operations are concerned with controlling, directing, and checking each of the diagnostic, prescriptive and treatment, or regulatory operations. Controlling includes evaluation. Case management is concerned with the integration of technologic operations to form a dynamic system of health service that is effective and judicious in the use of resources and that minimizes both psychological and physical stress for persons seeking and receiving the health service.

Nursing's professional-technologic operations

The general operations of health service practitioners become specific to nursing in terms of the proper object of nursing (persons with health-derived or health-associated self-care deficits or with dependent-care deficits associated with the health state of the dependent person) and the theories of self-care, self-care deficit, and nursing system. It is questionable whether the general operations of professional practice can be made specific to nursing or to any other practice field in the absence of understanding of the proper object of the field that lays out its domain and boundaries and understanding of the concrete entities (persons in time-place localizations, properties of the persons, changes in persons' properties or in their activities, and the products made), which become the foci of professional-technologic operations. The foregoing emphasizes the importance of nursing practitioners moving from a base in theoretically practical nursing science. The technologic orientations and operations of nursing practice as understood within self-care deficit nursing theory are listed in the box on page 267.

In nursing or medical practice, professional-technologic operations are sequential as previously indicated. This does not mean, however, that nursing diagnostic operations are completed before care prescriptions are made and care provided. This is illustrated in a case study developed by Susan G. Taylor in consultation with Jeanne Saathoff (pp. 59-68).[1] A 34-year-old man was hospitalized with diabetes mellitus out of control, a submandibular abscess, high fever, and a leg ulcer that resulted from a tick bite. An immediate decision was made for medical and nursing staff to take over the "regulation and production of self-care." All care measures to meet known components of the patient's therapeutic self-care demand, "including routine hygiene,

Technologic orientations and operations of nursing practice

1. The power of others to engage in self-care
   a. Diagnose the values of the constituent elements of self-care agency of the other in terms of:
      (1) Degree of development
      (2) Degree of operability
      (3) Adequacy as related to the operations required for meeting an existing or a projected self-care demand (2f below)
   b. Determine the presence or absence of a deficit relationship between existing powers of self-care agency and the action demands on it (2f below)
   c. Prescribe how self-care agency should be regulated
   d. Represent to the other need for and the rationale for and assist the other with:
      (1) The immediate exercise of self-care agency
      (2) The withholding of the exercise of self-care agency in a prescribed manner
      (3) The adjustment or development of one or more of the constituent elements of self-care agency in a prescribed manner in order to meet existing or projected self-care requisites
2. The continuous and effective meeting of the self-care requisites of others in accordance with 1a, 1b, and 1c
   a. Diagnose existing or projected self-care requisites
   b. Particularize the value(s) of each self-care requisite by determining the active conditioning effects of such factors as age, gender, developmental state, health state, sociocultural orientation, and available resources
   c. Determine the method(s) through which each existing or projected self-care requisite can be met
   d. Select the method(s) for meeting each self-care requisite that is both safe and effective in view of the age, developmental state, and health state
   e. Set forth the courses or systems of action required to use the selected method in meeting each particularized self-care requisite
   f. Calculate, in light of the foregoing, the totality of the courses of action required to meet existing and projected self-care requisites using selected methods (the therapeutic self-care demand) and then design the total action system
   g. Prescribe the role that the other can safely and effectively take in self-care in light of 1a
   h. Prescribe the role that the nurse (or a nonnurse) can and should take in meeting the therapeutic self-care demand of the other, including selecting and presenting valid and reliable ways of helping
   i. Perform and manage role operations to meet each self-care requisite of the other according to the selected or adjusted method(s), the determined action system, and the prescribed roles (2g and 2h)

were performed or initiated by the nursing staff." The health focus of care of nurses and physicians was (1) treating the infection and (2) regaining some control of the diabetes mellitus. With improvement in the patient's condition, the medical focus was shifted to "evaluating his general condition," including the use of intrusive medical diagnostic measures. "The nursing focus during this period was on support" because of the patient's anxiety about "procedure and outcomes." The nursing focus shifted "to one of evaluating and improving" the patient's "self-care system when he was able to attend to this" (p. 61).[1] This focus moved nurses back to nursing diagnostic operations related to the patient's self-care agency — his capabilities and limitations for self-care. The nursing diagnoses are expressed in a paragraph that is explanatory of the patient's self-care limitations and his past failures to know and meet components of his therapeutic self-care demand (p. 64).[1]

The initial decision that nurses would be the producers of continuing care to meet components of the patient's therapeutic self-care demand was based on the unexpressed nursing diagnosis that the patient was not able to engage in self-care because of the urgency for meeting his health-deviation self-care requisites and because his acute infection and hyperglycemia limited his ability to attend and his available energy. Health state, including acuity of illness, was the major dynamic variable in this first phase of nursing, affecting both the patient's self-care agency and the components of his therapeutic self-care demand.

The preceding example demonstrates the necessity for nurses to avoid conceptualizing the provision of nursing as a linear process moving from a complete, definitive nursing diagnosis to nursing regulation and evaluation. This experience may occur on occasion but is far from what should be expected.

Design operations and technologic nursing operations

Design operations are related to but different from the professional-technologic operations of nursing diagnosis, nursing prescription, and nursing regulation or treatment. Design operations and design units, described in Chapter 5 and illustrated with information from a typical case in Chapter 9, determine the jurisdiction of nursing, who is involved in the production of care, and the roles of these persons in the production of a continuous or periodic system of nursing. Nursing investigative, diagnostic, and prescriptive operations result in information and nursing judgments specific to Design Unit C (current or prior self-care or dependent-care system), Design Unit D (components of the therapeutic self-care demand), and Design Unit E (self-care roles — what patients can do, should do, or should not do). Design Unit F (design of the nursing system) results in a creative design for the system of nursing to be produced based on patient roles in self-care and the methods of helping that have validity in relation to the nature of patients' limitations for engagement in self-care. See Chapter 5 for the five general roles of adolescent or adult patients for incorporation into the design of nursing systems.

Nursing system design takes place before the production of nursing treatment or regulation to meet patients' therapeutic self-care demands and to regulate the exercise or development of their self-care agency. In the case presented earlier, nurses decided that the patient would have no active role in the production of self-care because of the acuity of his illness. The exercise of his self-care agency was being regulated by their decision. The decision necessitated the selection of *doing for* as the method of helping necessary to meet the patient's therapeutic self-care demand resulting in a system of nursing that was wholly compensatory for the patient's limitations of energy, awareness, and motivation to engage in self-care.

Thus nursing design operations in design Unit F follows nursing diagnosis and nursing prescription and precede the operation of nursing treatment or regulation focused on meeting patients' therapeutic self-care demands and regulating the exercise or development of their self-care agency. The design of the nursing system to be produced for a patient is subject to change as nursing diagnoses and nursing prescriptions change.

TECHNOLOGIC NURSING SYSTEMS

Nursing systems are series and sequences of practical actions of nurses that may be conjoined with practical actions of nurses' patients or their significant others to meet some or all components of patients' therapeutic self-care demands and to regulate the exercise or development of their powers of self-care agency. A system is anything that can be viewed as a single, whole thing. Nursing systems are constituted from actions that are performed because they are judged to have value in bringing about conditions or correlations that do not presently exist. Nursing systems have no permanent concrete existence. They are understood from their action elements and the persons with specialized properties who perform the actions. Technologic nursing systems are produced in conjunction with contractual and interpersonal systems.

Nursing process

Nursing process is a term used by nurses to refer to the professional-technologic operations of nursing practice and to associated planning and evaluative operations. These operations are conceptualized and named in various ways in works that develop the idea of nursing process.

Nursing conceptualized as process within the frames of reference developed in this book is summarized in Fig. 10-1. **Process** is used in the sense of a continuous and regular action or succession of actions taking place or carried out in a definite manner. The object or goal that is sought defines the direction and nature of the actions. Achievement of the goal sets the limits on the duration of a process. The succession of actions that constitute the nursing process are deliberately selected and performed by nurses as they nurse specific patients. The process operations of nursing practice are understood as technologically oriented and as performed within the all-encompassing system of societal relationships and within the enabling interpersonal, interactional system of relationships. Nursing considered from a systems perspective is understood as constituted from three interrelated types of processes or subsystems

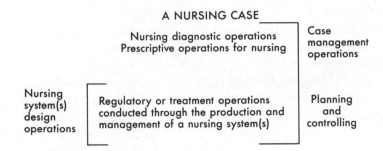

Fig. 10-1 The technologic process operations of nursing practice.

of action. The concern here is the technologic operations in relation to interpersonal and contractual operations.

Nursing diagnosis and prescription

Nursing diagnosis necessitates investigation and the accumulation of facts about patients' self-care agency and their therapeutic self-care demand and the existent or projected relationships between them. Nurses in practice understand or should understand that investigation should not go beyond what is needed for nurses to make valid judgments about existent conditions. Experienced nurses can quickly apprehend many facets of each practice situation and know the kind and amount of information they need as they proceed to nurse patients. In nursing, diagnosis is focused on persons who are accepted as having therapeutic self-care demands, the components of which are based in their particularized self-care requisites and as having the property of self-care agency, which may be in various stages of development and may be operable in whole or in part. Nevertheless, nurses require facts in order to make judgments that self-care agency, if it is developed and operable in individuals, will be exercised by them and will be adequate for meeting their therapeutic self-care demands.

Nursing diagnosis is a process of carefully examining and analyzing facts and nursing judgments about persons, their properties, their movements, or changes in properties to explain: (1) relationships between basic conditioning factors and existent self-care requisites and means for meeting them; (2) the patient's repertoire of self-care practices as related to known components of the therapeutic self-care demand; (3) limitation for deliberate actions that interfere with the estimative (investigative), judgment and decision making, and the production phases of self-care; (4) adequacy of knowledge, skills, willingness and other power components to perform self-care operations to meet each component of the therapeutic self-care demand; and (5) potential for the future exercise or for the development of self-care agency.

Diagnostic statements can be expressed in various ways with respect to the five types of explanations. However, it should be remembered that technically an explanation expresses a relationship between entities. In the type of nursing case described in Chapter 9 where information was sorted by design units diagnostic statements to describe the five explanations named in the preceding paragraph could be expressed appropriately as follows:

1a. All universal self-care requisites and means for meeting them are conditioned by the results and effects of the two cerebrovascular accidents (health state factors).

1b. There is a set of health-deviation self-care requisites associated with the condition of insulin-dependent diabetes mellitus with the continuing possibility to probability for the emergence of additional requisites of this type.

1c. There are health-deviation self-care requisites of a monitoring (watching or checking) nature related to the emergence of evidence of changes in vital functions.

1d. Developmental self-care requisites are for protection of human integrity and maintenance of a sense of self.

2, 3, 4. There is a complete deficit for engagement in estimative, judgment and decision making, and production of self-care operations in knowing and meeting the therapeutic self-care demand. This deficit is associated with the absence of self-management capabilities and limited cognitional functioning resultant from the effects of two cerebrovascular accidents.

5. There is no known potential for the future exercise or development of self-care agency because of the results and effects of the cerebrovascular accidents.*

Prescriptive operations specify (1) the means to be used to meet particularized self-care requisites, and the courses of actions, care measures, to be performed in using the means to meet the requisite; (2) the totality of care measures to be performed to meet all components of the therapeutic self-care demand, including a good organization of the care measures from the various components; (3) the roles of nurse(s)' patient and dependent-care agent(s) in meeting the therapeutic self-care demand; and (4) roles of nurses, patients, and dependent-care agents in regulating the exercise or development of self-care agency.

Diagnostic and prescriptive self-care operations that relate to patients' therapeutic self-care demands and self-care agency are summarized in Tables 10-1 and Table 10-2, respectively. These operations are expressed within the context of interpersonal and contractual operations of nursing practice.

In nursing diagnostic and prescriptive operations, as well as in regulatory and treatment operations, patients' and families' abilities and interest to collaborate with nurses affect what nurses can do. Patients, members of their families, or others who are acting for patients may or may not be interested in the need or psychologically

---

*A contrasting case in terms of potential for development of self-care agency is reported by Smith MC: An application of Orem's theory in nursing practice, Nurs Sci Q 2:159-161, 1989.

Table 10-1 Operations related to determining patients' therapeutic self-care demands

Interpersonal and contractual operations	Technologic-professional operations			Type of operation
Enter into and maintain effective relationships with patient, family, or significant others				
Reach an agreement (implicit or explicit) with the patient or family to seek answers to the questions: What is the patient's therapeutic self-care demand at this time? In the future?				
Collaborate with the patient or family	Determine the existing and projected self-care requisites, their particular values, and expected changes in their values:			Diagnostic of self-care requisites
Review with patient or family	*Existing requisites* Universal Developmental Health-deviation	*Current values*	*Projected requisites* Universal Developmental Health-deviation	*Projected values*
Collaborate with patient or family	Determine the methods through which each existing or projected self-care requisite can be met, i.e., methods that are valid and reliable in relation to the patient's age, developmental state, health state, and other conditioning factors			Preliminary–prescriptive

Review with patient or family	Select the methods that will be used for meeting each particularized self-care requisite, with knowledge of the safety and degree of effectiveness of each method	Prescriptive of methods
Review with patient or family	Lay out the procedures or care measures required for using the selected method(s) for meeting each of the requisites	Prescriptive of measures
Review with patient or family	Calculate the ideal therapeutic self-care demand and identify self-care requisites with high priorities:	Prescriptive of the ideal therapeutic self-care demand for some duration
	Self-care requisites *Values* *Methods* *Measures for meeting* Universal Developmental Health-deviation	
Reach agreements with patient or family about the constituent parts of the therapeutic self-care demand, and give the final prescription of the therapeutic self-care demand to the patient or family	Make adjustments as required in the therapeutic self-care demand to bring it into accord with what is possible (and necessary) to accomplish	Final – prescriptive of the therapeutic self-care demand
Specify nurse, patient, or family roles in making adjustments	Identify factors that will require changes in the values of self-care requisites. Indicate how to calculate value changes and to make adjustments in methods or procedures as needed.	Specification of rules for making changes in the therapeutic self-care demand

Table 10-2   Operations related to self-care agency and its regulation

Interpersonal and contractual operations	Technologic-professional operations	Type of operation
Enter into and maintain effective relationships with patient, family, or significant others		
Reach an agreement (implicit or explicit) to seek answers to the questions: Can and to what degree can the patient engage in required self-care at this time? At a future time?		
Collaborate with patient or family	Identify and describe the patient's repertoire of self-care practices and the usual components of the patient's self-care system	Diagnostic of self-care agency Specific existent abilities
Collaborate with patient or family	Identify and describe limitations for deliberate action that interfere with the decision-making and productive phases of self-care, including medically prescribed restriction of activity	Specific existent limitations
Review conclusions with patient or family	Make inferences about the general abilities and limitations of the patient for engagement in the decision-making and productive phases of self-care; formulate and express as judgments	Specific existent abilities and limitations by phases of self-care
Collaborate with patient or family	Validate inferences through continued observation of what the patient does and does not do	Confirmed self-care abilities and limitations
Collaborate and reach agreements with patient or family	Determine the adequacy of the patient's knowledge, skills, and willingness to meet each self-care requisite using particular methods and measures of care	Adequacy of self-care abilities in relation to components of the therapeutic self-care demand
Inform patient or family of the judgment about the presence or absence of a self-care deficit	Make and express judgments about what the patient is able to do, not able to do, and should not do in meeting the prescribed therapeutic self-care demand at this time or at a future time	Diagnostic of the presence or absence of a self-care deficit— existing; projected

Table 10-2   Operations related to self-care agency and its regulation — cont'd

Interpersonal and contractual operations	Technologic-professional operations	Type of operation
Reach agreements about prescribed roles with patient or family, nurses, or dependent-care agents	In light of the presence and nature of a self-care deficit determine what the patient should do, should not do, and is willing to do in the immediate meeting of the prescribed therapeutic self-care demand	Prescriptive of patient role and nurse role (or dependent-care agent role) in meeting the therapeutic self-care demand
Reach agreements with patient about prescribed patient role and related nurse role	In the event of an existing or a potential self-care deficit determine the potential for the future exercise of or the continued development of self-care agency	Prescriptive of patient role and related nurse role in regulating the exercise or development of self-care agency

able to accept the need to collaborate with nurses or to become active participants in their own self-care or the care of their dependents. Thus it is important for nurses to make initial observations about patients and their families in order to provide themselves with information they can use to guide their interactions and communications with patients.

From this perspective, nurses should concern themselves with (1) identifying the personality characteristics of patients and others related to them that will significantly affect the nursing situation (e.g., passivity-activity) and (2) identifying and exploring patients' concerns that may block their active collaboration with nurses and their participation in health care. To obtain this information, nurses must make observations about and elicit subjective information from patients. Nurses should also be alert to situations where patients never question what nurses say and do. It is important for nurses to know whether patients are understanding and accepting, or uninvolved, or always accepting of what persons in position of authority say, or fearful or unknowing. Such information should be limited to what is essential to know in order to work with patients and families. Patients' interests in and concern for their integrated functioning, their acceptance of the reality of their states of functioning, and their need for particular care measures will affect what patients will and will not do. Meeting the universal self-care requisite for promotion of integrated functioning and normalcy is a first step toward patients' collaboration with nurses and their participation in self-care.

Regulation or treatment operations

These operations are performed for the attainment of nursing results for individuals. Nursing results are expressed as the continuous meeting of the patient's therapeutic self-care demand, the regulation of the exercise or development of the patient's powers of self-care agency, and protection of the patient's developed self-care capabilities or their potential for further developments. Regulation or treatment operations are periodic or continuous and may be performed by nurses in conjunction with patients or dependent care agents.

As nursing diagnosis and prescription proceed, nurses have degrees of knowledge about components of patients' therapeutic self-care demands and the presence, extent of, and reasons for the existence of a self-care deficit. They have a basis for allocation of roles for performing regulatory or treatment operations.

Designs for regulatory operations

Nurses have knowledge about the instrumental role that the patient can fill in the production and management of self-care (no role, some role). Nursing system design should: (1) set forth relationships among the components of the therapeutic self-care demand that will result in good regulation of the health and developmental state of the patient; (2) specify the timing and the amount of nurse-patient contact and the reasons for it; and (3) identify the contributions of nurse and patient to meeting the therapeutic self-care demand, to making adjustments in it, and to regulating the exercise or development of self-care agency.

Nurses should keep in mind certain matters as they design systems of nursing for patients. For example, some self-care actions, particularly those involving choice, decision, and will, cannot be performed for a patient by anyone else. The provision of appropriate support and environmental conditions may help the patient to gradually acquire competence in these matters. In relation to a patient's requirements for sleep, rest, and activity, nurses may be able to or help others to establish and maintain environmental conditions that are conducive to rest, sleep, or activity, including the control of demands placed on the patient. Nurses should also keep in mind that patients may want to do more than they are physically or psychologically able. Provisions to help patients set limits on what they are to do in self-care should be included in the nursing systems design. Some patients may not desire or be willing to engage in self-care, even when they are able by objective standards. Here again, nurses may need to foresee the desirability of providing environmental conditions that will encourage or induce patients to assume self-care responsibility.

Patients who want to perform beyond their capacities may test themselves and learn from experience that they cannot do what they had judged themselves able to do. In the same way, reluctant or unwilling patients, when confronted by nurses who want to and know how to assist them to become self-directing, can often move quickly to engage in decision-making and planning activities relating to self-care and to perform selected self-care tasks. In both of these instances, nurses and patients do not agree as to who shall do what. They are not cooperating in an agreed-upon manner (positive cooperation); they are engaged in a struggle (negative cooperation) (pp. 62-64).[2] This type of cooperation is valid only if nurses' judgments about patients' abilities are sound and if they are motivated by a sincere desire to conserve patients' energies or to help them assume their self-care responsibility. Nurses must be certain, however, that the basis for action is valid so that the situation will not dissolve into a battle of wills. In designing a nursing system, evidence that indicates the positive or negative cooperation will prevail should be taken into consideration. Thus, an important element in designing a nursing system for a patient and in planning for the complement of nurses required is the identification of the extent and intensity of nurse-patient interaction which is required in order to meet nursing requirements. The psychological effects of nursing in various types of health care situations on nurses should be thoroughly studied as one of the principal elements for determining more effective and efficient nursing system designs.

Designing an effective and efficient system of nursing involves selecting valid ways of assisting a patient. The immediacy of patients' needs for self-care, as well as the nature of their self-care limitations, may affect nurses' choices about ways to assist patients. The nurse uses two types of knowledge to design valid nursing systems for patients. One type of knowledge is factual and is derived from or related to the patient. It describes the patient from a nursing perspective and includes detailed descriptions of his or her abilities and limitations for self-care. The other type of knowledge is general and relates to accumulated information about types of therapeutic self-care demands and how the ways of helping can compensate for or overcome limitations for therapeutic self-care. It takes into account the health-related causes of these conditions and factors that affect the effective use of the ways of helping.

When what a nurse will do and what a patient will do in relation to the patient's self-care and in adapting to, compensating for, or overcoming self-care limitations are determined by the selected ways of assisting, a pattern or design of system emerges. The design of a nursing system for a specific patient will be more detailed in that the roles of nurse and patient will be described in relation to (1) self-care tasks to be performed in coordinated patterns and in particular time sequences, (2) making adjustments in the therapeutic self-care demands, (3) regulating the exercise of self-care agency, (4) protecting developed powers of self-care agency, and (5) bringing about new development in self-care agency (e.g., acquiring konwledge, developing specific skills).

In making decisions about how to help patients effectively extend their self-care capabilities, it is necessary for a nurse to have for recall a body of knowledge about self-care as deliberate action. Understanding based on previously presented information about the conditions essential for self-care (Chapter 6) may be extended by further considering that some self-care behaviors are internally oriented, whereas others are externally oriented. See Fig. 7-5, which indicates the directional flow of some of these behaviors.

The internally oriented behaviors required for self-care are:
- Learning activities related to the development of self-care knowledge, attitudes, and skills
- Application of knowledge in initiating, performing, and controlling self-care activitites
- Self-care action to control behavior, such as controlling an emotional reaction, facing the reality of one's state of health or disability, or restricting one's activities in order to rest or to keep a part of the body immobilized
- Action to monitor one's condition or responses

The externally oriented behaviors required for self-care are:
- Knowledge-seeking activity directed to printed material or to persons who possess knowledge about health, disease, and effective self-care practices
- Resource-seeking activity related to securing equipment, materials, facilities, and services necessary in self-care
- Resource-utilizing activities related to using supplies or equipment in performing self-care
- Activity to control factors in the external environment, for example, controlling the movement of air, the number of social contacts, or biological elements in the environment
- Activity to seek assistance to accomplish a self-care goal within an interpersonal situation, for example, requesting help in performing a self-care task, seeking validation of a judgment, or asking not to be left alone
- Expressive interpersonal activity, such as when a patient expresses feelings about health or self-care verbally or nonverbally but without a direct request for help
- Action to become aware of one's location in an environment or of environmental conditions

The internally oriented behaviors necesssary in self-care depend on awareness of self and environment, as well as on motivation and interest. The internally oriented self-care behaviors of a patient at any particular time always depend in part on acquired knowledge about the goals and practices of self-care. This knowledge may have been acquired in the family setting, in school, in social contacts with friends and associates, or through previous contacts with physicians and other health workers. The presence of limitations in awareness; in valid knowledge about the nature and meaning of self-care; in self-care skills, and in initiating, directing, and controlling behavior to accomplish defined goals of self-care affect a patient's internally oriented self-care behavior.

The externally oriented self-care behaviors are need-fulfilling behaviors with an external environmental orientation. Factors in the patient or in the environment may be instrumental in prompting a person to behave in one of these ways. Ability to engage in specific goal-seeking activities is a prerequisite for the externally oriented self-care behaviors listed earlier. In a nursing situation, the kinds of externally oriented behaviors in which a patient will seek to engage, or should be helped to engage, are related to the patient's self-care habits, perceived needs for care, objective requirements for care, and need to express feelings or impart or secure information. Environmental conditions, as well as the persons' capacity for various forms of deliberate action and existent self-care limitations, are relevant to these behaviors.

In summary, the nurse's knowledge of the patient's objective requirements for therapeutic self-care now and in the future when related to the patient's interests in, desire for, and concerns about self-care, and immediate and projected future capacities and limitations for self-care enable the nurse to make judgments about appropriate ways of helping the patient to provide therapeutic self-care and accomplish appropriate self-care agency goals. Thus an effective nursing system provides ways to relate behaviors of both nurse and patient to the accomplishment of nursing goals appropriate to the situation. Adjustment of nurse and patient behaviors to immediate conditions and to projected future conditions is accomplished through the selection of helping methods and definition of roles. The nature of the patient's specific limitations for self-care and the patient's degree of deficit for self-care are important and continuing considerations, as is the health care focus.

When a nurse selects a system of assistance for the immediate care of a patient, she or he may not have sufficient knowledge for making projections about how the selected forms of assistance should change with anticipated changes in the patient's condition. Nurses should systematically collect information about their patients to enable them to project requirements for changes in the initially selected system. Designing systems of nursing assistance for individual patients is not a common activity of nurses in health care agencies. Designing is an essential nursing activity, since a nursing plan has as its central focus the delivery of some selected system of nursing assistance.

Planning for regulatory operations

Planning as an aspect of the technologic nursing process is the movement from designs for nursing systems or for portions of such systems to ways and means for their production. A plan sets forth the organization and timing of essential tasks to be performed in accordance with role responsibilities. If a design is partial, the plan for using the design to guide nursing actions will also be partial. *Partial* is used in the sense of not complete, related to the duration of time that a person will be under nursing care. At times, nurses may not separate design and planning operations from diagnostic and prescriptive operations. In such instances, plans are short-term and are integrated with nurses' judgments and decisions about the specific task performance of nurses and patients.

Planning adds to the proposed nursing system specifications of the time, place, environmental conditions, and equipment and supplies required for the production of the system. Planning also produces specifications for the number and the qualifications of nurses or others necessary in order to produce a designed nursing system or a portion thereof, to evaluate effects, and to make needed adjustments. When planning is for the immediate performance of a selected self-care task, it may amount to a judgment by a nurse that, under prevailing conditions, "The patient can and should do this. I will remain here to support the patient. Betty will get the supplies needed." In scheduling the performance of self-care measures, nurses should take into consideration (1) the relationships among the components of a patient's therapeutic self-care demands, for example, arranging the performance of measures of self-care to enable patients to have periods of uninterrupted rest and sleep; and (2) the provision for assistance when patients need it, for example, in helping patients with elimination.

Regulatory care

Regulatory nursing systems are produced when nurses interact with patients and take consistent action to meet their prescribed therapeutic self-care demands and to regulate the exercise or development of their capabilities for self-care. A valid design for one or for a series of nursing systems to be instituted for a patient can be used as a guide in the production and management of nursing systems. The planning for implementation of the design and related procurement activities will determine when nurses should be with patients and when essential materials and equipment will be available and ready for use. In this, the third step of the technologic nursing process, nurses act to help patients meet their therapeutic self-care demands and regulate the exercise or development of their abilities to engage in self-care.

Systems of nursing oriented to regulation or treatment should be produced and managed for patients as long as the self-care or dependent-care deficits exist. Systems for regulatory nursing at times are replaced by systems of assistance provided by persons other than the nurse who are prepared to perform some measures of self-care for others. In such instances, nursing consultation and supervision should be available to both the person with the care deficit and the persons providing care. In all such situations, a professional nurse should participate in the development of the care system design whenever patients and families cannot.

Regulatory nursing systems are produced through the actions of nurses and their patients during nurse-patient encounters. Nurses during these encounters will take action to:

1. Perform and regulate the self-care tasks for patients or assist patients with their performance of self-care tasks
2. Coordinate self-care task performance so that a unified system of care is produced and coordinated with other components of health care
3. Help patients, their families, and others bring about systems of daily living for patients that support the accomplishment of self-care and are, at the same time, satisfying in relation to patients' interest, talents, and goals
4. Guide, direct, and support patients in their exercise of, or in withholding the exercise of, their self-care agency

5. Stimulate patients' interest in self-care by raising questions and promoting discussions of care problems and issues when conditions permit
6. Support and guide patients in learning activities and provide cues for learning as well as instructional sessions
7. Support and guide patients as they experience illness or disability and the effects of medical care measures and as they experience the need to engage in new measures of self-care or change their ways of meeting ongoing self-care requisites
8. Monitor patients and assist patients to monitor themselves to determine if self-care measures were performed and to determine the effects of self-care, the results of efforts to regulate the exercise or development of self-care agency, and the sufficiency and efficiency of nursing action directed to these ends
9. Make characterizing judgments about the sufficiency and efficiency of self-care, the regulation of the exercise or development of self-care agency, and nursing assistance
10. Make judgments about the meaning of the results derived from nurses' performance of the preceding two operations for the well-being of patients and make or recommend adjustments in the nursing care system through changes in nurse and patient roles

The first seven operations constitute direct nursing care, that is, the action system that makes up the treatment or the regulatory phase of nursing. These operations are performed by nurses at moments when patients can benefit from these seven operations. They are selected and performed by nurses in accordance with the presenting needs and conditions of patients. The last three operations are for the purpose of deciding if direct nursing care should be continued in the present form or if it should be changed. Nurses' performance of the first seven operations and facts about patients' presenting needs and conditions are recorded in patients' charts to document nurses' day-to-day direct care actions. The results and recommendations resulting from nurses' performance of the last three operations are recorded as progress notations. Such notations document the basis for nurses' judgments about the effects of patients' current self-care regimens, their self-care agency, and the sufficiency and efficiency of nursing.

The direct nursing care actions of nurses may be started during nurses' first encounters with patients during the period of initial nursing diagnosis. Assisting patients with self-care or performing some parts of the other direct care operations cannot be deferred until nursing diagnosis is complete or until there is a formalized design for a regulatory nursing system. Diagnostic, prescriptive, and design and planning operations may be sequentially performed in rleation to direct care actions.

To understand the production of regulatory nursing care, it is necessary to visualize the distribution and duration of nurse-patient encounters, the kinds of operations nurses engage in during these encounters, the nursing focus maintained by nurses in relation to known health care focuses, and the helping methods nurses select in relation to the presenting needs and conditions of the patient and existing environmental conditions. The need for the performance of some self-care tasks at particular times can be anticipated. The degree to which tasks to meet patients' therapeutic self-care demands and to regulate self-care agency can be programmed by time and place varies with the stability of patients' health states and their health care regimens. The number of nurses required to produce a system of nursing for a patient varies with the intermittent or continuous nature of patients' self-care requisites; degrees of physical helplessness and dependency on others; states of development; the degree of stability of health states; the familiarity or strangeness of the environments in which health care is received; and, of course, what individual nurses can and should do within a particular time period. The frequency and duration of contact between nurse and patient must be sufficient for the intermittent or continuous performance of some or all of the 10 operations required for the production of effective regulatory nursing care systems.

Nursing practice situations where patients require nursing over the twenty-four hours of the day range from those where a professionally qualified nurse is unable or just able to provide continuous nursing for one patient without assistance to those where one nurse can effectively provide care to a number of patients during the same time period with or without assistance. In ambulatory care, nurses may carry large case loads of patients, the number of patients being related to the frequency of required nurse-patient contacts and the length of visits. When nursing is provided through home visits by the nurse, the number of patients in a nurse's case load is affected by the frequency of visits, the kind and amount of care provided, and travel time. When more than one nurse is contributing to the production of nursing assistance, there are requirements for coordinating nursing operations, clarifying the goals being sought through nursing, and socializing patients to a number of nurses. In a situation of this type, patients may be unaware of their own roles and the roles of nurses with whom they have contact.

Control operations

Control operations include observation and appraisal to determine (1) if regulatory or treatment operations are performed periodically or continuously according to the design for the system of nursing under production for a patient; (2) if the operations performed are in accord with the conditions of the patient or the patient's environment for the regulation of which they have been prescribed, or if the prescription is no longer valid; and (3) if regulation of patient's functioning is being achieved through performance of care measures to meet the patient's therapeutic self-care demand, if the exercise of patient's self-care agency is properly regulated, if developmental change is in process and is adequate, or if the patient is adjusting to declining powers to engage in self-care.

Control operations answer certain questions. The first control operation asks the question: Is this person receiving regulatory nursing treatment? The second asks the question: Are regulatory and treatment operations valid in relation to prior conditions and/or current conditions? The third control operation asks the question: Are nursing results being achieved and to what degree? All questions demand investigation, including observation of what is presently existent or in process, and all demand a standard against which appraisals are made.

The standard for the first question is the role responsibility of nurses, patients, and others and the use of methods of helping implicit in the statements of role responsibilities for (1) performance of self-care measures or (2) for the regulation of the exercise or development of self-care agency. There are two standards for the second operation. The first is the continued existence of the human or environmental conditions they were prescribed to regulate. The second is the presence of new not previously existent conditions or the absence of prior conditions. The third operation has as its standard the therapeutic self-care demand prescribed and its potential for bringing about functional stability or desired functional change in the patient. It also has as its standard the patient's prescribed roles in self-care and the patient's potential for developmental or regressive change.

Control operations are professional-technologic operations of nursing practice that can be performed concurrently with regulatory or treatment operations of nursing practice. They can also be performed in separation from them at intervals during the period when the patient is being nursed and before discharge from nursing or transfer to another nursing service. The second volume of the report of the Horn and Swain study of criterion measures of nursing care (Manual, Health Status Measures of Nursing Care for Adult Medical-Surgical Hospitalized Patients)[3] provides nursing students and nurses with finely developed examples of measures for appraisal of nursing care. The process for developing these criterion measures of nursing care is described in a 1977 article by the nurses who formulated them (pp. 41-45).[4]

NURSING SYSTEMS IN CONCRETE PRACTICE SITUATIONS

Nursing systems were conceptualized in Chapter 3 and the process of creating designs for them was described in Chapters 5 and 9. A system is anything that can be viewed as a single, whole thing. The use of a systems perspective is helpful in both understanding and in creating complex entities such as the production of nursing.

The Nursing Development Conference Group's 1970 description of a nursing system as a tridimensional system formed from social, interpersonal, and technologic subsystems is an important contribution to nursing knowledge. The subsystems are viewed as interrelated but are separated analytically to understand the complexity of nursing situations.

The concrete elements of nursing systems are the persons who occupy the status of nurse and the staus of nurse's patient and the events that transpire between them. These persons are conceptualized as having attributes that legitimate their occupancy of the status of nurse and the status of nurse's patient. Legitimate patients have (1) a therapeutic self-care demand to be met, (2) self-care agency in some state of development and operability, and (3) a deficit relationship between (1) and (2); that is, self-care agency is not adequate in quality or operability for meeting the existing or projected therapeutic self-care demand because of health or health-related factors. Nurses have the attribute of nursing agency and are willing to exercise their nursing abilities for the benefit of others with health-derived or health-related self-care deficits. These attributes of patients and nurses are viewed as the variables of the technologic component of nursing systems. The relationships between and among the variables in concrete nursing situations are indexes of the nature and purposes of nursing systems.

Nursing systems exist as systems of concrete action produced from the deliberate, discrete actions of nurses and patients in nursing situations. Nursing system projections that nurses (or nurses and patients) make about future actions in regulating patients' self-care agency and in meeting their therapeutic self-care demands are design or care measure changes. Projected nursing systems can exist as prescriptions, that is, statements of the type(s) of nursing system that has been judged both effective and reliable in light of the nature of and the factors associated with existing or projected patient self-care deficits. Nursing systems come into existence when nurses and patients operate according to their role prescriptions.

The basic design

The basic design of a nursing system is that of a helping system. Nursing system design delineates the structuring of the elements in nursing situations. These elements include social positions and roles, role relationships, the individuals involved, and technologic elements (patient and nurse variables) (Fig. 10-2). The manner in which the elements are related reveals the structure of the system. The design of a nursing system begins when nurses select and use one or some combination of the methods of helping in nursing situations based on the nature and extent of the deficit. Methods of helping prescribe general roles for the helper and the one helped. The general roles of nurses and patients defined by methods of helping are identified in Table 10-3.

Nurses make judgments about valid methods of helping in nursing situations as they perceive factors in their patients and the patients' environments (including nurses and other persons) that are relevant to how patients can and should be helped through nursing. These judgments are made on a moment-to-moment basis,

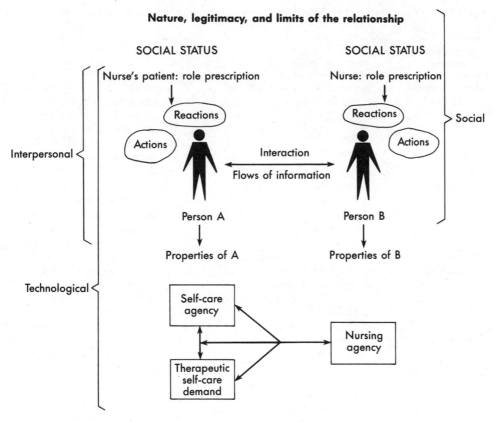

Fig. 10-2 Social, interpersonal, and technologic elements of nursing systems.

including the initial period of nurse-patient contact. Ideally, nurses see how patients should be immediately helped and foresee how they can and should be helped over some time period. The actual design of a concrete nursing system emerges as nurses and patients interact and take action in order to calculate and meet patient's therapeutic self-care demands, to compensate for or overcome the identified action limitations of patients, and to regulate the development and exercise of patients' self-care abilities.

Projected designs for nursing systems can be developed when nurses have the necessary knowledge, foresight, imagination, and creative abilities to make a structural design for nurse and patient actions for some projected time period. Nurses who function at the professional level should be skilled in making and projecting designs for nursing systems; all nurses must have some skills in designing or in making adjustments in the design of nursing systems. Projected designs for nursing systems for patients are analogous to an architectural blueprint. Projected and emerging designs of nursing systems make clear (1) the scope of the nursing

Table 10-3   Nurse and patient roles in nursing situations as specified by methods of helping

Method of helping	Nurse role	Patient role
Doing for or acting for another	A person who acts in place of and for the patient	Recipient of care to meet the therapeutic self-care demand and to compensate for self-care limitations Recipient of services relevant to environmental control and resources
Guiding and directing another	Provider of factual or techno-logic information relevant to the regulation of self-care agency or the meeting of self-care requisites	Receiver, processor, and user of information as self-care agent or as regulator of self-care agency
Providing physical sup-port	A partner, cooperating in per-forming self-care actions to regulate the exercise of or the value of self-care agency by patient	Performer of actions to meet self-care requisites or regula-tor of the exercise of or the value of self-care agency in cooperation with a nurse
Providing psychological support	An "understanding presence";* a listener, a person who can institute the use of other methods of helping if neces-sary	A person confronting, resolving, and solving difficult problems or living through difficult situations
Providing an environment that supports development	Supplier and regulator of essen-tial environmental conditions and a significant other in a patient's environment	A person who is confronted with living and caring for himself or herself in a way and in an environment that supports and promotes per-sonal development

Teaching	Teacher of:
	  Knowledge describing and explaining self-care requi-sites and the therapeutic self-care demand
	  Methods and courses of action to meet self-care requisites
	  Methods of calculating the therapeutic self-care de-mand
	  Methods of overcoming or compensating for self-care action limitations
	  Methods of managing self-care
		Learner engaged in the develop-ment of knowledge and skills requisite for continuous and effective self-care

*van Kaam A.: The art of existential counseling, Wilkes-Barre, 1966, Dimension Books.

responsibility in health care situations; (2) the general and specific roles of nurses, patients, and others; (3) reasons for nurses' relationships with patients; and (4) the kinds of actions to be performed and the performance patterns and nurses' and patients' actions in regulating patients' self-care agency and in meeting their therapeutic self-care demand.

Types of nursing systems

On the principle that nurses and/or patients can act to meet patients' self-care requisites, three basic variations in nursing systems are recognized: (1) *wholly compensatory* nursing systems, (2) *partly compensatory* nursing systems, and (3) *supportive-educative* (developmental) nursing systems.* This typology of nursing systems is associated with the question: Who can or should perform those self-care operations that require movement in space and controlled manipulation? If the answer is the nurse, the system of nursing is wholly compensatory because a nurse should be compensating for a patient's total inability for (or proscriptions against) engaging in self-care activities that require controlled ambulation and manipulative movements. If the answer is that the patient can perform some but not all self-care actions requiring controlled ambulation and manipulative movements, then the nursing system should be considered partly compensatory. If the answer is that the patient can and should perform all self-care actions requiring controlled ambulation and manipulative movements, the nursing system should be of the supportive-educative (developmental) type. Fig. 10-3 provides an overview of the basic nursing systems.

These three types of nursing systems describe what would be a good organization of the actions of nurses and patients under three conditions: (1) the patient has physiologic or psychological limitations for controlled movement in the accomplishment of required self-care, (2) the patient has a self-care requisite to limit energy expenditures because of health state, and (3) the patient lacks knowledge or skill or is not psychologically ready to perform self-care actions requiring controlled movement that must be performed only once or performed continuously for some time but are technically complex and require informed judgments and decisions at each step of execution. The types are also paradigms of nursing systems that vary over a range. Max Black's description of range words and range definitions is a useful guide for understanding the process for identifying the three types of nursing systems as well as in identifying possible subtypes (p. 29).[5]

---

*It should not be assumed that there is a direct correlation between these types of nursing systems and hospital patient service units referred to as critical or intensive care, intermediate care, and self-care units. In some self-care units nursing may not be provided; at most there may be some general surveillance from nurses. In intermediate care units, wholly compensatory as well as partly compensatory nursing systems may be required by patients. The same may be true in intensive care units. These patient service units are organized according to the principle of the acuteness of illness and rapidity of expected change in the condition of patients and to patients' ambulatory states.

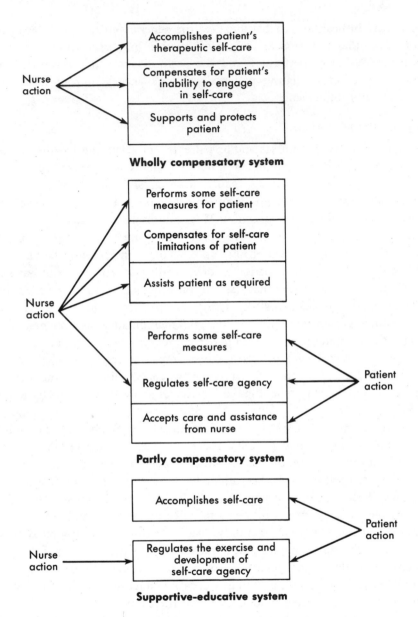

Fig. 10-3 Basic nursing systems.

These systems are derived from and relevant to individual nursing situations. When multiperson units such as families are served by nurses, the resulting nursing systems are usually combinations of the features of partly compensatory and supportive-educative nursing systems. It is within the realm of possibility that families or residence groups would need wholly compensatory nursing systems under some circumstances, but it is advisable at this stage of the development of nursing knowledge to confine the use of the three nursing systems to situations where individuals are the units of care or service.

Wholly compensatory nursing systems

The patient factor that is the criterion measure for identifying the need for a wholly compensatory nursing system is the inability to engage in those self-care actions requiring self-directed and controlled ambulation and manipulative movement or the medical prescription to refrain from such activity (a health-deviation self-care requisite). Three subtypes of wholly compensatory nursing systems are recognized. Each subtype is based on a complex of limitations for deliberate action that interferes with controlled movements necessary for deliberate actions, including self-care. Persons with these limitations are socially dependent on others for their continued existence and well-being. The subtypes are:

- Nursing systems for persons unable to engage in any form of deliberate action, for example, persons in coma
- Nursing systems for persons who are aware and who may be able to make observations, judgments, and decisions about self-care and other matters but cannot or should not perform actions requiring ambulation and manipulative movements
- Nursing systems for persons unable to attend to themselves and make reasoned judgments and decisions about self-care and other matters but who can be ambulatory and may be able to perform some measures of self-care with continuous guidance and supervision

Persons who fit the first subtype of wholly compensatory nursing are (1) unable to control their position and movement in space, (2) unresponsive to stimuli or responsive to internal and external stimuli through hearing and feeling, or (3) unable to monitor the environment and convey information to others because of loss of motor ability. These persons will be confined to one location in space, unless they are moved by others. They must be protected and cared for. The valid helping method is that of doing and acting for. Nurses and others should speak to these persons using a conversational tone, handle them gently, maintain continuous or frequent contact, and maintain environmental conditions that protect and support normal functioning.

Persons whose action limitations fit the second subtype differ from persons in the first subtype by being (1) aware of themselves and their immediate environment and able to communicate with others (communication powers may be normal or greatly restricted); (2) unable to move about and perform manipulative movements because of pathologic processes or the effects or results of injury, immobilizing measures of medical treatment, or extreme weakness or debility; or (3) under medical orders to restrict movement. These persons may be mentally competent and capable of making accurate observations. They may be involved in making judgments and decisions about self-care and perform self-care actions that do not require movement. They must exercise self-control and develop a style of living that promotes normalcy of outlook and continued personal development and must maintain their willingness to be cared for by others regardless of their reluctance to do so. Nurses use a number of methods of helping patients in the second subtype, with emphasis on maintaining a developmental environment and doing and acting for the patient. Patients with these limitations will suffer when neglected by nurses and others and when their interests and concerns are not solicited or are ignored. Psychological support, guidance and direction, and teaching are therefore valid methods also. Prevention of hazards and promotion of normalcy must be given special attention because of the possible deleterious effects of inactivity, restricted environments, and awareness of one's helplessness.

Persons in the third category differ from those in the first two subtypes in that (1) they are conscious but are unable to focus attention on themselves or others for purposes of self-care or care of others, (2) they do not make rational judgments and decisions about their own care and daily living without guidance, or (3) they can ambulate and perform some measures of self-care with continuous guidance and supervision. Persons characterized by such limitations bring about hazardous conditions for themselves and, at times, for others. They should be taken care of and protected, and others may need to be protected from them. The helping methods associated with this set of limitations include providing and maintaining a developmental environment, guiding and directing, providing support, and doing or acting for.

Wholly compensatory nursing systems have social and interpersonal and technologic dimensions that must be understood by nurses. These dimensions are related to the extremely restricted ability or inability of persons to manage themselves and to control environmental conditions. From the nursing viewpoint, nurses are not only major providers and managers of patients' self-care, they are also the makers of judgments and decisions about the self-care requisites of their patients and the designers of nursing care. Nurses have the responsibility to meet all three types of self-care requisites — universal, developmental, and health-deviation — for persons with the types of limitations described here. Nurses must be in close contact and communication with family members, know who is responsible for the patient's affairs, and be able to sort out the nursing responsibility for the patient from family members' rights and responsibilities. The social, interpersonal, and technologic dimensions of these nursing situations require that nurses be the major, and in some instances the sole, contributors to action systems produced to meet the self-care requisites of patients and protect patients' powers of self-care agency and their personal integrity.

Because of the labor involved in providing continuous care to persons with the action limitations identified here, persons other than nurses are frequently placed in positions of responsibility for patients requiring wholly compensatory nursing systems. Nurses have a social responsibility as members of the nursing profession to act to ensure safe and effective care to persons with extensive limitations of the self-care agency. This responsibility can be fulfilled when nurses are free enough as professionals to accept the responsibility and are creative and knowledgeable enough to design, put into operation, and manage effective care systems for these persons. They should also be knowledgeable enough to set the specifications for and guide and supervise others who can contribute to the operation of wholly compensatory care systems.

Partly compensatory systems

The second system is for situations where both nurse and patient perform care measures or other actions involving manipulative tasks or ambulation. The distribution of responsibility to nurse or patient for performance of care measures varies with (1) the patient's actual or medically prescribed limitations for ambulation and manipulative activities, (2) the scientific and technical knowledge and the skills required, or (3) the patient's psychological readiness to perform or learn to perform specific activities. The patient or the nurse may have the major role in the performance of care measures. A partly compensatory nursing system may take a number of forms. In one form, patients perform universal measures of self-care and nurses perform medically prescribed measures and some universal self-care measures. A second form is for these situations where patients are learning to perform some new care measures. In partly compensatory situations all five helping methods may be in use at the same time.

Supportive-educative systems

The third system is for situations where the patient is able to perform or can and should learn to perform required measures of externally or internally oriented therapeutic self-care but cannot do so without assistance. Valid helping techniques in these situations include combinations of support, guidance, provision of a developmental environment, and teaching. This is a *supportive-developmental system.* It is the only system where a patient's requirements for help are confined to decision making, behavior control, and acquiring knowledge and skills. There are a number of variations of this system. In the first, a patient can perform care measures but needs guidance and support. Teaching is required in the second variation. In the third, providing a developmental environment is the preferred method of helping. The fourth variation is in situations where the patient is competent in self-care but requires periodic guidance that he or she is able to seek; in this variation, the nurse's role is primarily consultative.

Nursing practice implications

The preceding descriptions of the three types of nursing systems are constituted from the differences in the roles of nurses and patients in meeting the patients' self-care requisites. One or more of the three types may be used with a single patient. For example, patients who are receiving nursing because of surgical treatment involving anesthesia and organ removal may progress from a supportive-educative system to a partly compensatory system to a wholly compensatory system, then back to a partly compensatory system and, finally, to a supportive-educative system before being discharged from nursing. Other patients, especially those in ambulatory care services, may take part in supportive-educative nursing systems, shifting at times to partly compensatory nursing systems. Nurses should select the type of nursing system or sequential combination of nursing systems that will have optimum effect in achieving the desired regulation of patients' self-care agency and the meeting of their self-care requisites.

Through nursing, patients with extensive action limitations may develop the capabilities needed to design and manage their own self-care and to guide and direct a helper in the provision of care. With nursing consultation and medical supervision, other patients may become able to identify their self-care requisites and to design, provide, and manage their own self-care toward the regulation of the effects of pathology (pp. 422-427).[6-7] The descriptions of the three types of nursing systems and the criterion measures for determining the kind(s) of system(s) needed should be used in examining information about patients' self-care abilities and limitations before prescribing nurse and patient roles. They can also be used to determine whether or not nurse and patient roles in active nursing situations are in accord with patients' self-care abilities and limitations. This further development of the conceptual structure of the theory of nursing systems articulated in Chapter 3 provides nurses with knowledge that can guide their decision making and evaluative actions in situations of nursing practice.

The utility of the basic design of nursing systems has been pointed out in relation to the specification of nurse and patient roles and the assisting techniques that the nurse would need to use. Thus the three nursing systems suggested for the purposes of this text could serve as a guide in the development of a typology of nursing situations for use within health care agencies or communities. Each patient presents specific requirements for assistance that describe his or her need for one or a combination of the three nursing systems. Professional nurses are responsible for accumulating information about patients that describes commonalities and differences in their nursing requirements, including both requirements for assistance with self-care and overcoming obstacles of self-care. The commonalities among specific types of patients, if identified in terms of factors that specify roles and requirements for specific assisting techniques, would indicate the health agency or community requirement for particular systems of nursing assistance. This information is important in planning for the number and kinds of nurses and nurses' assistants needed to provide a nursing service that will be adequate for a particular population. It is also important for nursing education.

NURSING SYSTEMS AND DEPENDENT-CARE SYSTEMS

With changes in health care systems come expectations that persons with major health deviation self-care requisites and major adjustments in the particularization of universal self-care requisites and the need for the use of specialized technologies in meeting them can be cared for in their homes. Situations vary from very young infants born prematurely to children and adults with catastrophic illness and terminal and chronic illness to debilitated elderly persons. Some hospitals, nurses, physicians, or whole communities do not attend to or make provision for ensuring the availability of nursing to individual families with these tremendous care responsibilities. On the other hand, there are outstanding examples of movement to provide not only nursing in the home but also other support services for the persons needing health care and their families.

Family members in positions of responsibility for ensuring the continuing self-care of others in their homes must develop the knowledge and skills and the interpersonal capabilities and maintain their willingness for providing dependent-care. These persons continue to bear responsibility for their own health and well-being as persons who are self-care agents. Some nurses in hospitals see themselves as responsible for preparing not only patients but also their family members or friends who will bear dependent-care responsibilities for the return home. Nurses have come to see more and more clearly the need to make appraisals, not just of dependent-care capabilities but also of the health states of persons who are taking on dependent-care responsibilities, including the probable effects of the burden of care on them. This problem is addressed by Taylor and Robinson-Purdy in a reported study "to describe the development of self-care, dependent-care, and professional nursing care systems for hospitalized, about to be discharged patients with physical illness or injury" (pp. 4-16).[8] This paper, an important approach to descriptive studies, identifies, for example, significant limitations of nurses, failures of nurses to assess prospective care givers, the importance of patients and care givers coming together to talk about and plan for care at home, and factors that result in unrealistic estimates of dependent-care agents about their capacities to provide dependent-care. The study introduces approaches for continued exploration of this nursing and family problem.

Nurses' contributions to the design of dependent-care systems and planning for their operation and maintenance should be an important consideration in endeavors to develop nursing services that meet needs of communities. The articulation of nursing systems with dependent-care systems is an important consideration whenever there is a need for periodic nursing that is conjoined with a wholly compensatory system of dependent-care (Chapter 9, example) or with combined systems of self-care and dependent-care.

UNITS OF SERVICE IN NURSING PRACTICE

A nurse's unit of service may be an individual or a multiperson unit. **Unit of service** is used in the sense of whether persons are provided with nursing as individuals or as members of multiperson units. Nurses recognize that only individuals have self-care requisites and developing or developed powers of self-care agency. It is the societal and interpersonal relationships of individuals and their interactions that focus nurses' attention on families and groups as units of service.

The difference in the objective focus of the nurse in the two units of service is illustrated in Fig. 10-4. When the unit of nursing is an individual the nurse sees the individual as the one in need of care; the nurse also sees the individual as having the position of family member with relationship to other family members. When the unit of service is a multiperson unit, the nurse's objective focus is the unit and she or he may work with individuals within the unit knowing that the health and well-being of individuals will contribute to the welfare of the unit.

Multiperson units

For nursing purposes multiperson units can be classified as follows:
- Dependent-care units, for example, parents and a seriously ill child or an adult caring for a chronically ill parent.
- Structured, enduring units, such as families or households.
- Structured but less enduring units, such as residence groups of various types including (1) groups constituted as therapeutic communities within health care agency settings or (2) residence groups living in homes in a community.
- Persons who meet as a group at specific times. These persons have similar types of self-care requisites and need to learn so that they will become able to meet particular components of their therapeutic self-care demands. Included are work groups exposed to particular hazards, self-help groups, prenatal or postnatal groups, weight control groups, and groups of patients in nursing clinics.

Nursing practice for multiperson units of service place demands on nurses for knowledge about the structure and functioning of groups, for knowledge about group processes, and for skill development in working with groups of persons. Nurses should remember that persons who are members of groups have functions and operations that are not functions and operations of the group as such. Nurses must develop skill in being able to see persons in groups both as individuals and as group members. In the framework of the theory of nursing systems in multiperson situations of practice, group processes and interactions would replace the interpersonal system that is

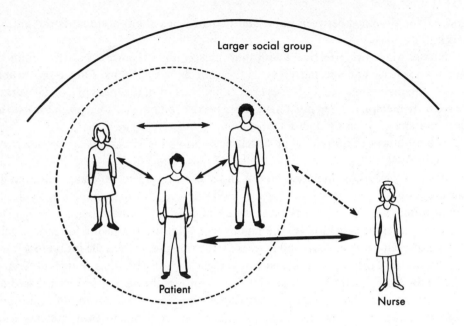

Individual type nursing situation

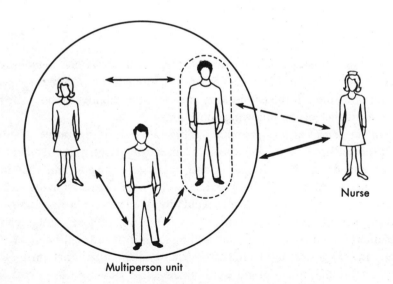

Multiperson unit type nursing situation

Fig. 10-4 The object of the nurse in individual and multiperson nursing situations.

created and develops between nurse and patient when the individual is the unit of service.

Nurses who work effectively with multiperson units require specialized foundational knowledge and specialized skills for working with groups. They must be able to take and maintain a nursing focus as distinguished from the focus of a social worker or a family therapist. They must have the expertise to help and to avoid harming the unit and any of its individual members.

Some features of individual and multiperson nursing situations are summarized in Table 10-4.

Nurses express considerable interest and some nurses have mistaken ideas about families as units of service or nurses. In a 1989 article, Taylor sets forth with clarity the position of family within the framework of self-care deficit nursing theory. The positions developed include (1) the family as a conditioning factor for individuals' therapeutic self-care demands and power of self-care agency when the individual is the unit of service of the nurse, (2) dependent-care units within families as units of service, and (3) the family as the unit of service. The family as the unit of service is based on the premise that the "family has certain functions related to self-care and dependent-care [of all its members] that exceed or are different from meeting each individual's self-care requirements" (pp. 131-137).[9] Multiperson units are divided into two groups for purposes of a discussion about rationales for their consideration as units of service by nurses. The groups are identified as groups whose members *do* and *do not reside in the same place.* They will be referred to as residence and nonresidence units.

Residence units

Nurses's decisions about accepting as their unit of service persons who live together as a family, in a household, or as a therapeutic community within an institution or a home in the community are based on judgments about the presence of one or a number of the following conditions.

A need for protection and prevention. This rationale is operative whenever the goodwill, personal energies, and coordinated endeavors of unit members must be mobilized and directed to designing and operationalizing a plan that meets the following specifications. The plan provides for (1) continuous knowing and meeting the therapeutic self-care demands and regulating the exercise or development of the self-care agency of one or more members of the unit whose care is complex or burdensome, (2) at the same time safeguarding the health and well-being of other unit members, and (3) protecting the unit as a structured and functional entity. Examples include serious illness of one or more unit members, or the addition of twins or triplets to the unit.

Regulation of a hazard. This rationale is operative whenever the continuous knowing and meeting of the therapeutic self-care demand and the exercise or development of self-care agency of one or more unit members is *adversely affecting the*

Table 10-4 Characteristics of individual and multiperson nursing situations

Type of nursing situation	Characteristics		
	Therapeutic self-care demand and self-care requisite	Action limitation and action requirement	Purpose of nursing
Individual	The therapeutic self-care demand is constituted from some mix of universal, developmental, and health deviation requisites.	There are all types of health-derived or health-related limitations for engagement in care.	To develop or regulate the exercise of self-care or dependent-care capabilities To compensate for action limitations so that the therapeutic self-care demand will be met effectively and continuously
Multiperson unit Community groups, including work group situations	Some self-care requisites are common to all persons who constitute the group. Methods for meeting these self-care requisites are developed and have a known degree of effectiveness. The environment in which group members work or live affects the nature of the common self-care requisites as well as the methods for meeting them.	Action limitations are limitations of interest, motivation, knowledge, or skill on the part of group members. There is a requirement for organized, cooperative effort to bring about the conditions and acquire resources to meet self-care requisites common to group members.	To promote the development or exercise of essential self-care or dependent-care capabilities To promote habitual performance of essential measures of self-care or dependent care under known prevailing conditions To bring about the development and maintenance of cooperative efforts essential for group welfare

Continued.

Table 10-4 Characteristics of individual and multiperson nursing situations—cont'd

Type of nursing situation	Characteristics		Purpose of nursing
	Therapeutic self-care demand and self-care requisite	Action limitation and action requirement	
Family or residence group situations	The interrelatedness of members and their living environment affects the values of the self-care requisites of individual family or group members. Meeting the therapeutic self-care demand of one or more individuals affects if and how the therapeutic self-care demands of other members can be met.	Action limitations are limitations of interest motivation, knowledge, and skill on the part of group members. There is a requirement for organized, cooperative effort to meet the therapeutic self-care demands of individuals within the group and to promote the well-being of the group as a unit.	To promote development by family or group members of the capability to view the family or group as a unit of structure and operation To promote the development or exercise of essential self-care or dependent-care capabilities To promote the development of the capability on the part of some or all group members to (1) plot out the interrelatedness of the therapeutic self-care demands of members, (2) design a plan for meeting individual and group needs, and (3) secure and maintain the required human effort and material resources

health or well-being of other unit members as well as the *structured and functional integrity* of the unit. Such conditions prevail when one or more dependent-care systems within the unit are complex, burdensome, of long duration, and draining of both the material and human resources of the unit.

Need for environmental regulation. This rationale is operative whenever the *conditions of living* of a family, a household, or a residence group, including environmental features, are not conducive to or obstruct the meeting of the universal and developmental self-care requisites of all members of the unit. A wide range of situations here can be described in terms of social and psychosocial climate and physical and biologic environmental conditions. In such situations nurses need to look for features that can and should be regulated and not dwell on features that are harmful but cannot be regulated at present or in the immediate future.

Need for resources. This rationale prevails whenever the *material* or *human resources* necessary to meet the therapeutic self-care demands of one or more or all members of a unit are not available at all or are insufficient in quality or quantity. A striking example is that of a young father with an infant and a toddler to care for and no resources for food or child care assistance.

In all the preceding situations nurses may have as their unit of service both individuals who are members of families or households or residence groups and the unit itself. What nurses do as nurses in such multiperson situations should remain within the domain and boundaries of nursing. Problem identification, resolution, and solution with unit members as well as use of the five ways of helping are proper approaches by nurses.

Nonresidence units

Nurses work with already formed *nonresidence groups* or organize them for purposes of learning and teaching. Group situations, for example, self-help groups or instructional groups, facilitate learning and developmental change. Instructional groups conserve the time and energies of nurses as they help people who have similar components of their therapeutic self-care demands and similar learning problems related to their self-care capabilities.

RULES OF NURSING PRACTICE

Rule is used to mean a principle that governs the conduct of nurses in practice situations by specifying proper ways of thinking or acting to achieve nursing results for patients. *Rule* is not used in the sense of regulation but in the sense of instructive and prudential rules (pp. 93-136).[10] Some general rules of nursing practice are presented. It should be understood that some rules, even general rules, do not hold under all conditions and circumstances.

Rules are organized in five sets and relate to initial and continuing contacts of nurses and their patients, the production of nursing, and nurses' relationships among themselves and with other health workers.

Set one: initial period of contact

1. Enter nursing situation in accordance with held credentials for nursing practice and occupational-professional status.
2. Initiate contacts with potential or actual patients in accordance with social norms, with receptiveness, and in a manner that is adjusted to patients' overtly perceptible states of health and well-being.
3. Convey in initial contacts with patients and their families what knowledge you have about reasons for patients being under health care for confirmation or the raising of questions that will provide historical or current information about patients' health care situations.
4. Determine in initial contacts with patients the presence or absence of gross evidence of a self-care deficit (see Chapter 7) and whether immediate regulatory nursing care to meet one or a number of self-care requisites takes precedence over engagement in detailed nursing diagnostic procedures.
5. Accept each patient as having continuing requirements for self-care and from some capacity to no capacity for its provision.
6. Determine in initial contacts with patients or with persons acting for them who has been the continuous provider of care to meet patients' therapeutic self-care demands and then come to an agreement about who will be the care agent(s) during the processes of nursing diagnosis and nursing prescription. Possibilities include the following:
   a. Patients will continue to meet the usual components of their therapeutic self-care demands. Patients will have appropriate guidance and directions from nurses if there are needs for adjustments.
   b. Patients will continue under a system of dependent care. Dependent-care agents will have appropriate guidance and direction from nurses if there are needs for adjustments.
   c. Patients and nurses together will maintain the continuing system of care to meet the usual components of patients' therapeutic self-care demands, making adjustments as needed.
   d. Nurses become the agents who maintain patients' continuing systems of self-care or dependent care.
7. Know the parties to, the conditions of, and the place of self as nurse in the agreements under which nursing is provided to patients for some specified or unspecified duration of time.
8. Confirm one's relationship as nurse to patients, expressing the bases for the relationship, role responsibilities as nurse, and manner and procedure of working with patients and patients' families.

9. Elicit patient or family expectations of the nurse(s) and their insights about their immediate roles in the nursing situation as a basis for confirming that roles are understood or for negotiating roles.
10. Assess one's legitimacy as nurse in the situation and one's willingness and fitness to proceed with the provision of nursing.

Set two: continuing contacts

1. Initiate and maintain the amount and kind of interpersonal contact and communication with patients that is essential for achieving nursing results with respect to knowing and meeting patients' therapeutic self-care demand and regulating the exercise or development of their self-care agency.
2. Keep the number and timing of contacts with patients adjusted to patients' capabilities for self-protection and the attainment of nursing results.
3. Initiate and maintain contact and communication with family members of patients or with persons legally responsible for patients to help them understand the nursing aspects of patients' health care situations now and in the future.
4. Accept patient-initiated contacts with you as nurse as requests for nursing and respond to them with social and nursing appropriateness.
5. Assist patients to become able to initiate contacts with you or designated nurses whenever specific conditions are perceived or whenever patients or their dependent-care agents are unknowing about how to proceed with matters related to patients' therapeutic self-care demands.
6. If you need to be replaced temporarily or permanently make sure that the nurse is as competent as you.
7. Initiate the cessation of contacts with patients when they are ready for discharge from nursing care with provision for nursing consultation and supervision as the need exists or arises.
8. Initiate and conduct referrals of patients (and their dependent-care agents) to agencies providing home nursing when patients cannot be discharged from nursing but are transferring to their homes.
9. Develop and transmit nursing care summaries when patients are transferring to residence care institutions, including hospitals and nursing homes.

Set three: quality of interpersonal situations with patients

1. Relate and attend to patients in ways that will protect, preserve, or promote their integrity as human beings, promote well-being, and foster continuing movement toward maturity.
2. Recognize patients' degrees of socialization to their roles in the health care situation.
3. Approach and work with patients as persons who are at specific stages of growth

and development, from particular families, with orientation to self and family, with likes and dislikes, and with values, habits, and life-styles, and who may or may not view or value themselves as self-care agents or have positive orientations to health.

4. Relate and attend to patients with knowledge of their self-management capabilities based on evidence of their (a) levels of awareness of self and environment, (b) degrees of physical strength and vigor, (c) control of movements, (d) affective state, (e) long- and short-term memory, and (f) cognitive functioning.

5. Become insightful about the expressed perceptions, the overriding interests and concerns, and the fears of patients that interfere with fulfilling their role functions with respect to self-care or to the exercise or development of their self-care agency.

6. Work with patients and members of their families to help patients become active participants in their own care whenever and to the degree that self-care is possible and at the same time compatible with health results being sought.

Set four: production of nursing

1. Engage in nursing diagnosis initially and on a continuing basis to obtain and organize data and make and verify judgments about patients' self-care abilities and self-care limitations, self-management abilities within their environmental situations, and the number and characteristics of existent and emerging self-care requisites as a basis for calculating patients' therapeutic self-care demands.

2. Calculate and prescribe patients' therapeutic self-care demands or components thereof.

3. Express and document nursing judgments about the presence, reason for, and extent of patients' self-care deficits.

4. Determine patients' potential for the initial or continuing development of self-care agency or its redevelopment when necessary.

5. Prescribe means for the regulation of exercise or development of self-care agency.

6. Recognize, express, and document the value of effective nursing for the life, well-being, and health of patients with the understanding that, at times, nursing may be essential for life and for maintaining human integrated function or for preventing deterioration of functioning, that nursing may be helpful in maintaining or promoting states of health and well-being of patients, or that nursing should be a limited adjunct to patients' ongoing system of self-care or dependent care.

7. Design, operationalize, and manage systems of nursing for patients, keeping

nurse and patient roles and methods of helping adjusted to changes in patients' self-care agency and in their therapeutic self-care demands.

8. Manage self-as-nurse and features of the environmental setting toward maximizing high-level coordination with patients and their families and toward economy in use of time, energy, and resources.

9. Seek nursing consultation for self and patients with respect to matters of nursing diagnosis, prescription, and regulation whenever you as nurse or patients and their families are unsure about what should be done to attain nursing results or the progress being made in attaining them.

10. Maintain a professional level of documentation of nursing operations performed and results attained.

Set five: relationships with nurses and other care providers

1. Know and communicate with other nurses who participate in the production of nursing for one's designated complement or case load of patients.

2. Ensure that nursing consultation is available as needed, and keep abreast of rules and procedures for obtaining specialty nursing consults.

3. Maintain and use open channels of communication with the attending physicians of patients under nursing care as needed for nursing purposes and for the achievement of health results for patients.

4. View and accept medical orders written by physicians for their patients as prescribed medical diagnostic or treatment measures that are within the domain of medical care but may need to be incorporated into these persons' therapeutic self-care demands and their systems of self-care or, when under nursing care, into a nursing system.

5. Maintain and use open channels of communication with other health workers participating in the care of persons under nursing care as needed for nursing purposes and to attain health results by patients.

The rules expressed in the five sets are general and useful as guides in all types of nursing situations. They provide nursing students with structures for organizing knowledge. They also provide bases for developing more detailed specifications for practice by nurses in various practice settings or specialty areas of nursing who work consistently with particular nursing populations.

REFERENCES

1. Orem DE, and Taylor SG: Orem's general theory of nursing. In Winstead-Fry P, editor: Case studies in nursing theory, New York, 1986, National League for Nursing.

2. Kotarbinski T: Praxiology, an introduction to the sciences of efficient action, Trans. Olgierd Wojtasiewicz, New York, 1965, Pergamon, pp. 62-64.

3. Horn B, and Swain M: Development of criterion measures of nursing care, vol II, Manual for instrument of health status measures, Ann Arbor, Michigan, University of Michigan, 1977, US Department of Commerce, National Technical Information Service PB-267 005.

4. Clinton JI et al: Developing criterion measures of nursing care: case study of a process, Journal of Nursing Administration, vol. VII, Number 7, pp. 41-45, September 1977.
5. Black M: Problems of analysis: philosophical essays, Ithaca, NY, 1954, Cornell University Press, p 29.
6. Rita M, Meyer S, and Torzeinski Morris D: Alcoholic cardiomyopathy: a nursing approach, Nurs Res 26:422-427, 1977.
7. Meyer M: Application of the Orem Self-Care Deficit Theory to Nursing Practice. Paper given at a conference on Nursing Theories: Adaptation and Self-Care, St. Louis University Medical Center, Oct. 25, 1978.
8. Taylor SG, and Robinson-Purdy AU: Assessing self-management and dependent care capabilities of hospitalized adults and care givers in preparation for discharge, Clinical and Cultural Dimensions Around the World, pp. 4-16. Papers and abstracts presented at the first international self-care deficit nursing theory conference, the School of Nursing, University of Missouri, Columbia, October 15-18, 1989, Kansas City, Missouri, The Curators of the University of Missouri.
9. Taylor SG: An interpretation of family within Orem's general theory of nursing, Nurs Sci Q 2:131-137, 1989.
10. Black M: Models and metaphors, Ithaca, NY, 1962, Cornell University Press, pp. 93-136.

SELECTED READINGS

Branch M: Self-care black perspectives. In Riehl-Sisca J, editor: The science and art of self-care, Norwalk, 1985, Appleton-Century-Crofts, p. 181-188.Chamarro LC: Self-care in the Puerto Rican community. In Riehl-Sisca J, editor: The science and art of self-care, Norwalk, 1985, Appleton-Century-Crofts, pp. 189-195.

Choi T, Josten L, and Christensen ML: Health specific family coping index for noninstitutional care, Am J Public Health, 73:1275-1277, 1983.

Hanchett ES: Orem's theory of self-care deficit and community health nursing and community assessment and intervention according to Orem's theory of self-care deficit. In Nursing frameworks and community as client, Norwalk, 1988, Appleton & Lange.

Horn BJ, and Swain MA: Development of criterion measures of nursing care, vols 1 & 2, US Department of Commerce, National Technical Information Service, Pub Nos 267-004 and 267-005, Springfield, Virginia, 1977, University of Michigan and National Center for Health Services Research.

Nickel-Gallagher L: Structuring nursing practice based on Orem's general theory, a practitioner's perspective. In Riehl-Sisca J, editor: The science and art of self-care, Norwalk, 1985, Appleton-Century-Crofts, pp. 236-244.

Nursing Development Conference Group: Nursing knowledge and nursing practice. In Orem DE, editor: Concept formalization in nursing: process and product, Boston, 1979, Little, Brown & Co., pp. 233-300.

Taylor SG: An interpretation of family within Orem's general theory of nursing, Nurs Sci Q 2:131-137, 1989.

CHAPTER 11

Nursing practice and nursing administration

Nursing one individual over time is quite different from the day-to-day provision of nursing to two or more persons during the same time period. The practitioner of nursing focuses on the patients within his or her case load as individuals to be nursed. The complement of individuals to be nursed by a single nurse with or without assistance during the same time period is determined according to some governing principle or plan used by health service institutions or agencies that have provisions for offering nursing as one of their health services. The complement of persons for whom a health service agency has contracted to or is in the process of contracting to provide nursing or agrees to admit on an ad hoc basis for purposes of receiving nursing (and other health services) is the focus of **nursing administration.**

The nursing administrator focuses on populations or subpopulations that have requirements for nursing and can benefit from nursing. Whereas the nursing practitioner focuses on individuals with diagnosed health-derived or health-associated self-care deficits in their time-place localizations, nursing administrators must ensure that existent and future populations are provided with nursing. The nursing practitioner provides nursing. Nursing administration knows members of populations real or projected in terms of types and configurations of requirements for nursing, not as individuals, except when questions of adequacy of nursing arise. Nursing practitioners know the members of health agency populations they are to nurse as individuals whose nursing requirements are specific to them and must be diagnosed. **Population** is used as a class word—a word used to refer to all the people served or to be served by a health care institution or agency.

NURSING SERVICE IN THE COMMUNITY

Many communities in the United States and elsewhere expect nursing to be available on a communitywide basis. The pattern for nursing as a community service to individuals and families was set in the United States during the latter part of the nineteenth century. That pattern has changed since the developmental years, but modern nursing practice can be traced back to the three types of nursing service identified as hospital nursing, private-duty nursing, and district nursing.

What quality and quantity of nursing service are available to a modern community? What are the costs involved in providing this service to the community? What must patients pay for nursing, and how and where can they obtain this assistance when it is required? These important questions must be answered, partly by the citizens of the community and partly by nurses. Nursing, like the other services established in a community for the health, welfare, and safety of its citizens, must be planned for, maintained, and developed in keeping with community needs. If a community is to have nursing available, it must have nurses; and each community, therefore, must answer the question: How can this community fulfill its needs for nurses?

The strength and effectiveness of nursing as a health service in the community depends on the values of the community. The provision of nursing makes heavy demands on community resources. Many persons in a community need nursing at the same time—in their homes, in hospitals and clinics, in nursing homes and homes for the aged, in child-care institutions and clinics, and in a variety of other facilities providing health service. A community may require large numbers of nurses to supply the demands for nursing that exist at the same time, and often in the same place, throughout the twenty-four hours of each day and each day throughout the year. From both the community's and patients' point of view, nursing is a costly service and frequently may be in short supply. A community that is convinced that nursing is an essential health service will be more likely to engage in activities and programs necessary for providing nursing than will the community that holds no such conviction. In addition, many communities face the problem of finding candidates for nursing careers and preparing them for nursing practice.

The types of nurses needed and the educational facilities available for preparation for nursing practice also must be considered in providing adequate nursing in the community. Before World War II, nurses were educated almost exclusively in schools maintained and controlled by local hospitals. The level of preparation for all nursing personnel was essentially the same. Since that time, the increasing demand for nurses, the shortage of nurses, and the increasing complexity of health care has resulted in the preparation of persons for work in nursing in all the existing forms of occupational education and training. The number and qualifications of persons employed to provide nursing often differ from the required number of nurses qualified to give nursing.

Nurses' failure to develop or implement standards of nursing practice at the local community level has resulted at times in ineffective nursing and undesirable conditions of practice. Licensed nurses may not be prepared, able, or willing to design, provide, and manage systems of nursing assistance for patients and to supervise other nurses and auxiliary workers who contribute to the daily provision of nursing for individuals. Nursing practitioners often are not present or are so infrequently or remotely available that patients have little or no contact with them. As a result, technically prepared nurses, practical nurses, and nursing aides are placed in positions they are unprepared to fill.

The growing interest of American nurses in the development and implementation of standards of nursing practice to enhance the quality of nursing provided in community health agencies and hospitals should bring about improved conditions for both the consumers and practitioners of nursing.

The development of criterion measures of nursing care along with instruments and procedures for use in measuring the quality of nursing provided in a health care facility is making an important contribution to nursing. The previously mentioned work of Horn and Swain and their associates is an example of such work. Continued effort to ensure that the nursing provided in particular settings is in accord with patients' self-care deficits is needed. This effort, however, should be accompanied by efforts to provide qualified nurses with opportunities to engage in nursing diagnosis and prescription and in the design, production, and management of effective nursing systems for individuals and groups.

The settings in which nursing is provided varies by types of health care agency. The setting affects both nursing administration and nurses' practice of nursing. The place in which a patient is nursed is a variable that requires consideration. Place is of importance for several reasons. Some of the reasons can be best expressed as questions. Is the patient away from his or her usual place of residence and from an accustomed environmental setting? If so, what is the patient's outlook? Is the experience stress-producing, accepted, or even comforting to the patient? A patient's response to being a patient in a hospital, an extended care facility, a nursing home, a community health center, a clinic, or an outpatient department of a hospital is influenced by his or her knowledge and attitudes regarding health care.

Although they provide modern diagnostic, treatment, and rehabilitation facilities, hospitals may become so routine oriented that individual patients and their need for nursing are submerged by routine practices. The task of each nurse in a hospital nursing situation is to make certain that each patient is provided with nursing care that conforms to the nature of and reasons for the patient's self-care deficit and that the hospital system is adaptable to the nursing system for the individual patient. Routines are necessary, but they are not necessarily valid or justifiable if they interfere with the accomplishment of health goals and nursing goals for patients.

Other resident care facilities, such as extended care facilities and nursing homes, present some of the same advantages and disadvantages to nursing that the hospital presents. Routine service, large numbers of persons to be given care during the same time period, inadequate numbers of nurses, nurses with inadequate preparation, or the absence of nurses often militate against effective nursing in extended care facilities and nursing homes. Courtesy, kindness, and help from nurses and others in assuring patients that health care facilities and services are for their benefit are important in securing effective use of community facilities.

Other community facilities, such as clinics or day or night care health centers, serve patients who are at home for some part of the day. Nursing care of patients who come to these centers must take into consideration the possible need to adjust factors in the home environment to the patient's system of self-care or the need for the patient to make adjustments to the home situation. Hazards of travel, the time required for travel, available modes of travel, and costs require consideration.

Patients who are given nursing care in their own homes are in their accustomed environments. The environment is new for the nurse, however. A nurse who nurses patients in their homes may be a staff member of an agency that provides home care services. The agency may be a community health agency or a hospital that provides home care services. Such nurses have available to them equipment provided by the agency and may call on the agency for other types of health care services needed by persons receiving nursing.

Persons who are in permanent or temporary residence in health care institutions such as hospitals, who may require nursing as well as other forms of health care, will require a range of services due purely to their status as residents. Fig. 11-1 identifies services that health care institutions, such as hospitals and nursing homes, should provide for persons under health care, health care providers and other workers, and visitors. Whenever and wherever numbers of persons come or are brought together in common facilities (e.g., clinics), preventive public health services are essential for their protection. Ideally, an institution will maintain a supportive and developmental environment for all who come within its walls. The responsibility for the continued provision and maintenance of preventive public health services rests primarily with health care institution executives and administrators. All residence care and health care workers and other personnel, however, as well as patients and visitors, should participate in the fulfillment of this responsibility. Public health services are concerned with the protection of populations.

NURSING ADMINISTRATION

Nursing administration is defined as the body of persons who function in situational contexts to collectively manage courses of affairs enabling for the provision of nursing to the population currently served by an organized health service institution or agency and to populations to be served at future times. To achieve this goal, administrators exercise powers given them by the governing bodies of institutions or agencies, the purpose of which are accomplished in whole or in part through nursing. Nursing administration in its various situational contexts within a health service agency or insitution is a managerial organ within the formal structuring of positions and role responsibilities.

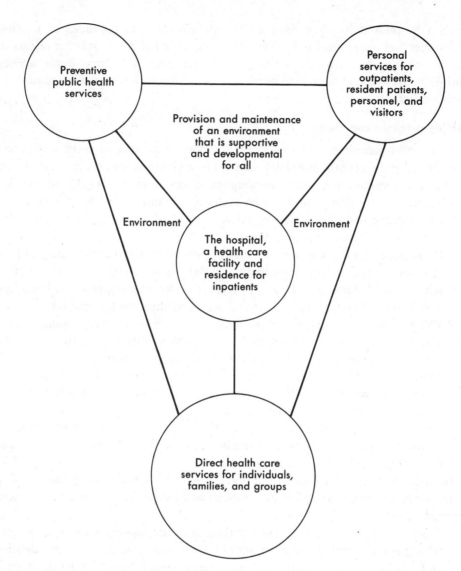

Fig. 11-1 Service operations of hospitals and health care facilities.

Location

The situational contexts in which persons who constitute nursing administration hold positions and function are identified in terms of distance from governing boards and chief executive officers or institutional administrators measured against distance from nurses engaged in the production of nursing for individuals or groups. Nursing administrators located in positions directly concerned with ensuring the day-to-day, minute-by-minute production of nursing for a subpopulation of a larger population (as on a hospital unit) often combine in one position the functions of nursing practitioner and operational unit administration. This holds not only for residence care institutions but also for home health care agencies where nurse agency administrators function to provide nursing consultation within their areas of nursing specialization.

Nursing-oriented functions

To function effectively, nurses who fill positions in nursing administration must have antecedent and continuously developing knowledge about nursing and about the organized enterprise that offers nursing as a community service. Knowledge requirements for nursing administrators includes at a minimum the following:
- Organized knowledge of the practical science of nursing, theoretically and practically practical nursing science
- Knowledge of practice models for nursing persons with types and configurations of types of requirements for nursing, validated and emerging models
- Knowledge of forms of education preparatory for nursing practice, including preparation of nursing specialists and legal qualification for practice
- The purpose of the institution or agency of which they are an organic part
- The extent to which and the manner in which nursing contributes to the continuing attainment of the institution's or agency's purpose
- The nature and extent of their received powers to manage courses of affairs that ensure the continuing provision to nursing to a population or a subpopulation served by the agency or institution
- Knowledge of the domain and boundaries of nursing in concrete practice situations, as well as the domain and boundaries of health professionals whose work articulates with nursing

In their positional locations within organized health service enterprises, nursing administrators use their knowledge of nursing and nurses (as well as other kinds of knowledge) to
- Produce nursing descriptions of populations or subpopulations served by identifying and classifying combinations of factors associated with self-care deficits, and factors relevant to contractual and interpersonal features of nursing practice
- Analyze the nursing descriptions to make judgments about the types of nursing practice models that would have to be juxtaposed or interlaced in the production of nursing for members of populations with the described types of self-care deficits
- Estimate the time requirements for nursing and the periodic or continuous nature of required nursing systems and the amount and quality of nursing effort required
- Consider desirable and undesirable locations for members of populations with types and configurations of requirements for nursing

- Consider (1) the capabilities that nurses must have to practice nursing for members of populations with types and configurations of requirements for nursing, and (2) desirable and undesirable mixes of nurses and assistants to nurses in the provision of nursing
- Consider and work with nursing practitioners in developing and testing desirable case loads for nurses or combinations of nurses and assistants considering both number of patients constituting a case load and the mix of patients by the types and configurations of their nursing requirements

Managerial orientations and operations

The foregoing nursing-oriented functions of nursing administration as well as associated managerial operations are understood within the larger framework of the functional systems of service enterprises developed in Chapter 2 in the section titled *Service Enterprises* and in Fig. 2-1.

Nurses through their production of nursing in the role of nurse perform one of the essential operational functions of a health service agency, but they also contribute to the executive and governing functions through what they do in the effective production of nursing. In the role of employee, nurses direct appropriate contributions to governing and executive functions. These contributions should be elicited and facilitated by nursing administration.

Nursing administration contributes to the operational function of the production of nursing through the suggested nursing-oriented functions. These six functions provide the ground work for administrators' performance of executive functions at their various locations in health service enterprises and in making appropriate contributions to the governing functions. Nursing administration is charged with knowing what nursing is required by the subpopulations and populations served and bringing about and maintaining conditions that will ensure its production. Nursing administration is charged with:

- The creation of functional wholes as organizational members fulfill their role responsibilities; this involves the proper ordering of persons and material resources; a patient unit within a hospital where nurses work together and with nursing administration, collaborating with other health professionals is an example of a part of a larger functional whole.
- Ensuring that current decisions and actions about ways and means to provide nursing for a population and its subpopulations are in harmony with future requirements for the production of nursing and for the survival or growth of the health care enterprise.

In fulfillment of these responsibilities, nursing administration performs the managerial work operations of (1) objective setting in relation to the population to be served and to the health care enterprise; (2) analysis and organization of work to achieve objectives; (3) establishing standards for selection and selection of nurses, assistants to nurses, and other support personnel; (4) motivating and communicating; (5) producing designs for measuring performance and results; and (6) measuring performance and results.*

NURSING PRACTITIONERS AND NURSING

In hospitals or in other resident health care enterprises, nurses function in the same situational contexts as other health professionals who provide direct health services for patients. Also operating in these situations are persons filling positions that provide residence services of housekeeping, food service, maintenance service, temperature and air control services, etc. Nursing administrators and practicing nurses must know and protect the domain and boundaries of nursing as a field of practice and at the same time coordinate nursing activities with other health services and with residence services. Boundary maintenance is required in situations where patients are not in residence in health care settings, but the requirement is less extensive.

Nurses are in resident health care agencies and in outpatient clinics of hospitals or public health clinics to provide nursing. They are not there to serve as clerks or receptionists, or to take patients from one place to another unless nursing is required during the process of moving the patient. To justify their presence in health care enterprises, nurses must be nursing oriented; to be nursing oriented is to be patient oriented. Nurses must be able to practice nursing but also to represent nursing to patients, families of patients, other health workers, nursing administration, executive officers of the enterprise, and, when necessary, to members of governing boards. The ability to communicate about nursing and what is required to produce it under prevailing and changing conditions and circumstances is an essential quality of nurses functioning within health care enterprises.

Production of nursing

Nursing may be provided to individuals continuously or periodically over some duration of time. The continuous provision of nursing is envisioned most readily in settings such as intensive care units or in therapeutic environments for mentally ill individuals. The continuous provision of nursing means that the nurse is with or immediately available to persons under care. The nurse is an essential human element in the environment of the patient. It does not mean that nurses are continuously engaged in doing something for or with persons under continuous nursing care. The periodic provision of nursing is envisioned most readily in terms of patients' visits

---

*Some ideas presented in this section are further developed in Orem DE: In Henry B et al, editors: Nursing administration, a theoretical approach, Dimensions of Nursing Administration, Cambridge, 1989, Blackwell Scientific Publications.

to nurses in nursing clinics, in nurses' offices, or nurses home visits to patients. Duration of visits vary.

Time requirements vary in situations where nursing is continuously provided in order to know and meet patients' therapeutic self-care demands, regulate the exercise or development of patients' self-care agency, and maintain or bring about a state of patient well-being. The subtypes of wholly compensatory nursing systems described in Chapter 10 are all time demanding, but in different ways. Lack of stability along dimensions of human functioning of patients and the complexity of and lack of stability in the therapeutic self-care demands of patients make additional time demands on nurses.

The periodic provision of nursing usually occurs within the design of partly compensatory and supportive-developmental nursing systems. The nature of and reasons for patients' self-care deficits are indicators of time requirements. The age, state of maturation, conditions of living, interests and orientations, and potential for extending and developing their self-care agency are other indicators. Backscheider identified four factors or combinations of factors associated with both time requirements for nursing and kinds of nursing results for an adult nursing clinic population (pp. 215-218).[1] The factors were expressed by Backscheider as "deficits for action" and included limitations for participating with nurses, limitations in actual provision of self-care, and limitations for extending and deepening self-care agency. The deficits were expressed as (1) action deficits in "operative knowing," as evidenced by patterns of concrete thinking; (2) motivational-emotional action deficits, as evidenced by patients from "high-stress, high-demand households"; (3) action deficits in consistency of performance and self-discipline; and (4) a deficit for action associated with quality of the health orientation, limitations of time, and location of care in the individual's priority schedule or value hierarchy.

In the production of nursing when nursing systems are periodic, nurses in leadership roles may work alone or with nursing assistants. These nurses may need and seek nursing consultation for both self and the person under nursing care. Nursing consultation should be available. When periodic nursing systems artic-ulate with dependent-care systems nurses, as well as nursing assistants, work with the dependent-care agents who may be members of the patient's family or friends. Nursing consultation may be needed to facilitate more effective relation-ships or to help individual dependent-care agents with specific nursing-relevant matters.

In the production of continuous systems of nursing over the twenty-four hours of each day more than one nurse is needed. The number of nurses is determined by the hours of nursing of each nurse and the arrangements with respect to the presence and responsibilities of nurses in leadership roles. The role responsibilities of nurses who provide nursing at different time periods to the same patient are sometimes ill defined. Failures of nurses to engage in nursing diagnosis and nursing prescription and to produce nursing that is in accord with known requirements can result in harm to patients and constitute malpractice. Nurses who care for the same patient at different times during the twenty-four hours of each day should function as a team. Such teams, when composed of nurses working at three different time periods, must overcome the difficulties of not meeting face to face at the same time and must ensure that there is essential agreement about stable elements or about how to handle changing elements in the design for the nursing system they are producing. Coordination of effort is not in opposition to the creative practical endeavors of each nurse.

The production of nursing demands the presence of nurses who know patients and their requirements for nursing. Nurses cannot know how patients can be helped through nursing in their time-place localizations if they are not with them. Nurses who do not engage in nursing diagnoses of patients have no basis for designing systems of care that reflect patients' requirements for nursing. In health care enterprises, because of free days for nurses and other reasons, there should be at least two nurses who know each person under nursing care. Although the foregoing statements may be judged as unrealistic, they are conditions to be worked toward by nursing administration. Nurse-nurse relationships in providing nursing of a subpopulation of patients during the same time period is of critical importance to both nurses and nursing administration.

Professionally realistic nurse teams

Team is used here in the sense of two or more nurses with different role responsibilities contributing to the nursing of persons constituting a single case load. Two types of teams are identified.

In the first type, the nurse in the governing and leadership role is an advanced, experienced nursing practitioner. The other nurses are qualified for entry to the professional level of practice of nursing who are gaining nursing experience under the guidance and direction of the advanced nursing practitioner. They are being introduced to increasingly complex nursing practice situations where the diagnostic and prescriptive and regulatory nursing operations are performed in conjunction with or are reviewed by the advanced nursing practitioner.

The role responsibilities of the nurses vary with the complexity of the nursing requirements of patients and the nursing systems to be produced for them. Nursing consultation may be required. The assignment of nursing assistants to the nurse team is based on the number and kinds of care measures that need to be performed regularly for persons constituting the case load that can be safely separated out for performance from the total system of regulatory or treatment nursing being produced by nurses (see Fig. 12-1).

This type of nurse team is indicated when patients' requirements for nursing are very complex, with some degree of instability of patients' therapeutic self-care demands and where nurses educated for entry to professional level practice are provided with a way to move toward this level of practice.

In the second type of nurse team, a nurse in the governing or leadership role is highly knowledgeable and experienced in the nursing of patients with particular and well-described types of self-care deficits. Other nurses working with this nurse would be technically prepared nurses, with ranges of experience depending on the types of cases within the case load. Diagnostic and prescriptive operations would be primary role responsibilities of the nurse in the governing and leadership role with time-specific contributions from technically prepared nurses. These nurses would be involved primarily with the continuing provision of treatment or regulatory nursing for patients constituting the case load. The assignment of nursing assistants would be based on the presence of the conditions identified for the first type of team.

This type of nurse team is indicated when patients' requirements for nursing are predictable within limits over some duration of time and when the technologies used in the production of nursing have a high degree of validity and reliability. This type of nurse team may require nursing consultation when special problems arise.

The suggestions about two types of nurse teams are made in light of the absence of career pathways for nurses prepared for entry to professional level practice and in light of the failure in some practice settings for nursing administration to differentiate the role responsibilities of professionally from technically prepared nurses and to safely separate out role responsiblities of vocationally prepared nursing assistants from total systems of nursing in production. Refer to role responsibilities of home health aide in the type of nursing case described in Chapter 9.

TIME REQUIREMENTS FOR NURSING

Nursing practitioners and nursing administrators should continuously acquire information about time requirements for nursing given particular types of nursing cases. Both must have the empirical knowledge and the nursing science base for using time requirements for nursing as a basis for planning for the production of nursing care.

Time requirements for nursing vary with the nature and causes of patients' self-care deficits associated with their therapeutic self-care demands and their self-care capabilities, their developed self-management capabilities, and their personal maturity and interests. Time requirements may also vary with patients' conditions of living, their family system elements, their potential for extending and deepening self-care agency, methods of helping used by nurses, and the arrangement of nurse and patient roles that are generative of particular types of nursing systems.

Attention is directed to variations in therapeutic self-care demands and self-care agency and to variations associated with the continuous and the periodic provision of nursing to individuals under the care of nurses.

Variations in therapeutic self-care demands

A therapeutic self-care demand has been described as a prescription for the self-care measures to be performed in order to meet identified sets of self-care requisites — universal, developmental, and health-deviation (Chapter 6). A person's therapeutic self-care demand is one of the two patient variables of nursing systems, the other being the patient's ability to engage in self-care, that is, self-care agency. A person's therapeutic self-care demand varies with age, developmental state, health state, and other factors.

Variations in therapeutic self-care demands of members of a nursing population and variations in the demands of individuals from time to time may be identified and described in terms of (1) the particular values of each one of the universal self-care requisites, (2) the particular values of the two kinds of developmental requisites, and (3) the presence of health-deviation self-care requisites and their derivation, for example, from a pathologic process, or as medically prescribed and associated with medical diagnoses or treatment measures, or as associated with regulation of the effects of medical diagnostic and treatment measures. Given particular values of specific self-care requisites, variations in therapeutic self-care demands may result from the methods selected for meeting them and from the measures of care (action systems) necessary for using a method in meeting a requisite.

Two possible variations in the mix of self-care requisites exist: (1) a combination of universal and developmental requisites and (2) a combination of universal, developmental, and health-deviation requisites. The eight types of nursing situations classified by health care focus (Chapter 8) suggest these two variations. Whenever the life cycle focus prevails, there is a mix of universal and developmental requisites. For example, in the event of mental retardation or other forms of retarded development with the absence of injury or overt disease processes, there would be a need for adjustments in the values of the universal and developmental requisites and for the use of appropriate methods for meeting them, for example, the selection and use of appropriate instructional methods and educational experiences and the appropriate regulation of living conditions to foster the retarded child's personal development, including involvement in self-care.

In the remaining seven types of nursing situations, health-deviation requisites are present in addition to universal and developmental requisites. These seven types of nursing situations also vary according to (1) the number and kinds of health-deviation requisites and the relationships among these requisites and (2) the degree to which the normal values and ways of meeting the universal and developmental requisites are changed.

For example, when persons have the condition that has the medical name of *chronic congestive heart failure,* the patient's health care focus, if it is therapeutic, is on self-management and meeting specific self-care requisites directed toward the regulation of the burden on the heart and toward the prevention of complicating conditions. Under the care of physicians and nurses and with assistance from family members, patients:

- Remain on a prescribed amount of bed rest
- Maintain a posture that prevents dyspnea
- Engage in some exercise, avoiding exertion that results in dyspnea
- Take precautions against contracting infections
- Act to regulate stress-producing conditions
- Control sodium chloride intake and use prescribed medications to regulate excretion of body fluids; monitor for effects and results
- Use prescribed medications to regulate cardiac functioning; monitor for effects and results
- Monitor for known complications and general sense of well-being or illness

This set of health-deviation self-care requisites includes ones that are essentially adjustments in the universal self-care requisites. The regulatory contribution to a person's well-being made by meeting each health-deviation self-care requisite and the interrelationships among the requisites must be understood by nurses if they are to help patients in managing themselves and in understanding and meeting their therapeutic self-care demands.

Nurses should have knowledge about recurring disorders of human structure and functioning, including knowledge of their natural history, in order to understand the associated health-deviation self-care requisites. This knowledge includes how the values of some or all of the universal self-care requisites may be affected. Specific pathologic processes usually affect the values of some but not all of the universals. When a disease becomes generalized (e.g., cancer) or when a person is critically ill, nurses must operate with continuing awareness that all of the universal self-care requisites may require continuing adjustment.

Variations in therapeutic self-care demands of individuals also result from the presence of factors that affect the choice of methods for meeting universal self-care requirements (and other requisites). Age, gender, states of development and health, and personal interests and concerns give rise to such factors. Methods selected for meeting each universal self-care requisite must be adjusted to certain conditions; for example, in maintaining a sufficient intake of food, the condition of being an infant or a child requires the use of methods that are effective for feeding infants or young children. A selected method must be able to surmount interfering factors, as in feeding by gavage when a person of any age cannot swallow.

Patients may also suffer conditions that interfere with the natural processes associated with meeting some or all of the universal self-care requisites, especially the requisites for maintenance of sufficient intakes of air, water, and food and for care related to excretory processes. Interference may be external to the individuals, for example, the quality of the atmosphere as related to air intake. In relation to food intake, interferences may be personal, as with food preferences or avoidance of certain foods on the basis of cultural or religious proscriptions. Interferences with food intake also may be due, for example, to structural anomalies such as cleft palate or disturbances of the neural mechanism of the swallowing reflex. In such situations, methods for meeting universal self-care requisites must be able to surmount interfering factors. Sometimes this requires the use of methods derived from medicine, for example, the use of the *surgical method of introduction of tubes and needles into the body*. Examples include feeding by gavage, feeding intravenously, and emptying the bladder by catheterization.

In summary, time requirements for nursing (or for self-care) vary with the internal composition of persons' therapeutic self-care demands, that is, with (1) composition by types of requisites, universal, developmental, health-deviation types; (2) the number of developmental and health-deviation requisites; for example, persons who suffer from one or two or more diseases or health disorders may have health-deviation self-care requisites associated with the regulation of each disease entity or with regulation of its effects; (3) the complexity of the methods or technologies used to meet the requisites; and (4) the sets of operations necessary to use the method or technologies in meeting each requisite. Nurses who provide nursing to particular nursing populations can estimate with considerable accuracy the time requirements for production of care.

Variations in self-care agency

In nursing practice, the capability of patients to engage in self-care can be assessed according to three scales — developmental, operational, and adequacy (pp. 203-210).[1] In taking this type of diagnostic approach to making judgments about the self-care agency of patients, nurses seek to determine the following with respect to self-care:

- What individuals have learned to do and do consistently
- What individuals *can and cannot do* now or in the future because of existing or predicted conditions and circumstances
- Whether what individuals have *learned to do* and *can now do* is equal to meeting all the current or projected demands on them to engage in self-care, that is, to meeting their therapeutic self-care demands now or at some future time.

Because self-care is learned behavior, nurses must take into account the readiness and capabilities of individuals for extending or deepening their abilities to engage in self-care. Variations in the self-care agency of patients as previously suggested can be understood and examined in relation to:

- Self-care measures that patients know how to perform and usually do perform (repertoire of self-care practices, usual components of the self-care system)
- Action limitations that restrict the performance of what patients know how to do with respect to self-care (limitations that interfere with the performance of the operations required for the decision-making and productive phases of self-care)

- Self-care measures to be performed to meet known self-care requisites for which patients have or do not have requisite knowledge, skill, or willingness (adequacy or limitation of knowledge, skills and techniques, or willingness to meet known self-care requisites using particular care methods)
- Patients' potential for extending or deepening their knowledge of self-care and mastering the techniques necessary to perform required self-care measures that are not within their existing self-care repertoires (potential for further developments to extend or deepen self-care agency)
- Patients' potential for consistent and effective performance of new and essential self-care measures, including the integration of essential self-care measures into the self-care system and daily life

To accumulate and validate knowledge about variations in the self-care agency of nursing populations, it would seem practical to approach the five possible variations separately. In particular nursing situations, nurses should consistently investigate the first three variations. If there is a lack of adequacy (third variation), the fourth and fifth variations, dealing with patient potential, should be investigated.

NURSING PRACTICE MODELS, POPULATION DESCRIPTIONS, AND MODELS

Development of practical sciences includes the stages of synthesis of nursing practice models (stage four) and the stage of description of nursing populations and synthesis of models for providing nursing to populations (stage five) (see Chapter 4).

A practice model is a carefully worked out design for the structure and formation of a nursing system or a segment of a nursing system for a type or subtype of nursing case when one or both patient variables (therapeutic self-care demand and self-care agency) have (or can be predicted to take on) certain qualitative or quantitative characteristics. A well-known example of nursing practice model is the design for nursing during the preoperative, intraoperative, and postoperative stages of nursing for persons undergoing major surgical treatments. Practice models are also illustrated through Joan E. Backscheider's work with educationally deprived adult clinic patients with *limitations of operative knowing* (one of the foundational capabilities and dispositions of self-care agency) (pp. 218-229).[1] Persons who think concretely and cannot deal with abstractions can be helped through nursing to master a regimen of self-care when their self-care limitation and its meaning for development of instructional systems for them is recognized by nurses, and appropriate instruction and other forms of help are instituted. The basis for use of a valid regulatory model is accurate diagnosis of limitations of operative knowing in persons under nursing care. Backscheider developed the foundations for a diagnostic model and an instructional model about what, when, and how to do something every day for oneself. The essential component of the instructional model is a communication element. Instructional models include content about self-care measures to meet components of therapeutic self-care demands and the courses of action to be performed. In nursing situations of this type, the self-care systems of patients often are articulated with partly compensatory periodic nursing systems. Backscheider's models are examples of (1) diagnostic and (2) instructional-developmental models addressed to the patient property of self-care agency.

Although practice models can be found in the nursing literature, many nurses use their own known only to themselves. Formalization and validation of practice models is work that can and should be done in nursing practice settings.

Population descriptions developed by nursing administration differ from the detailed nursing cases developed in stage three of practical science development (see Chapter 4). The descriptions of populations to be provided with the service nursing must be adequate for answering questions about the quality and amount of nursing required by time periods to serve the population of the agency. Nursing administrators should consider various approaches to description to find one that yields only essential information for judgment and decision making about kinds and numbers of nurses essential for the provision of nursing. The description also should yield information about both the physical and psychological demands on nurses who nurse members of described subpopulations.

Nursing administrators can review the kinds of data about patients currently and consistently available in the health care enterprises they serve. Nursing implications of available data can and should be identified. Moving from what is available to what is essential may save time, effort, and resources. One goal of nursing administration should be the immediate availability of descriptive nursing information about the population being served and projected populations. Nursing administration requires knowledge of developments in preventive health care and in medical diagnosis and treatment, the prevalence of types of diseases and injuries in the community and the major causes of death in the community, and changes in features of the community's health care system. The implications of this knowledge for nursing should be worked out in detail. Maintaining knowledge of what a community needs and what a health care enterprise can do in meeting a community's requirements for nursing is an essential task of every nursing administrator.

Models for the provision of nursing for populations are production models that relate nurses by qualification and nurse teams and case loads to subpopulations served by health care enterprises.

REFERENCE

1. Nursing Development Conference Group, Orem D, editor: Concept formalization in nursing: process and product, Boston, 1979, Little, Brown & Co., pp. 215-229.

SELECTED READINGS

Allison SE: Structuring nursing practice based on Orem's theory of nursing: a nurse administrator's perspective. In Riehl-Sisca J, editor: The science and art of self-care, Norwalk, 1985, Appleton-Century-Crofts, pp. 225-235.

Barnum BS: Contributions of nursing administration to the development of nursing as a discipline. In Henry B, et al: Dimensions of nursing adminstration, Boston, 1989, Blackwell.

Huckabay LM: Professional issues facing the field of administration of nursing services. In Henry B, et al: Dimensions of nursing administration, Boston, 1989, Blackwell.

Marz CE: North York referral intake and disposition system: an application of Orem's classification of nursing situations. In School of nursing, University of Missouri-Columbia, Clinical and cultural dimensions around the world, Papers and abstracts presented at the first international self-care deficit nursing theory conference, October 15-18, 1989, The Curators of the University of Missouri, pp. 107-126.

Nunn D, Marriner-Tomey A: Applying Orem's model in nursing administration. In Henry B et al: Dimensions of nursing administration, Boston, 1989, Blackwell Scientific Publications, pp. 63-67.

Nursing Department, Scarborough General Hospital: Self-care deficit theory material resources, Scarborough, Ontario, 1989, Scarborough General Hospital.

Underwood PR: Tools for implementation of self-care deficit theory, vol 1, San Francisco (no date), School of Nursing, Department of Health and Community Nursing, University of California, San Francisco.

Van Eron M: Clinical application of self-care deficit theory. In Riehl-Sisca J, editor: The science and art of self-care, Norwalk, 1985, Appleton-Century-Crofts, pp. 208-224.

CHAPTER 12

Education and nursing practice

Nursing practice is one of the six fields of endeavor necessary to keep nursing viable as an occupation and profession in social groups. As represented in Fig. 4-6 these fields are nursing practice, scholarly endeavors in nursing sciences and related sciences, theory formulation and development, nursing research, development and validation of nursing technologies and techniques, and teaching nursing. To understand the necessity for these fields of endeavor in nursing it is important to understand occupations and professions and to become able to conceptualize nursing as a profession.

NURSING, A MIX OF OCCUPATIONS

The term *occupation* is used to refer to the work, the kind of labor or activity, in which individuals who have been trained for it seriously and habitually engage often but not always as a means of earning a livelihood. Each of the six named fields of nursing endeavor singly or in various combinations can be considered as an occupational field. In concrete life situations of nurses the six named fields are usually combined. Some combinations encountered are:

- Nursing practice and scholarly endeavor in nursing science and related sciences
- Scholarly endeavors in nursing sciences and related sciences and nursing research
- Theory formulation and development and scholarly endeavor in nursing and related sciences
- Development and validation of nursing technologies and techniques combined with the first two combinations listed here
- Teaching nursing and scholarly endeavor in nursing sciences and related sciences and nursing practice

Nurses' combinations of occupational choices reflect their interests, talents, and values as well as the form of their educational preparation for nursing, their associations with nurses in particular occupational fields, their advanced nursing education, and their occupational experiences leading to understanding of nursing as a professional field.

It should be understood that in combinations the occupational fields support one another. Nurses who choose particular combinations must develop themselves in accord with foundational knowledge, skills, and orientations specific to each. As shown in Fig. 4-6, nursing knowledge (developed and validated as theoretically and practically practical nursing science as well as applied nursing sciences) is common to the six nursing occupational fields. Nursing science (practical science and applied science) informs the six occupational fields so that together they contribute to the existence and the advance of nursing as a profession. Although persons who engage in teaching nursing belong to two professions; the profession of nursing and the profession of education, they may align themselves more closely with one profession than the other. Ideally, however, they maintain a balance, understanding that they are engaged in education for the occupations and professions, namely, nursing.

NURSING, A PROFESSION

The term *profession*, like the term *occupation*, is used to refer to work pursuits. In this sense, it signifies fields in which individuals pursue years of study and training, achieve qualifying professional degrees from institutions of higher education, are tested to determine fitness to practice, and licensed to practice. In nursing, the term profession in this sense is the basis for distinguishing nurses prepared for entry to the beginning professional level of nursing practice who move themselves to become advanced professional practitioners from nurses prepared in technical-type programs preparatory for nursing. Profession is also used in the sense of all the persons engaged in a field of practice that requires the named qualifying characteristics.

Nurses must face and accept the matter of differences in their interests, differences in education preparatory for nursing, differences in their work or career orientations to nursing, and begin to be concerned about their contributions to the survival and advancement of nursing as a human service in social groups. What each nurse does and does effectively within one or some combination of occupational fields makes a contribution to the continued existence and acceptance of nursing in human society.

The professions exist in social groups so that members can identify, resolve, and solve or mitigate specific types of human problems of members of the society. In nursing the problems are ones that arise from the subjectivity of men, women, and children to health-derived or health-associated deficits for self-care or dependent-care of persons who must care for themselves or be taken care of by others. This is the domain about which professionally qualified and professionally advanced nurses must acquire knowledge through nursing practice, scholarly endeavors, and nursing theory formulation and development; validate knowledge through research; and develop and validate technologies of practice. The areas of theoretically and practically practical nursing knowledge are distinguished; and nursing knowledge, as it develops, is structured around the identified areas (see Chapter 4). The forms of the applied nursing sciences emerge.

Because a profession perpetuates itself and seeks to advance itself toward helping societies in resolving and solving existent as well as emerging human problems within its domain, each profession has members (1) engaged in providing professional services that are in accord with existent and emerging needs of the social group, (2) in the education of new members with qualifications and in the numbers required to provide services and in advanced education for present members, and (3) in the development of the practical and applied sciences specific to the domain of the profession. Thus it can be seen that all of nursing's occupational fields are essential for the survival and advancement of nursing in societies throughout the world. The international and intercontinental associations and collaborations among nurses continue to increase.

NURSES' SOCIAL AND PROFESSIONAL DEVELOPMENT

Nursing practice demands that persons who develop and continue to develop and refine the property of nursing agency (the human capability to nurse others) must develop themselves as persons who can:

- Establish contacts, negotiate agreements, and maintain contacts with persons who need nursing and those who seek it for them
- Interact and communicate with persons under nursing care and their significant others, with other nurses and care givers under ranges of conditions and circumstances that facilitate or hinder interactions and communication
- Direct interactions and communications toward the development of interpersonal, functional unities
- Perform with increasing developing skills professional-technologic operations of nursing — nursing diagnosis, nursing prescription, nursing regulation or treatment in a known range of types of nursing situations where patients' properties of self-care agency and therapeutic self-care vary within known ranges and the health care foci are clear cut. Skills include observational skills, reasoning skills, judgment and decision-making skills, and production of practical results in interpersonal and group situations. The focus of performance may be one or some combination of the three professional-technologic operations
- Seek nursing consultation as needed with respect to functioning as described in the fourth ability listed here
- Begin to extend capabilities for performing the basic operations of nursing practice (one, two, or all) to new types of situations within the range of nursing situations specific to four above or to new types of situations outside the range. Work under the direction of and with supervision from advanced nursing practitioners, functioning ideally as nurse assistants to them

- Know and represent to others types of nursing cases and situations of nursing practice outside your nursing practice capabilities
- Maintain a dynamic sense of duty in all nursing practice situations

Development of the personal capabilities to function in the described ways requires not only developed skills but also experiential and speculative knowledge organized around nursing considered as a human service and as a field of knowledge and practice.

Understanding nursing as a human service is facilitated by pursuit of knowledge in the liberal arts and humanities and knowledge of the history of health care and nursing in Western and Eastern civilizations. Orientation to languages and culture elements specific to culture groups is important for nursing students preparing for entry to professional practice. There is need to develop and extend experiential knowledge of social and interpersonal situations as well as development of social and interpersonal skills necessary for working with adults and children individually or in groups.

Functioning in the described ways also demands beginning and advancing understanding of nursing as a field of knowledge and practice. There is need for knowledge of the proper object of nursing that defines nursing's domain and boundaries. There is need for knowledge of the practical science of nursing with its theoretically and practically practical elements for beginning knowledge of the form of potential applied nursing sciences. Nursing knowledge is articulated with or supplemented by knowledge of the applied medical and public health sciences, all of which have connections to groups of foundational and basic sciences that are needed for understanding the practical sciences of nursing, medicine, and public health.

FORMS OF EDUCATION FOR NURSING PRACTICE ROLES

The needs of members of a social group for nursing is met by nurses who pursue careers in nursing practice. Ideally, nurses who practice nursing are at the same time scholars or students of nursing and of nursing-related disciplines. An adequate safe standard of practice cannot be maintained by nurses unless they keep their practice abreast of developments by reading and by participation in programs of continuing education. Engagement in nursing practice in any social group confronts nurses with a variety of conditions and problems associated with individuals, families, and larger community groups. Education preparatory for nursing practice must be enabling for nurses to enter and to become active participants in a variety of interpersonal and group situations.

Nurses' knowledge of nursing and their capabilities for effective performance of the operations of nursing practice will be in large part determined by the forms and quality of their education for practice as these relate to their individual capabilities, interests, and concerns. The cumulative effects of the historical emphasis on vocational-technical education for nursing has been a deterrent to nurses in becoming responsible professional practitioners of nursing and in the development of the practical science of nursing.

It is important that nurses have the freedom to bear the responsibilities of nursing practice. Nurses should understand the depths and breadth of their capabilities for nursing practice and their own legitimacy as nurses in concrete situations of practice. Nursing students and nurses should critically examine where they fit within the occupation and profession of nursing. Distinguishing roles and role responsibilities of persons prepared through different forms of work preparatory education should be understood by nursing students. How one moves in occupational-professional fields for the most part is determined by where one begins.

The traditional types of nursing educational programs are examined within the frame of reference of work preparatory education. Roles and role responsibilities of persons prepared in the different types of work preparatory programs are identified. Education that is preparatory for the role of nursing practitioner is described.

Overview

Schools of nursing have proliferated in the United States since the first schools were opened in the year 1873. Nursing education during the early period of its development was promoted by interested lay or professional people often associated with hospitals. Pioneer schools of nursing were modeled at least in part after the Nightingale School associated with Saint Thomas's Hospital in London, (pp. 7-9)[1] which was opened in 1860 under the sponsorship of Florence Nightingale and financed through the Nightingale Fund (pp. 225-238).[2] Since World War II, nursing has entered the so-called scientific age. Education for nursing has expanded to include a broader base in general studies, in the humanities and behavioral and social sciences, and in leadership and management. Traditional biologic and medical science content remains in nursing programs, sometimes with considerable expansion and restructuring of emphasis.

With the ever-increasing knowledge of humanity and the complexity of health care and medical technology, there has been a concomitant demand for nurses prepared at the university level. In addition, the enactment of social legislation (Medicare and Medicaid) has greatly increased the need for nurses and for personnel who assist them in providing and managing nursing. The number and types of workers who serve by providing self-care assistance has increased rapidly since 1940. Not all workers are prepared or licensed as nurses. Some persons with minimal knowledge and skills work without supervision from nurses. Nurses are limited by external and internal factors in what they can do to meet nursing requirements in a community. Limiting factors include time, prevailing conditions, interests, values, and abilities of the nurses of a community. Effective organization of nursing services is essential both in the provision of nursing and the maintenance of satisfaction among nurses. Modern nurses are no less capable than nursing leaders of the past. Finding ways to meet and keep up with changing requirements for nursing is the task of and a challenge to each nurse. Nurses have a substantial part in the process of moving communities toward standards of nursing practice that ensure safe and effective nursing. No other group can perform this task for nurses. Nurses, collectively, have a responsibility for the quality of the services they provide in a community.

Members of the younger generation of nurses have an education that has been enriched with modern science and technology and general studies. The young nurse may be in the formative stage of the art of nursing, but his or her foundation for its development may exceed that of nurses with years of nursing experience. Techniques and practices in current use are evaluated and sometimes questioned by younger nurses and nursing students. This is the role of each new generation, for in this way nursing practice is refined and enriched. Practices, since they tend to become fixed or institutionalized, are not easily changed, but without developmental change stagnation and deterioration of nursing effectiveness occur. Young nurses and nursing students should seek knowledge of valid but unrecorded nursing techniques from more experienced nurses who have attained nursing wisdom from thoughtful and effective nursing practice. Nurses who have developed techniques and have evidence of their effectiveness should contribute this information to the developing body of nursing knowledge. Developing, validating, and recording techniques of nursing practice are important tasks in the continued development of a body of nursing knowledge.

Educating nurses for limited roles in nursing was introduced in the United States. This is done in other fields and is a mark that a service is being extended to more and more persons. The content and length of programs of nursing education should vary according to the roles for which different types of nurses are being prepared. In the delivery of nursing in communities and in institutions the contribution that each type of nurse is to make to nursing should be defined, and provision should be made for coordinating efforts in the interests of both patients and nurses. Division of the work of nursing among several types of nurses without providing for the coordination of effort and results leads to chaos. The demand for nurses who are effective in appraising the needs of individual patients for nursing and in designing systems of nursing assistance is increasing, along with the demand for nurses who can effectively supervise nurses who are prepared for limited roles. Changes in nursing education and changes in nursing practice are interrelated.

Nurses must be able to fill their positions in a spectrum of health care services developed around technologies of health care and health care problems. The nurse is not a solitary worker. The days when only physicians and nurses made up health teams is over. Expansion of the spectrum of health services places demands on nurses for coordinating actions with persons from an increasing number and variety of health services. The specific character of nursing activities is closely related to the kinds of health problems that prevail in the community. For example, communicable disease, serious injuries from industrial accidents, and chronic illness result in needs for different types of nursing actions. Communities vary in the combinations of health problems that prevail, although certain health problems are common to all communities. The character of nursing activities is also affected by the way in which patients can be helped. The requirements of persons who are ill and are patients in hospitals or nursing homes sometimes result in heavy demands for continuing care by nurses and other types of personnel. Community health centers and health maintenance organizations bring an increased demand for nursing that emphasizes guidance and instruction in therapeutic self-care and help to patients so that they can identify and work with internal environmental conditions that interfere with their self-care actions. Some industrial and business firms employ nurses on a full-time basis to serve their employees' health needs. These nurses may give direct assistance to employees as the need arises, but they are primarily concerned with preventive measures related to the health and well-being of the firm's employees and their families. Many governmental, health, and welfare agencies also employ nurses in a variety of health-related activities. Regardless of the kinds of health and other problems that determine the specific work of the nurse, he or she is always recognized as a specialized worker with a distinctive social position and pattern of behavior. It has been indicated that the nurse's role in society focuses on (1) the maintenance of those self-care activities that individuals continuously need to sustain life and health, recover from disease and injury, and cope with the effects of disease and injury and (2) self-regulation of the individual's self-care capabilities.

Nursing students and nurses entering practice want to learn to nurse with effectiveness and in a way that is satisfying to persons nursed and to themselves. Since nursing is offered within social groups as an available human service, nurses must develop and advance in their knowledge of nursing and become skilled performers of the operations of nursing practice. These achievements are not possible without sound preparatory education for entry into nursing practice.

The membership and status or position of individual nurses in the occupation and profession of nursing depends on their educational preparation, type of license or certification to practice, and experience and recognition of practice capabilities by colleagues and peers. Education for nursing is work preparatory.

Work preparatory education

Three forms or types of work preparatory education are accepted in the United States. These usually are named as follows:
1. Vocational
2. Technical
   a. Low-level technical
   b. High-level technical or technological
3. Professional

Sometimes, and to confuse the matter, all forms of work preparatory education are referred to collectively as vocational education. The forms of work preparatory education serve different purposes and traditionally have been justified on the basis of economic considerations for the society and for individuals who pursue the specific forms of work preparatory education.

Persons enrolled in work preparatory programs ideally view themselves and are viewed by others as engaged in a form of personal development that is enabling for skilled performance within a selected occupational field. The time designation for achievement of skilled performance may be set as *upon program completion* or *after a stipulated period of apprenticeship under experienced individuals in the field.* In nursing, it is usually necessary for individual nurses to design and work out plans for their own apprenticeships. Career pathways in nursing are not well developed.

Skilled performance in nursing and other fields requires development and perfection of *perceptual skills* in receiving and processing sense information, the maintenance of alertness, and action to control factors that adversely affect attentiveness and vigilance. Skilled performance also demands *requisite knowledge for signal recognition,* that is, recognizing events that call for action, attaching meaning to signals singly or in combination, or making judgments that vagueness prohibits positive identification and that more information is needed.

For skilled performance in practical endeavors, individuals ideally psychologically structure or organize their knowledge in forms that can be readily drawn on as they (1) identify and observe the reality features of practice situations, (2) make judgments about features that can and should be changed or regulated, (3) make judgments and decisions about availability of appropriate and validated techniques for so doing, (4) make decisions about what kind and degree of change or regulation will be sought in specific features using techniques with high to low or no established validity and reliability, and (5) proceed to do and manage the work of changing or regulating features of the situation. How nursing students and nurses psychologically structure knowledge about nursing and nursing-related fields is affected by the forms of their work preparatory education and by the organization of nursing content and nursing-related content within their educational programs.

Skilled performance by a person in an occupational or professional field demands *motivation* to act for quality in performance, sustained endeavor, and management of self and work operations to achieve results within an effective time frame without harm to self and others and without waste of time or materials or human energy. Since all fields of endeavor demand performance of some *range of types of work operations*, skill performance requires the mix of skills necessary to perform specific work operations. Skills include perceptual motor skills, manipulative skills, verbal skills, and reasoning skills. Work operations can be typed according to the predominant skill or mix of skills required in their performance. Result and purpose achievement demand unification of actions to constitute a coordinated dynamic system. Skilled performance, therefore, demands knowledge of the fit of one work operation, one set of actions, within the larger framework of actions.

Forms of education in nursing

The form(s) in which nursing education should be offered continues to be questioned and is at times a public issue. The terms *professional, technical,* and *vocational* are emotion-arousing terms for some nurses. Past and present self-appointed experts on nursing practice and nursing education often did not and do not know or seek knowledge about the proper role functions of persons with different forms of work preparatory education or they disregard them as too difficult to implement. Persons tend to ignore or oversimplify the social, scientific, and economic rationales that legitimate the use of various types of workers in nursing.

Types of work preparatory education have different centers of organization and use different principles in the selection and organization of knowledge and learning experiences. The centers of organization of educational programs and rationales for program development are shown in Table 12-1.

Professional nursing programs preparatory for *entrance* to practice and for *movement* toward the professional (scientific) form of practice have as their organizing center human beings and the range of types of conditions and problems of persons who can benefit from nursing (form A in Table 12-1). Programs preparatory for entrance to practice subsume under form A the essential sets of process operations of nursing practice, the recurring type of problem situations for which there are developed valid and reliable technologies for achieving nursing results (form B in Table 12-1), and the related work operations necessary for result achievement. These programs also provide the science foundation for movement to a professional (scientific) level of practice.

True technical programs have as their centers recurring types of problem situations of persons who are seeking or are receiving nursing and the developed, validated, and reliable technologies for the identification, resolution, and solution of nursing practice problems (form B in Table 12-1).

Programs true to the vocational mode are organized around specific tasks or work operations that can be separated out from larger sets of series of operations without loss of effectiveness or production of adverse results within the whole system of action (form C in Table 12-1).

The variations in the work focuses of persons prepared in the three types of work preparatory programs are shown in Fig. 12-1. The illustration shows the interrelations of the three focuses within a single schematic situation of practice. It is easy to imagine the kinds of problems, errors, omissions, and outright harm to persons under care that arise in complex nursing situations when either a vocationally or technically prepared

Table 12-1   Forms of work preparatory education by organizing centers and rationales

Form	Center	Rationale
A	Conditions and problems of human beings that constitute the special domain of nursing	The proper object of nursing is identified, and nursing is established in a society. The practice discipline nursing is being developed. Individuals elect to prepare themselves to practice nursing, obtaining and maintaining a scientific base for practice in the practice discipline nursing and in nursing-related disciplines. Individuals elect to advance nursing as both a field of practice and a field of knowledge.
B	Recurring types of problem situations in the field of nursing practice and developed, validated technologies for identification, resolution, and solution of specific questions within the problem situation	Recurring types of problem situations in nursing are identified, described, and explained. Technologies of high validity and reliability are formalized. Individuals elect to do detailed technical work as outlined in standard operating procedures or as detailed by an expert practitioner. Individuals elect to perfect and to advance techniques of practice.
C	Work operations that can be safely selected out from a larger set(s) or series	Work operations can be isolated without adversely affecting the whole set or series of actions considered as a dynamic, coordinated system. Individuals elect to do repetitive, circumscribed work.

person is placed in a position of responsibility for the whole nursing situation without specific guidance and direction from a nurse who is functioning at the professional level of practice.

Nursing education in the United States from the period of its inception and initial growth has been beset with problems related to (1) the form in which it is offered and (2) its control by service agencies such as hospitals or by educational institutions. Nurses as well as the whole occupation and profession of nursing have been and continue to be adversely affected by issues of form and control of nursing education.

The question of how individuals with different forms of work preparatory education fit into the occupation and profession of nursing remains to be answered

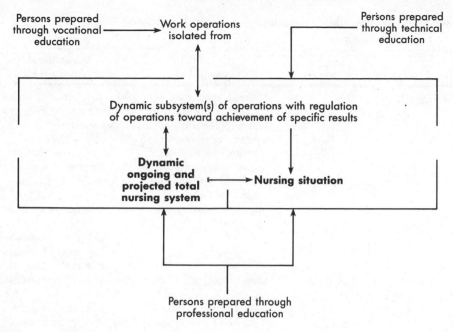

Fig. 12-1 Focuses of persons prepared in types of work preparatory programs.

in some educational and service settings. Clear answers to the question should be sought and used to ensure the welfare of individuals who enroll in the programs and individuals who seek nursing or related services. Table 12-2 may be of some help in sorting out role differences. In the table general roles associated with types of work preparatory programs are developed as roles and role responsibilities in nursing and in the personal care of individuals. Students in various types of work preparatory programs have a right to precise information about the social, economic, and occupational features of the programs in which they are enrolled. Sometimes these features are glossed over or misrepresented, or enrolled students are unable or unwilling to deal with information about them. It is reasonable to expect that students will be helped to understand how specific types of work preparatory programs will enable them to fill specific roles in the occupation and profession of nursing.

PREPARATORY EDUCATION FOR NURSING PRACTITIONERS

Authentic programs of education for qualifying individuals *for entry* to the profession as *nursing practitioners* and *for movement* to a professional (scientific) level of practice are offered at the senior college and university level. Persons who initiate, promote, operate, and finance such programs should understand the complex nature of education for the professions and the special requirements that arise from nursing.

Table 12–2   Roles and role responsibilities associated with forms of work preparatory
education

Form of education	General role	Role responsibility	Occupational-professional role
Vocational	Aide	*Nursing*: Performs assigned tasks selected out from the work operations of an ongoing nursing system	Aide to a nursing practitioner or a technically prepared nurse
		Self-care or dependent care: Performs tasks that are parts of self-care or dependent-care systems	Aide to persons who are responsible for and are managing: 1. Their own self-care systems 2. Dependent-care systems for dependent adults or children
Vocational-technical or technical	Technician	*Nursing*: Operationalizes, maintains, and manages dependent-care systems of therapeutic quality for helpless or near-helpless persons under stable conditions and circumstances	Practical or vocational nurse working with guidance and instruction from a nursing practitioner
		Conducts and manages subsystems of operations within a dynamic nursing system under control of a nursing practitioner	Technically prepared nurse working under standardized procedures or functioning as assistant to a nursing practitioner
High-level technical	Technologist	*Nursing*: Uses validated and reliable techniques in operationalizing and regulating dynamic subsystems of operations toward achievement of specified results in nursing systems, self-care systems, and dependent-care systems	Technologically prepared nurse with following functions: 1. Provides nursing, working within established protocols 2. Performs as associate of a nursing practitioner 3. Contributes a nursing component to ongoing self-care or dependent-care systems

Continued.

Table 12–2 Roles and role responsibilities associated with forms of work preparatory education — cont'd

Form of education	General role	Role responsibility	Occupational-professional role
Professional:			
1. Qualifying for entry to practice	Professional entry level of practice to experienced level of practice	Uses validated and reliable techniques in designing, operationalizing, and regulating dynamic nursing systems, including regulation of all subsystems	Nursing practitioner working within established protocols
		Operationalizes and regulates subsystems of operations within dynamic nursing systems, using validated and reliable techniques	Associate or assistant to a professional nursing practitioner
2. Advanced	Professional-scientific level of practice	Provides nursing diagnosis, including collecting data to the point needed for considered professional judgments	Professional nursing practitioner
		Provides creative design of nursing systems and subsystems of work operations	
		Provides design of techniques for attaining nursing results, in the absence of validated techniques	
		Operationalizes and manages nursing operations in complex nursing situations	
		Provides nursing consultation	

Broad components of professional education are recognized and expressed as preprofessional and professional program components.

PREPROFESSIONAL COMPONENT

- Course sequences in the liberal arts and humanities
- Course sequences in basic sciences or disciplines of knowledge necessary for understanding the courses of the professional component and for doing prescribed course work in them

PROFESSIONAL COMPONENT

- Foundational courses in the disciplines of knowledge essential for understanding courses in the professional field
- Courses in the professional field
- Continuing education courses

These broadly expressed components of professionally qualifying education are one indication of the complexity of education for the professions. Diversity of disciplines of knowledge and the need for systems of organization of content based on the function the organization is designed to serve are primary concerns of program developers.

Mastery of subject matter areas of a discipline involves a process of knowing that includes not only content but a style of thinking. Content includes concepts and their relationships. The thinking style is established by the modes of inquiry and the level of data leading to (1) the insights expressed by the concepts and to (2) relationships among concepts.

In development of programs of professional education for nursing practice, understanding the fields and areas of knowledge of the practical science nursing provides rationales for the selection of foundational courses. The points of articulations between subject matter areas of nursing science and foundational courses should be made explicit through teaching. The question of what is an adequate sequence of courses in nursing must be answered before making final decisions about foundational courses.

A major problem in education for entry to nursing practice is the development of courses in the professional field that are constituted from subject matter that is nursing. All too often courses that carry a nursing title are constituted primarily from content from the biologic, behavioral, and medical sciences. The offering of an adequate sequence of nursing courses is a major undertaking unless course designers are guided by a general concept of nursing and their understanding of nursing as a practice or science.

Nurses and nursing students should understand that the nursing sciences are but one of at least seven fields of knowledge that treat of nurses and nursing. The fields are identified as:

- Nursing's social field—dimensions of nursing as an institutionalized service in social groups under fixed and changing social, cultural, economic, and political conditions
- Nursing, a profession and occupation
- Nursing jurisprudence, or nursing and the law
- Nursing history
- Nursing ethics
- Nursing economics
- Nursing sciences, the practical and applied nursing sciences

Each one of the seven identified fields has its distinct structures and modes of inquiry. Some of them are constituted from a number of areas of knowledge. The modes of inquiry specific to the first six fields are those of the disciplines that are associated in the names with nurses or nursing, for example, law, history, ethics, and economics. The first two, nursing's social field and nursing, a profession and occupation, are associated with a number of social and behavioral sciences.

All seven fields of knowledge are drawn on in the development of courses in professional components of nursing education programs. This is essential if nursing students are to become able to think about and view themselves and their endeavors from the points of view of nursing as care, as help, as art, as knowledge, as an occupation and profession, and as a service.

There must be an adequate sequence of courses in the seventh field, the practical science of nursing. Subject matter from the other six fields is at times incorporated into courses in the nursing sciences. Or specific courses in a field may be offered, for example, a course in the history of nursing. The professional component of a program may include courses in the associated disciplines, for example, history or economics, and the professional component will no doubt include courses in sociology and ethics.

Another kind of knowledge must be considered in relation to education qualifying for nursing practice. This is *personal knowledge* arising from direct insights into self and others in personal relations. Phenix (pp. 193-211)[3] considers personal knowledge as a distinct sphere of knowledge.

Nurses in practice situations relate as persons to individuals under their care and to other involved individuals. The intersubjectivity of persons in practice situations may result, within the capabilities of individuals and the limits of time, in some personal knowledge of self and the other on the part of each involved individual. Furthermore, both nurses and patients need to reflect about the capabilities for action and about feelings and emotions experienced.

A number of disciplines investigate and contribute to the accumulation of knowledge about personal relations and personal knowledge of self and others. The work of Peplau,[4] Orlando,[5] and Travelbee[6] and other nurses contributes to this sphere of knowing from the perspective of nursing practice. I see this as a field of knowledge that should be developed as an applied science that would be associated with nursing

***Exercise* in recognizing subject matter by disciplines of knowledge**

1. Select one class period within a nursing course in which you are enrolled. During this class period identify the kinds of subject matter focused on by teacher and students during the class period as:
   a. Nursing content
   b. Content from other fields that is relevant to nursing
2. Distinguish nursing content to the degree that you can according to location in one of seven fields of knowledge about nurses and nursing identified in this chapter. If you identify nursing content as a part of nursing science, locate it in Figure 4-3 within one of the fields of nursing knowledge represented in the figure.
3. Name the sciences or disciplines of knowledge to which nonnursing content belongs.
4. To the degree that you can, identify how content from nonnursing disciplines is linked to nursing content.

practice and nursing cases within the description of the practice science nursing (see Chapter 4).

Personal knowledge as described by Phenix[3] is an essential component of the cognitional orientation of nurses. Knowledge of what is being experienced by individuals within nursing practice situations is essential experiential knowing. The intersubjectivity of nurses and persons under their care is a given condition of nursing practice, as is the contractual relationship between nurse and nurse's patient. The personality organization of each nurse should be enabling for the nurse's relating of self to others on a person-to-person basis and at the same time enabling for working with them within a contractual relationship toward the attainment of nursing results.

Persons who institute, promote, and finance formal preparation for nursing practice should recognize that nursing is practical endeavor. Even in the late twentieth century not all persons recognize or accept that the deliberate actions of nurses in practice situations must be grounded in previously mastered knowledge and technique, based on insights accumulated through experience in practice situations, and be immediately guided by acquired current factual information about the reality of each practice situation that rounds out the knowledge that nurses have gained through experience.

Each nursing practitioner must be able to approach, communicate, collaborate, and work with persons under care and with persons who are legally responsible for the individuals under care. But each nurse must be able to make right judgments and decisions about actions to be taken in each situation of practice in the achievement of objectively based and desired nursing results. Persons who enter into situations of nursing practice with knowledge limited to routinely performed tasks or technologic subsystems to be operationalized and regulated are not prepared to practice nursing. They may be able to assist adequately prepared and responsible nurses *or* to assist individuals who are able to direct and manage their care but not able to perform actual care measures.

The mastery of a general comprehensive theory of nursing is a first step for nursing students who want to become able to maintain awareness of the relationship between what they know and what they do as nursing practitioners. The conceptual elements of a general theory of nursing constitute one essential aid for nursing students who want to (1) know what to attend to and observe in nursing practice situations; (2) develop appropriate nursing imagery, for example, about what will occur if nursing is not provided when particular combinations of conditions exist; (3) characterize and name what is observed; (4) attach general and nursing meaning to what is observed; and (5) know the limits and the range of possible courses of action that are open to nurses and nurses' patients under types and combinations of prevailing conditions and circumstances.

Thinking nursing and seeing and conceptualizing the whole structure and dynamics of nursing situations to the degree necessary for understanding them is distinct from viewing nursing as skilled performance of standardized sets of operations or skilled performance of tasks separated out from larger dynamic systems of operations. Nursing practice demands that nursing practitioners understand systems of work operations and defined tasks both in terms of the specific results that each one brings about and in terms of their contributions to the attainment of specified nursing goals for persons under nursing care. The product of the *actions* of nurses, their patients, and those who assist in task performance is or should be a unified, dynamic, and continuing system of action (a nursing system) through which patients' demands for self-care of a therapeutic quality are met and their capabilities of engaging in self-care are regulated. Nursing practitioners ideally see their role responsibilities in terms of the wholeness of nursing situations and in terms of the design, production, and management of dynamic, effective nursing systems.

Nursing practitioners understand the domain of nursing knowledge, and they also understand the world of the nurse and the concrete domain of nursing practice.

The domain of nursing practice can be described in terms of the populations who can be helped through nursing. Candidates for nursing are those with *deficit relationships* between (1) their current or projected capability for providing self-care or dependent care and (2) the qualitative and quantitative demand for care. The reason for the deficit relationship between care capabilities and care demand is associated with the health state or health care needs of those requiring care. For example, parents who are competent to provide effective child care for their 6-year-old son may not be competent care providers if their son sustains multiple injuries in an accident or undergoes a severe life-threatening episode of viral pneumonia. In both situations, the child requires medical care and nursing; nursing actions would be adapted to the child as an individual, to the child's health state, to the child's age and particular state of development, and to the diagnostic and treatment measures prescribed by physicians. The current or future roles of the parents in the care of the child would be a nursing focus.

The domain of nursing practice can also be summarized in terms of the activities in which nurses engage when they provide nursing. Five activity areas of nursing practice are identified.

- Entering into and maintaining nurse-patient relationships with individuals, families, or groups until patients can legitimately be discharged from nursing
- Determining if and how patients can be helped through nursing
- Responding to patients' requests, desires, and needs for nurse contacts and assistance
- Prescribing, providing, and regulating direct help to patients (and their significant others) in the form of nursing
- Coordinating and integrating nursing with the patient's daily living, other health care needed or being received, and social and educational services needed or being received

The domain of nursing practice is thus a composite of persons characterized by conditions that generate nursing requirements and the actions that nurses perform when they provide nursing to these persons.

NURSES AS PRACTITIONERS AND SCHOLARS

To function effectively and to advance themselves in nursing practice, nurses must develop themselves as scholars or as students of nursing and nursing-related fields. Nurses qualified to function in some range of nursing practice situations must know authoritative sources in nursing and in fields that articulate with nursing within the frame of reference of types of cases. Clinical nursing specialists are necessarily advanced scholars in nursing and the other fields that define their specialty.

Nurses competent for the leadership and governing role in nursing patients with the nursing diagnoses expressed for the type of case described in Chapter 9 would know both the nursing and the related medical literature with respect to nursing persons with complete self-care deficit resulting from cerebrovascular accidents, including foundations in neurophysiology, the physiology of voluntary muscles, fluid and electrolyte balance, etc.

To move as a scholar or a student, it is necessary to identify within a field or a science the *areas* of knowledge to be investigated in relation to concrete practice problems about which knowledge is sought. Authoritative sources should be identified. Sources can be persons or reference works. Advanced practitioners and reference works in particular fields should be identified, their locations determined, and the relevant journals in particular fields identified.

To remain abreast in areas of nursing practice nurses must become conversant with periodical literature in nursing and in nursing-related fields. Related fields could be a specialty area of medicine, psychology, or physiology. For this reason, nursing practitioners should have a foundation(s) in the sciences of humans that are enabling for reading the literature in those fields and keeping abreast of changes in them.

Nurses prepared for nursing practice in technical-type nursing preparatory programs should seek and maintain contact with advanced practitioners in their particular areas of nursing. Concrete problems should be explored with them and authoritative references determined and pursued. Appropriate journals in nursing and nursing-related fields should be identified, access to them secured, and plans for reading developed and maintained.

All nurses should expend effort in resolving nursing practice problems, in clarifying and synthesizing knowledge, and in formulating and expressing insights achieved about problem solution. Discussions with colleagues, attendance at lectures, and discussions with advanced practitioners who are also advanced scholars may be helpful or necessary to resolve or solve concrete nursing practice problems.

NURSING DEVELOPMENT AND CLINICAL NURSING RESEARCH

Nurses engaged in the practice of nursing for individuals and groups are confronted with concrete practical problems of people that give rise to the occurrence of health-associated self-care and dependent-care deficits. Nurses in situations of nursing practice identify the absence of and the need for effective technologies for nursing diagnosis and for bringing about new conditions and correlations in practice situations. Refer to the listing of types of technologies in Chapter 4. An example of this nursing role follows.

The observation was made in a nursing clinic that some patients were not making progress in managing their conditions of diabetes mellitus, whereas other patients provided with the same kind of supportive-developmental nursing system became effective self-care agents. The question arose as to *why* certain patients were not making progress. These patients came to clinic, they appeared to participate and cooperate, but they were not effective in self-care. Asking the question *why* led to an investigation by the clinical nursing specialist of patients' behavior as they worked with the clinic nurse. The tentative diagnosis was made that these patients thought concretely and could not handle the content about regulatory care as it was being presented. This led to preliminary research toward answering two questions: Do these patients think concretely? How can nurses identify persons who think concretely? The goal of the investigations was to develop a diagnostic technology in the form of an assessment tool specific to one component of self-care agency grouped within the five sets of foundational capabilities and dispositions (see Fig. 7-3), namely, the capability of *operative knowing* (pp. 219-229)[7] This capability is shown within the substantive conceptual structure self-care agency in Fig. 7-4. In this example, nursing research and the development and validation of a diagnostic technology were linked together.

Other examples of practitioners' involvement in research arise from the questions patients ask about how to care for themselves and nurses' failures to find answers from nursing or medical specialists or from authoritative references. Nurses also engage in explanatory research to determine what patients do and do not do in meeting certain health-deviation-type self-care requisites.

The modes of thinking and the processes required for engagement in clinical research and in the development and validation of technologies differs from the mode of thinking and the processes of nursing practice. Nurses in practice must help themselves to understand and appreciate these differences in order to make judgments about feasible occupational combinations and about what they can do at particular times. All nurses in practice see combinations of phenomena that they do not understand but should understand for purposes of effective nursing. Ways and means to channel unsolved problems of nursing practice to appropriate nursing research and development centers should be instituted.

REFERENCES

1. Roberts MM: American nursing, New York, 1954, Macmillan, pp. 7-19.
2. Woodham-Smith, C: Florence Nightingale, 1820-1910, New York, 1951, McGraw-Hill, pp. 225-238.
3. See Phenix PH: Personal knowledge. In Realms of Meaning, New York, 1964, McGraw-Hill, pp. 193-211.
4. Peplau, HE: Interpersonal relations in nursing: a conceptual frame of reference for psychodynamic nursing, New York, 1952, GP Putnam.
5. Orlando IJ: The dynamic nurse-patient relationship, New York, 1961, GP Putnam.
6. Travelbee J: Interpersonal aspects of nursing, ed 2, Philadelphia, 1971, FA Davis Co.
7. Nursing Development Conference Group, Orem DE, editor: Concept formalization in nursing: process and product, Boston, 1979, Little, Brown & Co., pp. 219-229.

SELECTED READINGS

Arons AB: Achieving wider scientific literacy, Daedalus, Scientific literacy, 112:91-122, 1983.
Collège de Bois-de-Boulogne: Guide de la démarche de soin selon Orem, Montreal, 1987, Décarie Editeur, Inc.
Nursing Development Conference Group: Nursing knowledge and undergraduate nursing education. In Orem DE, editor: Concept formalization in nursing: process and product, Boston, 1979, Little, Brown & Co., pp. 284-295.
Piemme J, and Trainor M: A first year course in a baccalaureate program, Nursing Outlook 25:184-187, 1977.
Taylor SG: Curriculum development for preservice programs using Orem's theory of nursing. In Riehl-Sisca J: The science and art of self-care, Norwalk, 1985, Appleton-Century-Crofts, pp. 25-32.
Whelan EG: Analysis and application of Dorothea Orem's self-care practice model, J Nurs Educ 23:342-345, 1984.

Obstacles to and other factors that affect meeting universal self-care requisites

Several years ago, I participated in a survey of a nursing home population to identify (1) reasons for admission to the home and (2) factors that would condition the kind and amount of nursing required. One finding of the survey was that every resident in the nursing home had one or more health disorders, the effects and results of which established the conditions under which each universal self-care requisite had to be met and affected the choice of methods or technologies that could be used in meeting the requisite. The nursing question posed was: How can these requisites be met under prevailing conditions by a nurse, a dependent-care agent, or a self-care agent?

This question led to an investigation of the possible ranges of conditions that could affect the importance of and the actual meeting of universal self-care requisites, including the need for specialized methods or technologies to overcome obstacles, the circumstances under which action to meet them must be undertaken. Preliminary survey lists of factors were developed to establish conditions and circumstances under which meeting each universal requisite would be of special importance or that would in some way limit how and to what degree they could be met. Preliminary survey lists for three requisites — maintain a sufficient intake of air, water, and food — were expanded through exhaustive surveys of standard and authoritative reference work followed by validation of and revision of listings. Janet L. Fitzwater and I accomplished this work, with collaboration of Evelyn Vardiman in developing the project on the requisites for maintaining sufficient intake of water and food. This work extended from 1977 to 1983.

The listings of factors that can condition the meeting of each universal self-care requisite is presented. There is greater detail for requisites focused on intakes of air, water, and food because of the more detailed investigations of factors for these requisites. Universal requisites differ according to the concrete entities with which they deal, thus, the form of expressing factors that affect the need to and the ways of meeting them differ. The requisites focused on air, water, and food are concerned with the *movement of these entities from the environment into the individual*. The requisite on excrements is concerned with *movement of materials from individuals to their environment.* The requisites related to activity and rest and solitude and social interaction are concerned with *balance establishment and maintenance.* Preventing hazards is concerned with *avoidance or elimination.* Being normal or promotion of normalcy is concerned with *living within human norms and one's human potential* and this includes maintaining functioning within these norms to the degree possible under existing conditions and circumstances.

MAINTAINING A SUFFICIENT INTAKE OF AIR

Factors that interfere with meeting this requisite are organized by broad types (groups), subtypes (Roman numerals), characterizing features of factors (A,B,C . . .), and conditions associated with characterized factors (1, 2, 3a, b, c, . . .).

Group one — environmental interference, the availability and composition of air

I. Composition and oxygen partial pressure of atmospheric air not in accord with physiologic requisites
   A. Low oxygen partial pressure in atmospheric air
      1. At heights of approximately 12,000 feet resulting in arterial hypoxia in all persons
      2. In air in confined spaces resulting in arterial hypoxia
   B. Increase in carbon dioxide beyond 10% to 20% in inspired air, resulting in decreased respiratory minute volume and convulsive seizures
   C. Presence of irritant gases that stimulate nasal branches of the fifth cranial nerve, causing abrupt temporary inhibition of respiration
II. Availability of air
   A. Environments where air has been infiltrated by substances, such as smoke, or displaced by heavier-than-air gases
   B. Mechanical cutting off of available air by external blocking of air passages

Group two — interferences with the process of pulmonary ventilation

I. Interferences with air flow
   A. Obstruction of air passages by foreign objects and materials
      1. Presence of deliberately placed or inspired foreign objects in nose, nasopharynx, larynx, trachea, bronchi
      2. Presence of blood in air passages resultant, for example, from
         a. Bleeding from nose or nasopharynx
         b. Bleeding from the trachea, for example, bleeding caused by a low-lying tracheostomy tube, which erodes the innominate artery
         c. Lung hemorrhage
      3. Presence of food or fluid or vomitus in larynx or trachea associated with
         a. Failure of the glottis to close during swallowing or gagging due to paralysis of the adductor fibers of the vagi
         b. Passage of food and fluid from esophagus to trachea through a fistulous connection

B. Abnormalities that interfere with air flow and increase airway resistance
  1. Obstruction of upper respiratory passages by
     a. Swelling of mucosa of mouth, nose, pharynx or larynx with exudate, occlusion of airway and difficult breathing associated, for example, with respiratory infections, hay fever, or other allergic reactions
     b. Polyps, nodules, enlarged adenoids and tonsils
     c. Deformities such as deviated nasal septum, laryngeal atresia
     d. Abscess formations such as peritonsillar abscess, sublingual abscesses, retropharyngeal abscesses
     e. Laryngostenosis, tracheal stenosis
  2. Dysfunctions that interfere with air flow
     a. Inability of the glottis to open because of paralysis of the abductor fibers of the vagi
     b. Laryngospasm
     c. Depression or suppression of the cough reflex and sneeze reflex, resulting in failure to clear air passages
     d. Diffuse narrowing of the bronchial tree that interferes with air flow and increases airway resistance (generalized obstructive lung disease)
        (1) Reversible as in bronchial asthma or in infections with excessive secretions
        (2) Irreversible as with fibrosis following infections, chronic bronchitis
II. Factors associated with changes in lung compliance and vital capacity of lung
  A. Gross structural and positional factors restricting lung compliance and vital capacity
    1. Total thoracic cage motion limitations as in kyphoscoliosis
    2. Immobility of costovertebral joints, as in spondylitis
    3. Assumed positions of the body that interfere with lung expansion
  B. Pressure factors associated with decreased lung compliance
    1. Change from natural negative intrapleural pressure to positive intrapleural pressure with pneumothorax
       a. Open pneumothorax with atelectasis
       b. Closed pneumothorax with atelectasis
    2. Increased pressure on unaffected lung in tension pneumothorax due to deviation of the mediastinum toward the unaffected lung
    3. Increased intra-abdominal pressure with restriction of movement of the diaphragm
  C. Alterations of lung tissue affecting lung compliance or vital capacity
    1. Increase in rigidity of the lung parenchyma with decreased lung compliance, for example, that associated with pulmonary hypertension
    2. Reduction of number of available lung units with decreased lung compliance associated, for example, with lesions of lung tissue due to biologic and chemical agents
    3. Decreases in lung compliance ranging to atelectasis associated with deficiencies of surfactant in the lining of the alveoli
       a. Premature infants
       b. Newborns who are not premature
       c. Adults with adult respiratory distress syndrome

       d. Individuals who undergo pulmonary-circulatory interruptions, as in use of heart-lung machines

    4. Decrease in elasticity of lung parenchyma with increased compliance and decreased vital capacity, as in obstructive pulmonary emphysema

  D. Voluntary restriction of chest expansion during respiration because of associated pain, as in pleurisy and fractured ribs

  E. Muscular and neuromuscular factors associated with decreased lung compliance or vital capacity
    1. Paralysis of muscles of inspiration, especially the diaphragm
    2. Paralysis of accessory muscles of respiration
    3. Spasm of respiratory muscles with temporary cessation of breathing, as in generalized convulsions
    4. Fibrotic muscles
    5. Specific neuromuscular disorders
       a. Progressive muscular dystrophy
       b. Myotonic dystrophy

III. Interferences with optimal alveolar ventilation with or without diffusion impairment
  A. Nonfunctional alveoli associated with intracellular accumulations obstructing the air sacs (aveoli)
    1. Pulmonary edema
    2. Intra-alveolar bleeding
    3. Interstitial pneumonia
    4. Proteinosis
    5. Microlithiasis
  B. Decrease in number of alveoli and total alveolar surface area due to destruction of septa of alveoli as in emphysema
  C. Loss of alveoli and pulmonary capillaries due to removal of, destruction of, or pathologic changes in lung tissue
    1. Pneumonectomy, lobectomy
    2. Pulmonary infarction
    3. Fibrosis of lung; diffuse scarring of lung due to pulmonary hypertension (restrictive pulmonary diseases)

IV. Interferences with maintenance of gaseous equilibrium between alveolar air and pulmonary blood
  A. Alveolar hypoventilation, general or regional, associated with, for example, conditions that decrease expansibility of the lung
  B. Thickening of the alveolar and capillary membranes that separate blood and alveolar air (more restrictive of O_2 than CO_2 diffusion)
  C. Low ratio of pulmonary blood flow to ventilation as in
    1. Cardiac failure and dyspnea
    2. Vasospasm, thrombosis, embolus
    3. Congenital cardiovascular anomalies affecting pulmonary circulation
    4. Acquired cardiovascular dysfunction disorders (e.g., ischemia of heart muscle)
    5. Cardiac asthma
  D. Lowered oxygen capacity of pulmonary blood flow associated with

1. Low hemoglobin content of blood as in anemias of all types
2. Hemoglobin combined with something other than O_2 (e.g., carbon monoxide)
3. Altered hemoglobin that cannot combine with O_2, for example, methemoglobin as in poisoning with chlorates, nitrates, acetanalid, ferrocyanides

V. Factors affecting the central neural and neurochemical regulatory mechanisms of respiration
  A. Interferences with the automatic rhythmic activity of the medullary respiratory center with its inspiratory and expiratory centers
    1. Interferences with neuronal functioning within the centers associated with
      a. Depression of the medullary respiratory center relative to high concentrations of CO_2 or to anoxia
      b. Tissue changes in the center associated with tumors, inflammatory disease, vascular accidents, edema
      c. Inadequate blood to respiratory center
    2. Interferences with normal periodic inhibition of activity in inspiratory center so that expiration can occur
  B. Interferences with chemical regulatory receptors (as in the carotid and aortic bodies) and mechanisms that adjust ventilation to keep alveolar CO_2 partial pressure constant and raise O_2 partial pressure when it falls to dangerous levels

Group three — Changes from normal respiration associated with selected physiologic and psychological states

I. States characterized in part by temporary cessation of breathing, for example
  A. Generalized convulsions with continued spasm of the respiratory muscles giving way to clonic movements of these muscles (breathing ceases and is followed by air entering the lungs in short, convulsive gasps)
  B. Breath-holding spells in young children where crying and screaming are followed by apnea for as long as a minute

II. Absence of respiration
  A. Apnea in apparently healthy infants, characterized by (1) an episode of apnea during sleep with change in color and (2) unresponsiveness to gentle stimulation. Mouth-to-mouth resuscitation or prolonged vigorous shaking is necessary to restore breathing
  B. Apnea in sick preterm hospitalized infants subjected to low levels of somatic and vestibular stimulation (as from touching and rocking) or associated with temperature instability in infant or environment
  C. Apnea in the first 24 hours of life secondary to sepsis
  D. Apnea associated with cardiorespiratory diseases, such as hyaline membrane disease, patent ductus arteriosus
  E. Apnea due to metabolic causes, such as hypocalcemia, hypoglycemia

III. States characterized in part by experiences of respiratory distress or by changes in depth and frequency of breathing, for example
  A. Anxiety states with persons experiencing difficulty in breathing, tightness in the throat, a feeling of smothering or suffocating sometimes with pronounced hyperventilation (symptoms of fear, anger)

    B. Hysteria and emotional disturbances with persons experiencing distressing dyspnea, sensations of smothering, needs for more oxygen, tightness of chest muscles

    C. Pulmonary or cardiac pathologic states with the experiencing of dyspnea by the individual

        1. On exertion

        2. At rest

    D. Periodic breathing in preterm infants

    E. Dyspnea and cyanosis in newborn associated with hypoplasia of mandible and glossoptosis

IV. States characterized in part by decreased respiratory rate with decreased pulmonary ventilation and vital capacity

    A. Cachexia

    B. Malnutrition

 V. States where there is a marked increase in the work of breathing, for example, physiologic states characteristic of

    A. Injury

    B. Acute illness

This listing should be used as an exploratory tool and should be subjected to continuing validation and updating as new scientific findings emerge. It provides a basis for organization of nursing approaches already identified and validated. The question for investigation is: What can and should nurses do to help patients maintain an adequate intake of air when X condition is present? What should individuals be helped to do for themselves?

MAINTAINING A SUFFICIENT INTAKE OF WATER AND FOOD

Factors that interfere with meeting this requisite are organized by broad types (groups), subtypes (Roman numerals), and categories of factors (A. B. . . .) and named factors within the categories (1, 2, 3a, b, c . . .).

Group one — interferences with taking and holding water and food in the mouth

 I. Conditions and circumstances that interfere with having access to water and food

    A. Conditions of communication

        1. Limited ability or inability to communicate needs or desires for water and food, for example, early developmental stage, low levels of cognitive development, limited or loss of awareness, speech defects or disturbances of speech pattern, aphasia

        2. Modes of communication not understood by persons who can procure water and food, for example, speech in a foreign language, sign language

        3. Failure to communicate needs for water and food to appropriate persons, for example, lack of knowledge about how to proceed, reluctance to ask for water or food, fear of persons who can procure water and food

    B. Conditions of access

        1. Inability to procure water and food for self

   2. Inaccessibility of provided water or food
   3. Water and food not available when needed or desired
 II. Characteristics of available water and food that provoke reluctance or refusal to take in or hold water or food in the mouth
   A. Water, food deviate from cultural norms
      1. Source of water not in accord with customary source
      2. Unfamiliar foods or unfamiliar preparation of food
      3. Food not in accord with religious or cultural prescriptions
   B. Water, food deviate from personal standards of acceptability
      1. Available food is disliked
      2. Water or food is displeasing to sight, smell, taste
      3. Texture of food is displeasing
      4. Water or food is repugnant according to individual's standards of acceptability
   C. Water, food is incompatible with structural or functional conditions of individual's or general health state
      1. Incompatible with existent powers of mastication or deglutition
      2. Incompatible physiologically, as in allergy
      3. Not in accord with nutritional state or with digestive or metabolic powers
III. Internal and external conditions that interfere with attending to or suppress the desire for or the willingness to take in, receive, or hold water and food in the mouth
   A. Interferences with attention
      1. Loss of interest in drinking and eating
      2. Sensory deprivation, sensory overload
      3. High level anxiety with narrowing of the perceptual field and agitation
      4. Confusion, stupor, coma
   B. Interferences with desire for or willingness to take in water or food
      1. Human conditions that interfere with desire or willingness
         a. Satiety, anorexia
         b. Obtunded sense of thirst
         c. Nausea, vomiting, regurgitation of gas or small amounts of food from stomach
         d. Fear of choking
         e. Limited ability or inability to perceive color or texture or aroma of food or to taste food
         f. Visual or auditory hallucinations
      2. Absence of psychic stimuli that promote salivation — sight of food, smell, sound of cooking, hearing descriptions of food
      3. Behaviors that are not in accord with the reality of human requirements for water and food
         a. Negation of feelings of hunger with failure to eat or drink
         b. Refusal to eat when food is available
         c. Self-concept that negates the need for a sufficient intake of food
         d. Bulimia
      4. Behaviors not in accord with the real characteristics of water and food, such as delusions about the characteristics of water or food, distorted perceptions of water and food, or olfactory hallucinations

5. Environmental conditions that can adversely affect the desire for water or food or willingness to eat or drink
   a. Social conditions — absence of preferred social situations for eating, strained relationships, aesthetically displeasing conditions
   b. Biologic conditions — infestation with vermin, unsanitary conditions, aesthetically displeasing conditions
   c. Physical conditions — offensive and disturbing noise level, undesirable climatic conditions, inadequate light levels, aesthetically displeasing conditions

IV. Conditions and circumstances that interfere with the natural processes of taking in and holding water and food in the mouth
   A. Developmental and constitutional states, such as absence of suck or weak suck in infants
   B. Anomalies of the mouth and face, including cleft lip, cleft palate, mandibulomaxillary discrepancies, developmental defects of the tongue or lips
   C. Painful and obstructive conditions — inflammations and lesions, soft tissue swellings, intraoral tumors, tumors of face and neck
      1. Stomatitis, gingivitis, glossitis, fissures of tongue
      2. Tumors of mucous membranes, tongue, bony structures of mouth
      3. Oral abscesses
      4. Mumps (parotiditis)
   D. Excessive flow of secretions from mouth and nose
      1. Excessive flow of saliva as in Parkinson's disease, use of specific pharmacologic agents, increase in blood acidity
      2. Excessive flow of nasopharyngeal secretions and lacrimal fluid, as in upper respiratory infections
   E. Difficulty to inability to open or close the mouth
      1. Temporomandibular joint disorders
      2. Surgical procedures that temporarily prevent opening or closing the mouth, for example, wiring of teeth in occlusion
      3. Neurologic conditions that affect, for example, ability to open mouth, maintenance of occlusion
   F. Surgical procedures on the mouth, jaw, and tongue that involve excision and reconstruction restricting the taking in and holding of water and food in the mouth, for example, surgery of the lips, resections of maxillae or mandible, resection of hard or soft palate, hemiglossectomy or total glossectomy
   G. Soft tissue changes in the mouth
      1. Effects of dietary deficiencies and restricted or no oral water intake on the tissues and organs of the oral cavity
         a. Sore mouth associated with degeneration of connective tissue of gums and peridontal ligaments and atrophy of tongue epithelium
         b. Increased sensitivity of periodontal tissue to local irritants and trauma
         c. Dehydration of tissues
      2. Atrophy of oral mucosa in older people with resultant abnormal taste perception and burning sensation in mouth

H. Positions of the body that interfere with taking in and holding water and food in mouth, including Trendelenburg position and prone position

I. Unwillingness to open mouth to eat based on false beliefs about consequences

Group two — interferences with mastication

I. Conditions that interfere with the crushing and breaking up of food
  A. Conditions of the teeth and jaws including
    1. Malocclusion of jaws and teeth
    2. Absence of teeth — incisors, molars
    3. Temporomandibular joint disorders, such as ankylosis of joints — stiffening or fixation, dislocation of joint
  B. Conditions of the masticatory muscles including
    1. Weakness with fatigue of muscles after limited movement as in myasthenia gravis or the asthenia of metabolic disease
    2. Weakness and atrophy of muscles associated with muscular dystrophy
    3. Atrophy as in myotonia and long-standing myasthenia
    4. Partial or total paralysis associated with lesions of the brain stem
    5. Disturbances of motor functioning affecting coordination
  C. Pain associated with mastication, as with soft tissue and bone lesions
  D. Diminished amounts or absence of saliva hindering the moistening of foodstuffs and lubrication of the mucosa of the mouth
  E. Habitual bolting of unchewed food
II. Conditions and circumstances that interfere with the mixing of food with saliva
  A. Conditions and circumstances related to salivary flow and its composition
    1. Diminished or arrested salivary secretion (asialism) associated with, for example,
      a. Body dehydration
      b. Not taking water and food by mouth
      c. Cessation of salivary function associated with inflammation of the salivary glands producing dry mouth (xerostoma)
      d. Vitamin A deficiency
      e. Use of atropine and other cholinergic blocking agents
      f. Fear, depression, anxiety, excitement
    2. Blockage of salivary ducts by calculi, tumors, inflammatory conditions
  B. Conditions of the muscles of the tongue and cheeks that interfere with placement of food between the dental arches and collection of food into a mass or bolus
    1. Conditions of the tongue
      a. Microglossia, aglossia, macroglossia and ankyloglossia
      b. Resection of part of tongue, removal of tongue
      c. Paralysis of half of tongue with atrophy that occurs with occlusion of vertebral artery
      d. Paralysis of extrinsic and intrinsic muscles of the tongue
    2. Conditions of the facial muscles, including weakness, atrophy, and paralysis
  C. Bolting of unchewed food

Group three — interferences with deglutition

I. Conditions and circumstances that interfere with the movement of chewed and moistened food or liquids from the mouth to the space between the base of the tongue and the posterior wall of the pharynx (oral, voluntary phase of swallowing)

A. Inability to initiate or regulate voluntary action as in stupor and coma

B. Interferences with the events of the oral phase of swallowing: closing of the lips and jaw; elevation of the tip of the tongue to the hard palate subsequent to the separation out of a bolus of food or the taking in of liquid; pushing the dorsum of the tongue upward and backward against the palate moving the bolus of food or liquid into the pharynx; closing of the nasopharynx by the elevation of the soft palate

  1. Disturbances of motor functioning that interfere with

    a. Compressing the lips (orbicularis) and compressing the cheeks (buccinator)

    b. Elevation of the mandible — temporal muscle, masseter, and internal pterygoid muscle

  2. Anomalies of the lip, palate, and tongue

  3. Partial or total paralysis of the tongue; resection or removal of tongue

  4. Painful and obstructive conditions intraoral or of the face and neck

II. Conditions and circumstances that interfere with the arrival of food or liquid in the pharynx, movement through the pharynx and through the pharyngoesophageal sphincter into the esophagus (reflex pharyngeal phase of swallowing)

A. Obstructive conditions and painful conditions of the pharynx

  1. Pharyngeal pouch associated with loss of support of the muscle fibers

  2. Obstructing tumor masses and foreign objects

  3. Abnormalities of the cricoid pharyngeal sphincter including spasm, delayed onset of relaxation, premature contractions with shortening of relaxation

  4. Inflammatory conditions and lesions of the soft tissues

B. Disturbances of the neural mechanisms of the swallowing reflex

  1. Central lesions — pons, thalamus, frontal cortex, medulla

  2. Lesions of receptors in the mouth and pharynx and afferent fibers of the glossopharyngeal nerve and superior laryngeal branch of the vagus

  3. Lesions of the pharyngeal muscles

C. Lesions that hinder the movement of the larynx cranialward and ventrally

D. Lodging of food in the pharynx due to size of bolus or consistency of food

III. Conditions and circumstances that interfere with the passage of food and liquid through the esophagus and through the lower esophageal sphincter into the stomach (reflex esophageal phase of swallowing)

A. Obstructive conditions including, for example

  1. Atresia

  2. Stenosis, congenital or secondary to disease or injury

  3. Esophageal webs

  4. Compressed esophagus with the opening to pharynx thrown out of axis by pharyngeal pouch

  5. Obstruction of lumen by foreign bodies, tumors

B. Anomalies, including absence of esophagus, tracheoesophageal fistula, esophageal diverticula

C. Painful conditions and conditions involving the integrity of the tissues of the esophagus
   1. Acute or chronic esophagitis associated with
      a. Compromised lower esophageal sphincter
         (1) Primary incompetence
         (2) Surgical removal or destruction, all leading to reflux
      b. Hiatal hernia; congenital short esophagus; columnar-lined lower esophagus
      c. Diseases such as schleroderma; neoplasms
      d. Pregnancy
      e. Secondary to factors including
         (1) Vomiting
         (2) Intubation
         (3) Anesthesia
         (4) Prolonged hiccups
         (5) Stress reaction
         (6) Recumbency that is forced, or associated with unconsciousness of long duration
         (7) Central nervous system lesions
         (8) Terminal phase of an illness
         (9) Use of alcohol secondary to irradiation and concurrent chemotherapy for persons with pulmonary small cell carcinoma
   2. Ulceration of the esophagus
   3. Esophageal varices
   4. Perforation of the esophagus
      a. As complication of esophagitis, peptic ulcers, neoplasms, presence of foreign bodies
      b. Spontaneous rupture during vomiting or coughing, or associated with gluttony
   5. Vertical lacerations of esophagus at gastroesophageal junction with severe hemorrhage
D. Disturbances of the neural mechanisms of the swallowing reflex: central lesions, lesions of receptors, neuromuscular lesions of esophagus and efferent nerve fibers
E. Motility changes and motor dysfunction associated with old age, use of alcohol, diminished or absent peristalsis when smooth muscle is replaced by dense fibrous tissue, as in scleroderma
F. Gastroesophageal reflux in newborn infant due to normal low resting pressure of the gastroesophageal sphincter

This listing of interferences should be subjected to refinement and continuing validation and should be kept in accord with scientific developments.

PROVIDING CARE ASSOCIATED WITH ELIMINATIVE PROCESSES AND EXCREMENTS

The factors that were identified as focusing attention on the meeting of this universal self-care requisite or on methods of meeting it were organized under categories of change, affective reactions, care performance, and environment.

Group one — bowel evacuation

  I. Changes in bowel evacuation patterns, feces, and bowel integrity
    A. Change from individuals' patterns of evacuation — constipation, diarrhea
    B. Changes in the form, color, and other characteristics of feces
    C. Changes in bowel integrity — functional or structural changes
      1. Incontinence
      2. Obstruction of bowel — partial or complete
      3. Structural changes in bowel, for example, from infection, tumors, surgical intervention
  II. Feelings and emotions associated with bowel evacuation
    A. Discomfort or pain
    B. Anxiety or fear associated with bowel elimination pattern or characteristics of feces
  III. Care performance
    A. Required movements of body are difficult or impossible to execute
    B. Discomfort or pain associated with execution of required movements
  IV. Environment
    A. Resources for receiving and disposing of feces are not readily available or adequate or safe
    B. Resources for after care of body parts for sanitary and aesthetic purposes are not available or adequate or safe
    C. The social and physical environment does not provide privacy for bowel evacuation or after care
    D. Prevailing practices about bowel evacuation and after care are not congruous with those of the individual

Group two — urination

  I. Changes in pattern of urination, in urine, and in the integrity of organs
    A. Change from individual's normal pattern of urination
    B. Qualitative and quantitative changes in urine
    C. Changes in structural or functional integrity of organs
      1. Incontinence
      2. Paralysis of bladder
      3. Obstruction of urethra, bladder neck, ureter(s)
      4. Structural changes in ureters, bladder, urethra resultant from injury, pathology, or surgical interventions
  II, III, IV. See under bowel; adjust for urination and urine

Group three — perspiration

  I. Change from usual pattern of sweating under specified conditions and circumstances
    A. Diminished or absent
    B. Increased
  II. Reactions and feelings associated with

A. Diminished or absent sweating

B. Excessive sweating

III. Care performance

A. Required movements of body are difficult or impossible to execute

B. Discomfort or pain associated with execution of movement

IV. Environment—resources for care not available or adequate

Group four—menstruation

I. Change from normal pattern of menstruation or suppression

A. Change in time and duration of bleeding or amount of bleeding

B. Suppressed menstruation

II. Feeling and emotions associated with menstruation or its absence

A. Discomfort or pain

B. Anxiety or fear associated with changes in pattern of menstruation

III. Care performance

A. Required movements of the body are difficult or impossible to execute

B. Discomfort or pain associated with use of care measures or with required movements

IV. Environment

A. Resources for care are not available, adequate, or safe

B. Prevailing care practices are not congruous with those of the individual

MAINTAINING A BALANCE BETWEEN ACTIVITY AND REST

Factors were organized into two groups with subgroups. The main organizing groups were factors of human and environmental origin. Factors call attention to needs for special concern for meeting the requisite and the methods for use in meeting it.

Group one—human factors

I. States that interfere with balancing activity at rest

A. Debility and weakness

B. Emotional states of apathy or excitement

C. Wakefulness

D. Narcosis, comatose states

E. Overriding interests and concerns about some matter or affair of daily living

F. Disability

G. Inactivity or immobility prescribed for therapeutic purposes

II. Specific conditions that interfere with balancing activity and rest

A. Dyspnea on exertion

B. Uncontrolled pain

C. Continuous discomfort

D. Sensory overload; sensory deprivation

E. Anxiety or fear associated with being

1. At rest or active
2. Alone or in contact with other persons

Group two—environmental factors

I. Social environment—what significant others want, permit, recommend, or demand
II. Resources and time are inadequate to
    A. Engage in productive work, recreation, preferred activities
    B. Change from one activity to other types of activities
    C. Change from being active to a resting state
    D. Obtain sufficient rest and sleep
    E. Maintain needed or desired physical conditions
III. Physical environment
    A. Climatic conditions that militate against activity or rest
    B. Noise that interferes with either rest and sleep or activity requiring concentration
    C. Unaccustomed noiselessness or personal need for it
    D. Personal preferences about light and darkness for rest and sleep
IV. The environmental situation
    A. Crisis situation in family or residence
    B. Disaster conditions resulting from earthquakes, hurricanes, floods, fires
    C. Disaster conditions from war

MAINTAINING BALANCE BETWEEN SOLITUDE AND SOCIAL INTERACTION

Factors that signify need for attention to meeting this requisite and that affect methods of meeting it were organized under conditions of living and human and environmental conditions.

Group one—conditions of living

I. Isolation from other persons
    A. Minimal, infrequent contact to no contact because of location of residence
    B. Self-imposed isolation in a nonrestricted social environment
    C. Imposed isolation within the social group
II. Continuous demand for interactions with other persons throughout waking hours
III. Continuous involvement in provision of care associated with acute or chronic illness or injury

Group two—human factors

I. Personal factors
    A. Characteristics of temperament and personality
    B. Chronological age and developmental stage
    C. Anxiety to fear of being alone or being with others
    D. Personal characteristics, including physical features, that elicit avoidance behaviors from others

II. Specific interferences
   A. Sensory impairments
   B. Inadequate communication skills
   C. Lack of skill and habit formation for being alone
   D. Continuous seeking of contacts with others

Group three—environmental factors

I. Persons for social contact and interaction are
   A. Pleasing, displeasing
   B. Preferred, not preferred
   C. Available, not available when needed
II. Physical environmental conditions and resources facilitate or hinder
   A. Social contacts and interactions
   B. Solitude

PREVENTING HAZARDS TO LIFE, FUNCTIONING, AND WELL-BEING

Factors that signify need to attend to meeting this requisite or affect methods for meeting it are organized in groups of human and environmental factors

Group one—human factors

I. States
   A. Intense emotional states that restrict attention and awareness
   B. States of sleep and reverie
   C. Light to deep coma
   D. Debility and weakness
II. Specific interferences
   A. Disabilities that interfere with control of position and movement in space
   B. Limited awareness of self and environment in a specific time frame, regardless of cause
   C. Lack of knowledge of specific hazards or means to control or avoid them
   D. Modes of cognitive functioning that do not deal with abstractions and do not take into account what has not happened or has not been experienced
   E. Absence of reasonable concern about hazards
   F. Excessive concern about and fear of hazards

Group two—environmental factors

I. Physical hazards
   A. Atmospheric and weather conditions
   B. Geologic hazards
   C. Physical hazards in the home, work situation, or recreational situations
II. Social conditions
   A. Dependents of individuals who are
      1. Indifferent to fulfillment of responsibilities to take care of their dependents

2. Overprotective of dependents, not allowing freedom necessary for development
B. Abandonment
C. Exposure to personal abuse
   1. Psychological
   2. Physical and psychological
III. Resources — resources necessary for life and health are not available or adequate
IV. Social group
A. Does not act to prevent the occurrence of or control of known hazardous conditions
B. Does not communicate information to members about existent hazards and measures to prevent or mitigate their effects
   1. Under usual conditions of living
   2. Under disaster conditions

PROMOTING NORMALCY

Factors when present that focus attention on the needs to meet this requisite or on methods for meeting it are organized under groups of human and environmental factors.

Group one — human factors

I. States
A. Arousal states that result in restriction of knowledge or incorrect knowledge of self, environment, and situations of action
   1. Sleep and reverie
   2. Light to deep coma
   3. Intense emotional states that restrict attention and interfere with perception
B. States of cognitive development (or modes of thought) in which persons do not deal with abstractions or that which has not been experienced
C. States of physical disability that interfere with sensation and perception and ability to control position and movement in space
D. Imposed states of restricted physical activity, resulting in a limited environment
II. Specific factors
A. Impairments of communication, reasoning, or memory
B. Absence of or defects in bodily parts visible, not visible
C. Anxiety to fear or anger associated with changes in self and in life-style
D. Reluctance to refusal to attend to existent conditions in self or environment
E. Overriding interests and concerns that rule out attention to conditions in self or environment that should be regulated
F. Diminished powers to manage and care for self and to fulfill role responsibilities
G. Unsatisfying conditions of living

Group two—environmental factors

   I. Social
   - A. Exclusion from or rejection by family or intimate social group
   - B. Exclusion from the larger society

  II. Conditions and resources not supportive of personal developments and not adequate to maintain satisfying conditions of living

Glossary

act That which is done by a person; the deed.

action The process of a person doing something, usually involving more than one step and occupying some time.

agency The power to engage in action to achieve specific goals.

agent The person who engages in a course of action or has the power to do so.

agreement The act of two or more persons who unite in expressing a mutual purpose.

basic conditioning factors Conditions or events in a time-place matrix that affect the values or ways of meeting persons' existent self-care requisites or bring about new self-care requisites or affect the development, operability, or adequacy of persons' capabilities to care for themselves or their dependents; conditions or events in a time-place matrix that affect the values of nurses' powers of nursing agency.

case In nursing, a concrete instance of a person requiring and receiving nursing.

case load In nursing, the number of persons that a nurse provides with nursing individually or in multiperson units during the same time duration.

case management operations In nursing practice the series of actions performed by a nursing practitioner to plan and control; that is, direct, check, and evaluate the professional practice operations of nursing diagnosis, prescription and regulation to form an effective, dynamic system of service to nurses' patients.

communicate To make common to parties or objects involved nontangible things such as information.

community A social group sharing common characteristics or interests based in the intersubjective spontaneity of group members and an intelligently devised social order and perceived or perceiving itself as distinct in some respect from the larger society in which it exists.

conceptualization The level of cognitional activity in which ideas from acts of understanding based on data of sense or data of consciousness are formulated and expressed as concepts to give an outward form to what is understood.

concrete Concerned with actual things or instances; constituting an actual thing or instance.

content In human experiences that which is experienced as distinguished from the act.

contract A promissory agreement about specific matters between two or more competent parties creating a mutuality of agreements and obligations expressed in ascertainable terms.

control The process of keeping things within the bounds of what is essential, correct, and proper.

coordinated Combined in harmonious relations; unified for action.

criterion A measure used in the making of a correct judgment about something that is accomplished.

deliberate action The doing of something by a person on the basis of the person's practical judgment of what is the appropriate thing to do.

dependent care The practice of activities that responsible maturing and mature persons initiate and perform on behalf of socially dependent persons for some time on a continuing basis in order to maintain their lives and contribute to their health and well-being.

dependent-care agency The developed and developing capabilities of persons to know and meet the therapeutic self-care demands of persons socially dependent on them or to regulate the development or exercise of these persons' self-care agency.

dependent-care agent   A maturing adolescent or adult who accepts and fulfills the responsibility to know and meet the therapeutic self-care demand of relevant others who are socially dependent on them or to regulate the development or exercise of these persons' self-care agency.

dependent-care system   Courses and sequences of action that are being or have been performed by dependent-care agents to meet the particularized self-care requisites of socially dependent persons for whom they are responsible.

design   A proposed way of making or doing something with a setting forth of the disposition of individual elements or details of elements in the process of production.

design unit   In nursing practice, a distinct result achieving component of a total pattern for the production of nursing for a patient.

development   A sequence of dynamic and increasingly differentiated arrangements and patterns toward realization of the hidden or latent possibilities of a thing.

diagnostic operations   Nursing practice operations that result in reflective judgments about what is, what are the distinguishing characteristics of what is, what is its nature, and why is it as it is. These operations follow or are concurrent with investigations of patients' self-care agency, self-care requisites, and conditioning factors that provide the data on which nurses' reflective judgments are based.

empirical   Derived from or guided by experience.

form   The particular condition in which something appears, including its internal structure, disposition of details, boundary lines, and unity of the whole.

health   A descriptor of living things with respect to their structural and functional wholeness and soundness.

hierarchy of values   Possible concrete objects of choice of individuals (excluding concrete objects of aversion) that are understood by them as being arranged in a particular order that influences choice and practical action.

insight   An instance of persons apprehending in data the answers to a question for investigation proceeding from an accurate presentation of the problem, to cues, to images, to knowing.

intersubjectivity   Person-to-person togetherness: mutual or reciprocal action or influence.

judgment   The mental act of asserting (affirming or denying) something on the basis of sufficiency of evidence and acts of reflective understanding.

meaning   The idea that a word, statement, facial expression, bodily movement, or situation in a time-place matrix convey to persons or is intended to convey; social and cultural changes are changes in meaning that are understood and accepted by members of communities.

mode   Appearance, form of disposition of a thing, or one of its essential properties or attributes.

model   Interlocking sets of terms and relations that are useful in guiding investigations, framing hypotheses, and in writing descriptions; a model also is identified as a postulated representation of an unobservable entity or process with the elements used in the representation partly understood from their presence in another entity.

nursing administration   The body of persons who are responsible for and function in governing and executive positions in formally constituted organizations to ensure the provision of nursing to the whole of or segment of the populations served by health service enterprises, the members of which have legitimate nursing requirements.

nursing agency The developed capabilities of persons educated as nurses that empower them to represent themselves as nurses and within the frame of a legitimate interpersonal relationship to act, to know, and to help persons in such relationships to meet their therapeutic self-care demands and to regulate the development or exercise of their self-care agency.

nursing diagnosis A deliberate process through which nurses in nursing practice situations carefully examine and analyze facts and judgments about persons who are their patients, and about properties and activities of these persons, to explain and state the nature and causes of their therapeutic self-care demands; the state of development, the operability and adequacy of their self-care agency; and the presence and extent of self-care deficits existent or projected.

nursing design A professional function performed both before and after nursing diagnosis and prescription through which nurses, on the basis of reflective practical judgments about existent conditions, synthesize concrete situational elements into orderly relations to structure operational units. The purpose of nursing design is to provide guides for achieving needed and foreseen results in the production of nursing toward the achievement of nursing goals; the units taken together constitute the pattern to guide the production of nursing.

nursing practice Nurses' responsibility for and regular engagement in nursing one or more persons (singly or in groups) in these persons' time-place localizations.

nursing practitioner A person professionally educated and qualified to practice nursing who is engaged in its regular provision to persons individually or in multiperson units at the beginning or advanced or scientific level of professional practice.

nursing prescription A deliberate action process through which nurses make practical judgments about what can and should be done to meet their patients' particularized self-care requisites and to regulate the exercise or development of their self-care agency under existent or projected changed conditions and circumstances.

nursing process A reference term used by nurses to subsume the professional operations of nursing practice, including work management operations.

nursing regulation or treatment Nurses' use of valid and reliable measures to continuously meet their patients' particularized self-care requisites in order to keep their functioning and development within ranges compatible with life and with normal functioning and development; it also includes use of measures to ensure that patients' developed or potential powers of self-care agency are protected and the exercise or development of self-care agency regulated.

nursing situations A combination of concrete circumstances involving both persons with health-related self-care or dependent-care deficits and nurses at some place in some time frame with nurses acting to the advantage of the persons with self-care or dependent-care deficits.

nursing systems Series and sequences of deliberate practical actions of nurses performed at times in coordination with actions of their patients to know and meet components of their patients' therapeutic self-care demands and to protect and regulate the exercise or development of patients' self-care agency.

object   That toward which or because of which action is directed or taken.

operation   A particular process of a mental or a practical nature necessary in some form of work or production.

order   A relation in a set of elements or members of a class (individuals, facts, objects of any kind) that arranges the elements of the set or the members of a class in a particular way.

organized   Formed as or into a whole consisting of interdependent or coordinate parts toward ensuring harmonious or unified action.

pattern   A combination of qualities or acts forming a consistent or characteristic arrangement.

phenomenologic   Pertaining to the study and description of observed or observable facts, occurrences, or circumstances in all areas of experience.

plan   The specification of the organization and timing of essential tasks to bring a design for something to be produced into actuality. Specifications relate to time and place of action and duration of actions; requisite environmental conditions and equipment and supplies; number of persons required at particular times and places; and control measures to be used.

population   All persons who have some characteristics in common such as residence in the same geographic area or being served by the same health care institution or agency.

postulate   To set forth a proposition accepted as true as a basis for a specific chain of reasoning, a specific argument, or a specific system of thought.

premise   A proposition or one of several propositions supporting or helping to support a conclusion.

prescriptive operations   In nursing practice, the action sequences engaged in by nurses to make practical judgments about and to specify in relation to qualitative and quantitative features of identified self-care requisites the ways in which they can and should be met and when and how to use the ways of meeting them; this is a prescription of the therapeutic self-care demand. Also included are nurses' prescriptions about what should be done to protect patients' capacities for self-care and ways and means to develop their powers of self-care agency or regulate their use.

process   The series and sequences of actions or operations involved in the accomplishment of something moving from a beginning stage to the stage of the actual making or production or changing of something (the end or goal sought).

production   Performance of detailed operations to bring into being or make services or objects or arrangements of persons or things; production requires exertion of effort and the exercise of skill and creativity conjoined with knowledge of what is to be done and made and the means to be used.

professional-technologic operations   In the health services, the processes of diagnosis, prescription, regulation or treatment, and case management performed by professional practitioners within their respective fields in their provision of health care to persons who seek or use their services.

proper object   That which persons in a specific field of art or science study, observe, or endeavor to bring to some new condition or form.

properties   Characteristics or attributes of things.

public health   A field of knowledge and a field of practice concerned with ways and means of enhancing and conserving the health of members of a community.

relation   A connection between a pair of reciprocally dependent things.

regulate   To control, direct, or adjust in accordance with a principle or rule.

regulatory nursing system   In nursing practice, a deliberate action process of ensuring that patients' calculated and prescribed therapeutic self-care demands are met, and their powers of self-care agency are protected and the exercise or development of self-care agency is regulated.

rules of nursing practice   Principles that specify proper ways of thinking and acting and govern the conduct of nurses in nursing practice situations; rules may be general, applicable in all nursing situations, or specific to types of nursing cases. When principles or rules are institutionalized by a health service agency to be followed by all nurses they are identified as regulations or policies.

self-care   The practice of activities that maturing and mature persons initiate and perform, within time frames, on their own behalf in the interests of maintaining life, healthful functioning, continuing personal development, and well-being.

self-care agency   The complex acquired ability of mature and maturing persons to know and meet their continuing requirements for deliberate, purposive action to regulate their own human functioning and development.

self-care capabilities   Constituent developed abilities that together form the self-care agency of persons for effectively performing, within appropriate time frames, the investigative, judgment and decision making, and regulatory or treatment operations necessary to keep their own functioning and development within norms compatible with life, health, and well-being. The performance of the three self-care operations rests on developed and exercised knowledge, skills, and motivations specific to self-care, and sets of foundational human capabilities and dispositions.

self-care deficit   A relation between the human properties therapeutic self-care demand and self-care agency in which constituent developed self-care capabilities within self-care agency are not operable or not adequate for knowing and meeting some or all components of the existent or projected therapeutic self-care demand.

self-care limitations   Restricting human and environmental influences within time frames on persons' performance of the investigative, judgment and decision making, and production operations of self-care.

self-care requisite   A formulated and expressed insight about actions to be performed that are known or hypothesized to be necessary in the regulation of an aspect(s) of human functioning and development continuously or under specified conditions and circumstances. A formulated self-care requisite names (1) the factor to be controlled or managed to keep an aspect(s) of human functioning and development within norms compatible with life and health and personal well-being and (2) the nature of the required action. Formulated and expressed self-care requisite constitutes the formalized purposes of self-care. They are the reasons for which self-care is undertaken; they express the intended or desired results – the goals of self-care.

self-care systems   Courses and sequences of action that are being or have been performed by individuals to meet their particular self-care requisites.

self-management capabilities   Abilities of individuals at various stages of human development to control their position and movement in space and to manage their own affairs.

service   The providing of resources or courses of action (activities) required by persons or organizations.

situation   A state or condition that represents a combination of concrete circumstances arranged with reference to relations of circumstances to one another; this includes relations among properties and circumstances of persons involved that affect these persons to their advantage or disadvantage.

societal   Pertaining to large groups of persons associated together for various purposes or to these persons' activities or customs.

standard   A rule, pattern, or model for guidance in doing or making something so that what is done or made will be of a particular quality.

state   A form of existence; the named combination of circumstances affecting a person or thing at a given time.

structure   The arrangement of parts of a whole; something that is composed of parts.

system   Anything that can be viewed as a single whole thing; an orderly arrangement resulting or understood from discovered connections among things.

technology   A practical means for bringing about or producing something.

therapeutic   Contributory to: support of life process; normal human functioning and development; prevention, cure, or control of disease and injury; prevention of disability; structural or functional compensation for disability; promotion of well-being.

therapeutic self-care demand   The summation of care measures necessary at specific times or over a duration of time for meeting all of an individual's known self-care requisites particularized for existent conditions and circumstances using methods appropriate for (1) controlling or managing factors identified in the requisites the values of which are regulatory of human functioning, for example, sufficiency of air, water, food; and (2) fulfilling the activity element of the requisite, for example, maintenance, promotion, prevention, and provision.

theory   A coherent set of propositions used as principles to form a frame of reference for a field of inquiry and from which laws can be deduced.

thing   A particular, concrete unity, identity, whole; grasped by considering the individuality and unity data.

treatment or regulatory operations   In nursing practice, deliberate courses of action of nurses specified within individuals' therapeutic self-care demands that are performed to keep human functioning and development within norms compatible with life, health, and well-being; operations also include those actions selected by nurses for purposes of regulating patients' development or exercise of self-care capabilities and the overcoming or compensating for self-care limitations.

unit of service   A term used to designate whether nurses provide nursing to persons as individuals or as members of multiperson units. In the first instance, the individual person is the focus or object of nurses' attention; in the second instance, the multiperson unit with its members is the primary focus or object of nurses' attention.

value   The good, the desired as the possible object of rational choice of individuals; values become known from questioning if this or that is truly good and not just apparently good, or whether this or that is worthwhile.

well-being   A perceived condition of personal existence including persons' experiences of contentment, pleasure, kinds of happiness, as well as spiritual experiences, movement to fulfill one's self-ideal, and continuing personal development.

Bibliography

Ackerman NW: The psychodynamics of family life, New York, 1958, Basic Books.

Allison SE: The meaning of rest: some views and behaviors characterizing rest as a state and a process, an exploratory nursing study, doctoral dissertation, Teachers' College, New York, 1968, Columbia University.

Allport GW: Becoming: basic considerations for a psychology of personality, New Haven, 1955, Yale University Press.

Allport GW: Personality and social encounter: selected essays, Boston, 1960, Beacon Press.

Allport GW: Pattern and growth in personality, New York, 1965, Holt.

Andersen R and Anderson O: A decade of health services: social survey trends in use and expenditure, Chicago, 1967, University of Chicago Press.

Arnold MB: Emotion and personality, vol I: Psychological aspects, New York, 1960, Columbia University Press.

Arnold MB: Emotion and personality, vol II: Neurological and physiological aspects, New York, 1960, Columbia University Press.

Ashby WR: An introduction to cybernetics, London, 1964, Chapman & Hall.

Bailey NA: Toward a praxeological theory of conflict, Orbis 11:1018–1112, 1968.

Barnard CI: The functions of the executive, Cambridge, Mass, 1962, Harvard University Press.

Blocker CE, Plummer RH, and Richardson RC Jr: The two-year college: a social synthesis, Englewood Cliffs, NJ, 1965, Prentice-Hall.

Bronowski J: A sense of the future, essays in natural philosophy. Ariotti PR and Bronowski R, editors: Cambridge, Mass, 1977, MIT Press.

Brooks DL: Identification of selected nursing factors to determine the availability of learning experiences for students, master's thesis, Washington, DC, 1963, School of Nursing, Catholic University of America.

Buckley W: Sociology and modern systems theory, Englewood Cliffs, NJ, 1967, Prentice-Hall.

Dubos R: Humanistic biology, American Scholar, 34:179–198, 1965.

Dubos R: Man adapting, New Haven, 1965, Yale University Press.

Entralgo PL: Doctor and patient, New York, 1969, World University Library, McGraw-Hill (Translated by F Partridge).

Firth R: Elements of social organization, ed 3, Boston, 1961, Beacon Press.

Foucault M: The birth of the clinic: an archaeology of medical perception, New York, 1975, Vintage Books (Translated by AM Sheridan Smith).

Fromm E: The heart of man, New York, 1968, Harper & Row.

Galdston I: Medicine in transition, Chicago, 1965, University of Chicago Press.

Gilby T: Appendix I Structure of a Human Act. In Thomas Aquinas, Summa Theologica, vol 17, Psychology of Human Acts, Blackfriars, New York, 1970, Cambridge, and McGraw-Hill.

Hall LE: Another view of nursing care and quality. In Straub KM and Parker KS, editors: Continuity of patient care: the role of nursing, Washington, DC, 1966, Catholic University of America Press.

Hampton IA, et al: Nursing of the sick, 1893, New York, 1949, McGraw-Hill.

Harrison TR, et al, editors: Principles of internal medicine, ed 5, New York, 1966, McGraw-Hill.

Hartnett Sister Louise Marie: Development of a theoretical model for the identification of nursing requirements in a selected aspect of self-care, master's thesis, Washington, DC, 1968, School of Nursing, Catholic University of America.

Helson H: Adaptation level theory: an experimental and systematic approach to behavior, New York, 1964, Harper & Row.

Henderson V: The nature of nursing: a definition and its implications for practice, research, and education, New York, 1966, Macmillan.

Houssay BA, et al: Human physiology, New York, 1955, McGraw-Hill.

Illich I: Medical nemesis, New York, 1976, Pantheon Books.

Jaco EG, editor: Patients, physicians and illness: sourcebook in behavioral science and medicine, Glencoe, Ill, 1958, Free Press.

Johns EB, Sutton WC, and Webster LE: Health for effective living, ed 3, New York, 1962, McGraw-Hill.

Katz RL: Empathy, its nature and uses, New York, 1963, Free Press.

Knutson AL: The individual, society, and health behavior, New York, 1965, Russell Sage.

Kotarbinski T: Praxiology: an introduction to the sciences of efficient action, 1st English ed, New York, 1965, Pergamon (Translated by O. Wojtasiewicz).

Leavell HR, et al: Preventive medicine for the doctor in his community, ed 3, New York, 1965, McGraw-Hill.

Lewin K: Field theory in social science, selected theoretical papers, Cartwright D, editor, New York, 1951, Harper Torchbooks.

Lonergan BJF: Insight, a study of human understanding, New York, 1958, Philosophical Library.

McHale J: Global ecology: toward the planetary society, American Behavioral Scientist 11:29-33, 1968.

Macmurray J: The self as agent, London, 1957, Faber and Faber.

Mechanic D: Medical sociology: a selective view, New York, 1968, Free Press.

Monnig Sister M Gretta: Identification and description of nursing opportunities for health teaching of patients with gastric surgery as a basis for curriculum development in nursing, master's thesis, Washington, DC, 1965, Catholic University of America.

Nadel SF: The theory of social structure, Glencoe, Ill, 1958, Free Press.

Nagel E: The structure of science, New York, 1961, Harcourt, Brace & World.

Neff, WS: Work and human behavior, New York, 1968, Atherton.

Nursing Development Conference Group: Concept formalization in nursing: process and product, Boston, 1973, Little, Brown.

Nursing Development Conference Group: Concept formalization in nursing: process and product, ed 2, DE Orem, editor, Boston, 1979, Little, Brown.

Orem DE: Guides for developing curriculum for the education of practical nurses, Washington, DC, 1959, US Government Printing Office.

Orem DE: Discussion of paper, another view of nursing care and quality. In Straub KM and Parker KS, editors: Continuity of patient care: the role of nursing, Washington, DC, 1966, Catholic University of America Press.

Orem DE: Levels of nursing education and practice. Paper presented to the Alumnae Association of the Johns Hopkins School of Nursing, Oct 12, 1968, The Alumnae Magazine, 68:2-6, 1969.

Parsons T, Bales RF, and Shils EA: Working papers in the theory of action, Glencoe, Ill, 1953, Free Press.

Paul BD, editor: Health, culture, and community: case studies of public reactions to health programs, York, 1955, Russell Sage.

Plattel MG: Social philosophy, Pittsburgh, 1965, Duquesne University Press.

Roberts MM: American nursing, New York, 1954, Macmillan.

Selye H: In vivo: The case for supramolecular biology, New york, 1967, Liveright.

Sigerist HE: Civilization and disease, Chicago, 1962, University of Chicago Press.

Solomon DN: Sociological perspectives on occupations. In Becker HS, et al, editors: Institutions and the person, Chicago, 1968, Aldine.

Somers HM and Somers AR: Medicare and the hospitals: issues and prospects, Washington, DC, 1967, The Brookings Institution.

Sommerhoff G: Analytical biology, London, 1950, Oxford University Press.

Sorokin PA: Social and cultural dynamics, Boston, 1957, Extending Horizons Books.

Spalding EK and Notter LE: Professional nursing, Philadelphia, 1970, Lippincott.

Stewart DA: Preface to empathy, New York, 1956, Philosophical Library.

Teilhard de Chardin P: The human rebound of evolution and its consequences. In The future of man, New York, 1964, Harper & Row (Translated by Denny N).

Ullman M: Health deviations and behavior. In Orem DE and Parker KS, editors: Nursing content in preservice nursing curriculums, Washington DC, 1964, Catholic University of America Press.

U.S. Surgeon General's Consultant Group on Nursing: Toward quality in nursing: needs and goals, Report, Public Health Service, Washington, DC, 1963, US Department of Health, Education, and Welfare.

van Kaam A: The art of existential counseling, Wilkes-Barre, Pa, 1966, Dimension Books.

Vernon MD: The psychology of perception, Baltimore, 1962, Penguin Books.

von Bertalanffy L: Robots, men and minds: psychology in the modern world, New York, 1967, Braziller.

Wallace WA: From a realist point of view: essays on the philosophy of science, Washington, DC, 1979, University Press of America.

Weiss P: You, I and the others, Carbondale and Edwardsville, 1980, Southern Illinois University Press.

Whipple DV: Dynamics of development: euthenic pediatrics, New York, 1966, McGraw-Hill.

Whitehead AN: Part three, philosophical. In Adventures of ideas, New York, 1964, New American Library.

Wiedenbach E: Clinical nursing, a helping art, New York, 1964, Springer.

Wiener N: Cybernetics, ed 2, Cambridge, Mass, 1961, MIT Press.

Willig S: Nurse's guide to the law, New York, 1970, McGraw-Hill.

Woolsey AR: A century of nursing, with hints toward the organization of a training school, and Florence Nightingale's historic letter to the Bellevue School, September 18, 1872, New York, 1950, Putnam.

Yovits MC, and Cameron S, editors: Self-organizing systems: proceedings of an interdisciplinary conference, May 5 and 6, 1959, New York, 1960, Pergamon.

Index